365 Favorite Chicken Recipes

(365 Favorite Chicken Recipes - Volume 1)

Maria Girard

Copyright: Published in the United States by Maria Girard/ © MARIA GIRARD

Published on December, 07 2020

All rights reserved. No part of this publication may be reproduced, stored in retrieval system, copied in any form or by any means, electronic, mechanical, photocopying, recording or otherwise transmitted without written permission from the publisher. Please do not participate in or encourage piracy of this material in any way. You must not circulate this book in any format. MARIA GIRARD does not control or direct users' actions and is not responsible for the information or content shared, harm and/or actions of the book readers.

In accordance with the U.S. Copyright Act of 1976, the scanning, uploading and electronic sharing of any part of this book without the permission of the publisher constitute unlawful piracy and theft of the author's intellectual property. If you would like to use material from the book (other than just simply for reviewing the book), prior permission must be obtained by contacting the author at author@shellfishrecipes.com

Thank you for your support of the author's rights.

Content

365 AWESOME CHICKEN RECIPES 9

1. Chicken Pozole Chilli 9
2. Chino Southern Pan Fried Dumplings 9
3. Hey, These Don't Taste Like Turkey Burgers 10
4. TUSCAN ITALIAN BRICK CHICKEN WITH ARUGULA AND SPINACH BREAD SALAD 10
5. ...and The Capon You Rode In On 11
6. 18 Minute Paella Valenciana Recipe (the Authentic) 11
7. 30 Minute Roast Chicken 12
8. 5 Spice Grilled Chicken Bahn Mi 12
9. A Happy Chicken Salad Roll, Herby & Nutty! 13
10. A Spring Riff On Shepherd's Pie 13
11. Add Exotic Flavor To The Table Taiwanese Style Sesame Oil Chicken Rice 14
12. Adobo Hot Wings 15
13. Air Fryer | Garlic Chicken Legs 16
14. All Day Duck Gumbo 16
15. All In One Salad 17
16. Alpine Turkey Burgers 18
17. Apple Chicken Salad With Hazelnut Curry Vinaigrette 18
18. Artichoke Turkey Panini With Basil Pesto Aioli 19
19. Asha Gomez's Kerala Fried Chicken 19
20. Asian Sesame Chicken & Broccoli 20
21. Asian Spiced Chicken Livers With Lemon Grass And Ramps 20
22. Asopao De Pollo (Chicken Stew) 21
23. Autumnal Zuppa 21
24. BBQ Chicken Bacon Ranch Salad 22
25. BBQ Whiskey Chicken Thighs 22
26. BBQ Pulled Chicken Lettuce Wraps 23
27. Baby Potatoes In Cheese Sauce 23
28. Baby Spinach, Arugula, And Fruit Salad With Balsamic Dressing 23
29. Bacon Blueberry Dog Biscuit 24
30. Bacon Wrapped, Spatchcocked Turkey In 80 Minutes 24
31. Baid Mutajjan – Middle Eastern Fried Hard Boiled Eggs 25
32. Baked Meat Cannelloni Cannelloni Di Carne Al Forno 25
33. Baked Pasta With Chicken Sausage 27
34. Baked Salt And Pepper Wings 28
35. Baked Pineapple Fried Rice With Cashew Nuts 28
36. Balsamic Chicken Sandwich With Peach Jam And Brandied Onions 29
37. Basil Chicken 30
38. Beer Can Chicken 30
39. Best Ever Turkey Chili 31
40. Best Stuffed Peppers 31
41. Bev's Chicken (or Pork Or Beef) Or Vegetarian Tortilla Casserole 32
42. Bibimpap 32
43. Big Mama's Fried Chicken 33
44. Bikini Bolognese 33
45. Bison And Chicken Sausage Chili 34
46. Blue Hubbard Squash Chili 35
47. Blueberry Sweet Tea–Brined Chicken Thighs From Todd Richards 35
48. Braised Mediterranean Cinnamon Chicken 36
49. Breaded Turkey Meatballs 37
50. Breakfast Salad 37
51. Broccoli Chicken Alfredo Skillet 38
52. Buffalo Chicken Frittata (or Egg Cups) 38
53. Buffalo Chicken Grilled Cheese Sandwiches 39
54. Buffalo Chicken Sausage Salad 39
55. Buffalo Chicken Soup 40
56. Buffalo, Blue Cheese Chicken Burgers 40
57. Burmese Chicken Salad 41
58. Butter Chicken 41
59. CHA! Hoisin Glazed Roasted Chicken Wings 41
60. CHA!Cho's 42
61. Cajun Honey Grilled Chicken 42
62. Cajun Spiced Chicken And Fettuccine 43
63. Calabrian Style Chicken 43
64. Can't Believe Its Not Beef! 44
65. Caprese Chicken Breasts 44
66. Cardamom Carrot Meatball Soup 44
67. Chai Spiced Chicken, Barley, And Chickpea Stew 45
68. Chcken Dupiaza 46

69. Cheater's Chicken Schnitzel 47
70. Cheesy Stuffing 47
71. Cherry Poppy Seed Chicken Salad 48
72. Cherry Tomato Hot Browns 48
73. Chestnut, Pork And Nut Stuffing My Family's Traditional Recipe 49
74. Chicken "Stoup" 50
75. Chicken & Cabbage Salad With Sesame Seeds, Scallions & Almonds 51
76. Chicken & Quinoa Stuffed Peppers 52
77. Chicken & Vegetable Ramen Noodles 52
78. Chicken Asparagus Penne Pasta 53
79. Chicken Avocado & Veggie Egg Rolls With Sweet & Sour Sauce 53
80. Chicken Bog 54
81. Chicken Breast With Cream Of Herb Sauce 55
82. Chicken Breasts & Thighs Pounded, Wrapped In Pancetta, Filled W/ A Cilantro, Feta, Mint Pesto And Covered In A Blood Orange Sauce 55
83. Chicken Breasts Over Fennel In Parchment 56
84. Chicken Cordon Club 56
85. Chicken Crepes With Ricotta, Parmesan And Spinach With Parmesan Bechamel 57
86. Chicken Curry 58
87. Chicken Curry With Moringa 59
88. Chicken Flautas 59
89. Chicken Fricassee 60
90. Chicken Liver Pate With Bourbon, Honey, And Sage 60
91. Chicken Liver Pâté 61
92. Chicken Liver Spread (née Pâté) 61
93. Chicken Marsala 62
94. Chicken Meatball Tikka Masala 62
95. Chicken Paillard With Lemon Salad 63
96. Chicken Paprikash With Rhubarb, Cherry, And Red Pepper 64
97. Chicken Pot Pie Provencal 64
98. Chicken Prosciutto Roll Ups 66
99. Chicken Salad With Wild Rice And Oranges 66
100. Chicken Skillet With Sweet Potatoes & Wild Rice 67
101. Chicken Sophia 67
102. Chicken Soup Pipian 68
103. Chicken Souvlaki Naan Plate 69
104. Chicken Stew 70
105. Chicken Thigh Surprise 70
106. Chicken Thighs Smothered In Gravy 70
107. Chicken Tikka Masala 71
108. Chicken Tsukune 72
109. Chicken Under A Brick With Pickled Peppers 73
110. Chicken Veggie Soup 74
111. Chicken Vermicelli Soup 74
112. Chicken Yellow Curry 75
113. Chicken And Dumplings 75
114. Chicken And Pinto Bean Sauté 76
115. Chicken And Shrimp Meatloaf With Whole Grain Mustard Dipping Sauce 76
116. Chicken And Steak Skewers With A Tahini Yogurt Marinade 77
117. Chicken And Veggie Curry 78
118. Chicken And White Bean Stew With Rosemary 78
119. Chicken Drumsticks Wrapped In Pancetta 79
120. Chicken In White Wine With Mushrooms 79
121. Chicken Rillettes 80
122. Chicken Stir Fry Wraps 81
123. Chicken Tikka Masala 81
124. Chicken With Black Truffles 82
125. Chicken With Fennel, Pernod And 40 Cloves Of Garlic 83
126. Chicken, Spinach And Pasta Al Forno 83
127. Chicken, Spinach, Tomato And Feta Pasta 84
128. Chicken, Chile And Tomatillo Soup 84
129. Chicken Pecan Quiche 85
130. Chicory Coffee Glazed Game Hen With Giardiniera Cabbage 86
131. Chile Verde With Chicken 87
132. Chinese Chicken Salad 88
133. Chipollini Cognac Chicken 88
134. Chutney Chicken Meatballs 89
135. Classic Chicken Coconut Curry 89
136. Classic Chicken Parmigiana 90
137. Coconut Chix Stix 90
138. Coconut Pecan Crusted Chicken Served With Sweet And Spicy Apricot Sauce 91
139. Collard Greens With Smoked Turkey Leg 92

140. Coq Au Vin 92
141. Cornish Hens With Potatoes, Porcinis And Tarragon En Papillote 93
142. Country Stuffing 94
143. Creamy Gnocchi With Braised Chicken And Winter Vegetables 95
144. Creamy Sun Dried Tomato + Parmesan Chicken Zoodles 96
145. Creamy Chicken With Lemon And Rosemary 96
146. Crispy Chicken Thighs With Chicken Fat Fried Rice 97
147. Crispy Grilled Chicken With Blueberry Barbecue Sauce 98
148. Crispy Roast Chicken With Truffle Butter 98
149. Crock Pot Chicken Stock 99
150. Crunchy Apple And Brussels Sprout Salad 99
151. Cumin And Mustard Roasted Chicken With Fruit 100
152. Curried Chicken Mulligatawny Soup 100
153. Curried Smoked Turkey Salad 101
154. Curried Turkey And Potato Hand Pies ... 102
155. Curried Peanut Chicken And Date Stew 102
156. Deep Dish Chicken Pot Pie 102
157. Deliciously Cheesy Crumb Chicken Casserole 103
158. Denny's Tetrazzini 104
159. Dinner Salad With Roasted Chicken Thighs, Caperberries And Roasted Lemons 104
160. Don't Tell My Cardiologist Thanksgiving Leftover Sandwich 105
161. Duck Confit 105
162. Duck Prosciutto 106
163. Duck A L'orange Tartlet 106
164. Duck! It's Baby Eggs In Onion Nests! 107
165. Easy Indian Chicken Curry 108
166. Easy Oven Baked Chicken Shawarma Recipe 108
167. Easy And Customizable Hasselback Chicken 109
168. Filipino Chicken Porridge (Arroz Caldo) 110
169. Filipino Chicken Adobo 110
170. Filipino Style Chicken Rice Porridge 111
171. Frogsicle Pops With Basil And Meyer Lemon 111
172. Fusion Sticky Rice With Star Anise Chicken, Shiitake, Edamame, And Sunchokes 112
173. Garlicky Parmesan Corn Flake Baked Chicken Tenders 113
174. Gin Brined Turkey 113
175. Ginger Chicken Meatballs With Bok Choy 114
176. Ginger Chicken W/ Braised Baby Bok Choy 114
177. Goat Cheese And Chicken Stuffed Peppers 115
178. Grandma Ray's Oyster Stuffing 115
179. Grandpas Chicken Noodle Soup From Scratch 116
180. Granny Karate's 'Korean' Chicken Remedy Soup (For The Bachelor's Lady's Cold) 116
181. Greek Chicken With Herbed Yogurt Sauce 117
182. Green Diva Casserole 117
183. Grilled Apricot, Honey, And Habanero Pepper Chicken Wings 118
184. Grilled Chicken Bread Salad 118
185. Grilled Chicken Tacos 119
186. Grilled Chicken And Mixed Greens Salad 120
187. Guinea Hen With Salsa Verde 120
188. Hainanese Chicken Rice 121
189. Hanoi Inspired Fried Chicken Wings 122
190. Harissa Turkey With Pomegranate Cous Cous 123
191. Harvest Stuffing 123
192. Hearty Chicken Harvest Dinner 125
193. Hill Country Honey Bacon Quail 125
194. Homemade Chicken Noodle Soup 126
195. Honey Vanilla Glazed Chicken Over Sweet Vanilla Rice 126
196. Honey And Garlic Chicken Stew 127
197. Hot Smoked Paprika, Oregano Flower & Pepper BBQ'd Chicken 127
198. Huckleberry Glazed Chicken Wings 128
199. Huli Huli Wings 128
200. In The Midwest, We BAKE Chicken (with Lime, Spices And Garlic) 129
201. Iranian/Persian Fesenjoon (walnut And Pomegranate Dish) With Rice 129
202. Italian Chicken And Vegetable Casserole 130
203. Italian Lemon Chicken Bowtie Pasta Salad 131

204. Italian Style Breaded Chicken 131
205. Japanese Cream Stew (クリームシチュ) 132
206. Jerk Chicken & Mango Kabobs 132
207. Judie's Beggar's Chicken 133
208. Kerala Chicken Stew 133
209. Kitchen Sink Chicken And Vegetable Curry 134
210. Korean Kimchi Quesadilla 135
211. L'Orengue De Pouchins (Chicken In Orange Sauce) 135
212. Lamb Sausage, Feta And Mint Stuffing ... 135
213. Lemon Pepper Chicken Salad Sandwich . 136
214. Lemoniest Roast Chicken 137
215. Lemony Chicken Noodle Soup 137
216. Librarian's Turkey 138
217. Lime Chicken Enchiladas With Roasted Red Pepper Herb Sauce 138
218. Lime Cilantro Chicken Milanese 139
219. Malawian Chicken Curry With Nsima 139
220. Malaysian Chicken Curry 140
221. Mamie's Brunswick Stew 141
222. Maple Mustard Chicken Thighs 141
223. Maple And Mustard Glazed Turkey With Killer Gravy 142
224. Matzo Ball Soup 143
225. Mediterranean Potstickers 145
226. Melissa Hartwig's Instant Pot Chicken Cacciatore With Zucchini Noodles 145
227. Melissa Hartwig's Instant Pot Sesame Chicken 146
228. Melly's Braised Holiday Chicken With Olives, Lemon And Apricots 147
229. Mini Duck Quesadillas W/Avocado Crema 147
230. Mini Persian Rice Cakes (Tachin) 148
231. Moroccan Chicken Tagine 149
232. Mung Bean Rice Mosh Polo 149
233. My Favorite Roasted Chicken, With Jerusalem Artichokes 150
234. My Version Of My Mom's Chicken Paprikash 150
235. Nana's Chicken Salad 151
236. Not My Grandmother's Chopped Chicken Liver 151
237. One Pan Roasted Chicken & Veggies 152
238. One Pot Sticky Coconut Chicken Curry . 152

239. Onion Marinated Grilled Chicken Breasts 153
240. Ostrich Stuffed Peppers 153
241. Our Family Fried Turkey 154
242. Overstuffed Chicken & Broccoli Quesadillas 155
243. Pad Thai From Kris Yenbamroong 155
244. Pad Thai With Chicken 156
245. Paella 157
246. Pan Roasted Chicken With Bacon, Rosemary And Lemon 157
247. Pancit 158
248. Panko Crusted Chicken With Chanterelle Gruyere Sauce 158
249. Parmesan Crusted Chicken With Herby Potatoes 159
250. Pasta Puttanesca W/ Chicken & Basil 160
251. Peachy BBQ Chicken 161
252. Peachy Sweet Wings 161
253. Pepita Crusted Chicken Cutlets 161
254. Peppy Chicken Liver Toasts 162
255. Perfect Pear Fall Salad 163
256. Perfect Roast Chicken 163
257. Perfect Thanksgiving Turkey & Gravy ... 164
258. Persian Saffron Roast Chicken & Barberry Rice 166
259. Pesto Stuffed Chicken Parmesan 167
260. Pho Sho 168
261. Pickle Fried Chicken 168
262. Pinaupong Manok (Chicken Steamed By A Bed Of Salt) 169
263. Pink Bolognese 170
264. Piri Piri Chicken Meatballs With Crispy Potatoes 170
265. Pollo E Peperoni (Chicken With Tomatoes And Red Peppers) 171
266. Portuguese Chicken Soup Aka Canja 172
267. Post Thanksgiving Turkey Ragu 172
268. Poulet À L'Estragon (Tarragon Chicken) 173
269. Pozole Blanco Con Pollo 174
270. Provençal Style Chicken In The Pot 174
271. Pulled Chicken Tacos With Pineapple Salsa 175
272. Pulled Chicken On Pan Fried Corn Cakes 176
273. Quick Sesame Ginger Stir Fry 177
274. RIVERBOAT LEMON LIME CHICKEN

275. Rachel Khoo's Sticky Malaysian Chicken With Pineapple Salad 178
276. Radish And Sausage Quiche 178
277. Rainbow Chard Barley Risotto With Chicken Sausage 179
278. Ramen Redux 179
279. Real Deal Buffalo Wings 180
280. Roast Chicken Legs With Grapes And Shallots 180
281. Roast Chicken Salad With Arugula And Pomegranate Seeds 181
282. Roast Chicken With Garlic Croutons 181
283. Roast Chicken With Oranges And Olives 182
284. Roasted Garlic Chicken 182
285. Roasted Fennel And Red Quinoa Salad, Chicken, Arugula, tomato, Sherry Vinaigrette 183
286. Salad With Pear, Magret De Canard, Jerusalem Artichokes And Hazelnut 183
287. Saliva Chicken Meatballs 184
288. Sangria Chicken 185
289. Sausage, Sauerkraut, And Spicy Mustard Potato Bowl 185
290. Savory Duck Buns Aka Kalua Manapua . 186
291. Scallion, Dijon And Chicken Ham Cake Salé 187
292. Sesame Chicken With Radicchio & Orange Salad 188
293. Shaken (not Stirred) Corn Dogs 189
294. Showstopper Stuffed Squash 189
295. Shoyu Chicken Over Rice 191
296. Shredded Chicken Gorditas 191
297. Shredded Red Chile Chicken Tacos 192
298. Smoked Chicken Salad With Peanuts And Apples 192
299. Smoked Corn Chowder With Crispy Duck Skin 193
300. Smoked Duck Breast With Creamy Wasabi Green Onion Dipping Sauce 193
301. Smokey Chicken, Rainbow Vegetable Saute And Cruncy Almonds 194
302. South Station Bourbon Chicken 195
303. Southern Chicken Dressing 195
304. Southwestern Chicken Salad 196
305. Special Stuffing 196
306. Spiced Smoked Tea Shortbread With Gingered Orange 197
307. Spiced Turkey Breast With Balsamic Grilled Peaches 198
308. Spiced Yogurt Baked Chicken On Roasted Broccoli 198
309. Spicy Chicken Vegetable Soup 199
310. Spicy Lemongrass Coconut Tacos 199
311. Spicy Thai Chicken And Sweet Potato Stew 200
312. Spinach Chicken Feta Thin Crust Pizza + Variations 200
313. Spinach Mushroom Pasta & Meatballs In Garlic Wine Sauce 201
314. Split Breast Of Chicken With Roasted Carrots And Potatoes 202
315. Spring Hill Ranch's New Mexico Green Chile Sauce 202
316. Sriracha Hot Wings 203
317. Sticky Blackberry Honey Hot Wings 203
318. Straight Up, Down Home Southern Fried Chicken With Honey 203
319. Stuffed & Seared Chicken Thighs With Refrigerator Door Mustard 204
320. Stuffed Tomato Chicken 205
321. Sumac Chicken With Cauliflower And Brussels Sprouts 205
322. Summer Grilled Chicken Cacciatore 206
323. Sunday Chicken Ragu 207
324. Sunday Chicken With Roasted Vegetables And Garlic Breadcrumbs 207
325. Super Easy Slow Cooker Chicken And Dumplings (with Gnocchi!) 208
326. Super Gingery Chicken And Herb Soup 209
327. Sweet Corn Chicken Stew With Mushroom 210
328. Tamale Pie 210
329. Tandoori Chicken Wraps 210
330. Tangine Gravy 211
331. Thai Curry Noodle Soup 212
332. Thai Inspired Chicken Coconut Soup 212
333. Thanksgiving Osso Buco 213
334. The Alchemist's Chicken (Chicken Roasted With Seville Oranges, Onions And Bay) 213
335. The BEST Chicken Thigh Recipe You Will EVER Have! 214
336. The Crispiest Cutlets 215
337. The Empy Nester Gourmet's Rich And

Creamy Roast Turkey Gravy 215
338. Tom Kha Teacups 216
339. Tomatillo Chicken Soup 216
340. Turkey Andouille Chili 217
341. Turkey Curry Meatballs 218
342. Turkey Lentil Chili 218
343. Turkey Soup 219
344. Turkey Veggie Meatballs With Spaghetti Squash 219
345. Turkey Green Curry 220
346. Turkey Meatloaf 220
347. Turkey Pot Pie With A Crispy Parmesan Crust 220
348. Turkey, Lentil, And Mixed Brown Rice Soup 221
349. Turmeric Yogurt Grilled Chicken 222
350. Ultimate Chicken Tikka Masala 222
351. Vanilla Carrot Broth 223
352. Vietnamese Classic Chicken Salad 224
353. Vietnamese Sticky Wings 224
354. West African Chicken Peanut Stew 225
355. White Chicken Chili 226
356. Whole Slow Cooker Poached Chicken ... 226
357. Wild Gochujang Wings 227
358. Wild Rice, Chicken And Almond Soup .. 227
359. Yellow Mole With Chicken And Masa Dumplings 228
360. A Simple Chicken & Rice Noodle Bowl . 229
361. Asian Chicken Salad 229
362. Basil Chicken With Brown Rice 230
363. Boxing Day Pate 230
364. Spicy Peanut Butter Bacon Cheeseburgers 231
365. Đuveč 231

INDEX 233

CONCLUSION 238

365 Awesome Chicken Recipes

***

1. Chicken Pozole Chilli

Serving: Serves 4-6 | Prep: | Cook: | Ready in:

Ingredients

- 4 chicken legs, cooked, bone and skin discarded (or just buy rotisserie chicken)
- 2 tablespoons coconut oil
- 1 medium onion, diced
- 2 cloves garlic, minced
- 1 chipotle in adobo sauce
- 1 teaspoon cumin, ground
- 1 can (14 oz) diced tomatoes, drained
- 1/2 cup chicken stock
- 1 can (15 oz) white hominy (pozole), drained and rinsed
- salt and pepper, to taste
- fresh coriander and flour tortillas

Direction

- Shred the chicken meat and keep on the side.
- Heat oil and cook onion 3-4 minutes, add garlic and cumin, drained tomatoes and chicken stock.
- Add drained and rinsed white hominy and chipotles.
- Adjust the seasoning.
- Add shredded chicken and cook 4-5 minutes.
- Serve with warm flour tortilla and cilantro.
- You can eat right away or refrigerate and reheat as needed it will taste even better.

2. Chino Southern Pan Fried Dumplings

Serving: Makes 12 | Prep: | Cook: | Ready in:

Ingredients

- 3 cups Shredded Cooked Chicken
- 1 Clove Garlic (minced)
- 1 1/2 tablespoons Sesame Oil
- 3 tablespoons Hoison Sauce
- 1 1/2 tablespoons Sriracha Sauce
- 1 teaspoon Rice Wine Vinegar
- 12 Dumping Wrapers (available @ Asian markets)
- Any neutral oil for frying

Direction

- - Add sesame oil and garlic to pan and sauté garlic over medium heat (2 min). Add the shredded chicken, hoison, sriracha and vinegar, mix all ingredients to combine flavors and heat up. Once hot, set aside in a bowl to cool (10 min)
- - To Make Dumpling - Fill a small cup with some water, put a dumpling wrapper on your work surface, place a heaping teaspoon of your filling into the center of the wrapper. Dip your finger into the cup of water and wet the entire rim of the wrapper. Bring the bottom of the wrapper to the top forming a half circle shape, press sides together. Starting from the left, make little 1/4 inch folds spacing each fold an equal amount till you reach the right side, the dumpling should plump in the center, press folds tightly together, repeat till all dumplings are formed
- - Heat 2 tbsp. of oil into pan on medium heat, add six dumplings to pan and brown on all sides till crispy, when browned add a small amount of water to pan (about a shot glass worth), cover for 20 seconds. Remove dumplings from pan and place on serving plate. Wipe pan clean and repeat.

3. Hey, These Don't Taste Like Turkey Burgers

Serving: Makes 3 or 4 burgers depending on size | Prep: | Cook: | Ready in:

Ingredients

- 1 pound ground Turkey, preferably dark meat.
- 1 cup fresh bread crumbs
- 1 bunch scallions
- 1 handful chopped parsley
- 1 tablespoon chopped dill
- 1 teaspoon dried oregano
- 1 heaping tablespoon dijon Mustard
- 2 teaspoons Worcestershire sauce
- 1 lightly beaten egg
- 1 teaspoon coarse salt
- 1/4 teaspoon Black Pepper

Direction

- Put turkey in a large bowl
- Chop scallions parsley dill, or any other herbs you care to use, in a food processor.
- Add crumbs and chopped and dry herbs to Turkey and combine well.
- Add mustard, Worcestershire sauce, beaten egg, and salt and pepper to bowl and mix well.
- Form into 3 or 4 patties and pan fry in a preheated cast iron or heavy nonstick pan, 6 to 7 minutes a side. Remember that turkey has to cook thoroughly. These will develop a crunchy outside and delicious smell while cooking.
- Lightly toast some buns of your choice, and add any toppings you like
- I like to serve these with roasted sweet potatoes or sweet potato fries and a big salad, but the choice is yours

4. TUSCAN ITALIAN BRICK CHICKEN WITH ARUGULA AND SPINACH BREAD SALAD

Serving: Serves 4 | Prep: | Cook: | Ready in:

Ingredients

- 3 1/2 pounds Chickens Butterflied (2) *Ask the butcher to do this
- 1/2 cup Olive Oil
- 1/3 cup Fresh Lemon Juice
- 4 pieces Garlic, minced
- 2 tablespoons Fresh Rosemary, minced
- 2 tablespoons Fresh Safe, minced
- 1 tablespoon Red Pepper Flakes
- 2 teaspoons Paprika
- 2 teaspoons Salt
- 2 teaspoons Pepper

Direction

- Cover the two bricks with foil
- Preheat the grill to medium-high heat.
- In a bowl, add all marinade ingredients and mix thoroughly.
- Place chickens skin side down in a large baking dish and season with salt and pepper. Pour marinade over the chicken. Cover the dish and chill at least 4 hours or overnight.
- Spray grill rack with nonstick spray. Heat the grill over medium heat. Remove chicken from marinade. Place chicken, skin side down, on grill. Place foil-wrapped bricks atop chicken. Cover and grill until skin is crispy and brown, about 15 minutes. Remove bricks. Flip chicken over using tongs. Replace bricks and cook, covered, until chicken is cooked through, about 20 minutes longer. Let chicken rest 10 minutes.
- While chicken is resting slice lemon in 4 quarters and place on grill. Cook until slightly charred, turning often, about 1 minute. Serve alongside for squeezing over chicken.

5. ...and The Capon You Rode In On

Serving: Serves 6 | Prep: | Cook: |Ready in:

Ingredients

- 1 8 to 9 pound capon
- 3 or 4 blood oranges (substitute valencia or other orange if necessary)
- 1 stick butter
- Fresh tarragon
- Sea salt plus fleur de sel for the table
- ground pepper
- 1 cup Homemade chicken stock (which came first?)
- 1/2 cup Wondra superfine flour
- cornstarch and water for a slurry

Direction

- Heat your oven to 450F
- Put your butter out to soften and then chop up the tarragon
- Cut the blood oranges into quarters or eighths to fit the capon cavity. Salt the cavity and stuff in the orange pieces
- Mash the tarragon into the softened butter. Using your freshly washed hands pull away the skin at the outside of the cavity and carefully push some of the butter herb mixture in. Don't tear the skin.
- Wash your hands again. Using kitchen string truss the chicken to your own preferred method. All you really want to do here is twist the wings around and keep them close to the body, and also to tighten the legs to the cavity. Be sure to close the flap. There's a name for that which I'm not going to mention. Okay, trussed up right? Now rub the outside of the bird with remaining butter and sea salt.
- Place Monsieur Capon in a roasting pan and put him in your oven. After 15 minutes lower the temperature to 350F. With a brush (silicone) baste the bird every 20 minutes or so with the buttery juices that are now dripping out. It's likely to take about an hour and a half to cook. But you will need to check the temperature to be sure it reaches 160. See notes below on instant reads.
- When the flesh tested away from the bone reaches 160, remove the capon to a platter and tent with aluminum foil for at least 15 minutes. It will get a "heat boost" and the juices will settle back in.
- While it's resting make your "gravy". Put your roasting pan on a gas burner and add the Wondra superfine flour. Scrape around a bit so that the flour colors. Add the chicken stock, and continue to stir. Make a slurry with water and corn starch, about half and half. Set that aside. Strain the stock and dripping mixture. Whisk in the slurry which will give it body and shine. Carve and serve.
- Notes: I'm almost as bad a therma-geek as Alton Brown. I check temperatures with a laser (no two oven dials are calibrated exactly---you can be off by 25?). I also use a Thermapen to test the meat. After using one for ten years I was happy to see Alton pull one out. Precise temperature control is your secret weapon as a good cook.

6. 18 Minute Paella Valenciana Recipe (the Authentic)

Serving: Serves 2 | Prep: 0hours5mins | Cook: 0hours20mins |Ready in:

Ingredients

- Jar of Ibérico Club's Paella
- Bag of Special Paella bomba rice
- Paella Pan

Direction

- Pour the content of the jar into the paella pan and bring to a boil on medium heat.
- Add the rice and spread evenly across the pan.

- Leave to simmer for 18 minutes on medium heat until the liquid is absorbed.
- Your delicious Paella Valenciana is ready! Let it stand for 3 minutes before serving.

7. 30 Minute Roast Chicken

Serving: Serves 4 | Prep: | Cook: | Ready in:

Ingredients

- 4 pounds chicken
- 1 1/2 tablespoons extra-virgin olive oil
- 2 teaspoons kosher salt
- Freshly ground black pepper

Direction

- Set the oven to 450° F. Immediately add a rimmed sheet pan. Once the oven comes up to temperature, set a 15-minute timer.
- In the meantime, spatchcook and season the chicken. Lay it breast side down on a cutting board. Use a pair of scissors or poultry shears to snip along one side of the spine, then the other, to remove it. (You can save this in the freezer for stock down the road.) Flip the chicken over and press down on the breastbone until you hear a soft crack. Pat the chicken dry with paper towels. Rub with olive oil, then season with salt and pepper.
- When the timer goes off, carefully remove the sheet pan from the oven. Quickly add the chicken, then get it back in the oven.
- Roast for about 30 minutes — until a meat thermometer inserted into the joint between the thigh and body reaches 165°F, or until a knife inserted in the same place produces clear (not pink) juices.
- Let rest for about 10 minutes, then carve. Serve on the sheet pan with bread and salad alongside.

8. 5 Spice Grilled Chicken Bahn Mi

Serving: Serves 4 | Prep: 1hours0mins | Cook: 0hours30mins | Ready in:

Ingredients

- Pickled Carrots and Daikon
- 1 cup Carrots, cut into matchsticks
- 1 cup Daikon, cut into matchsticks
- 3/4 cup White Wine Vinegar
- 1 cup Water
- 3 tablespoons Agave Nectar
- 1 tablespoon Salt
- 5 Spice Chicken Bahn Mi
- 2 Chicken Breast
- 2 tablespoons 5 Spice Seasoning
- 1 Jalapeno, cut into slices
- 3 tablespoons Cilantro Leaves
- 1 Cucumber, ends removed & cut into vertical slices
- 4 Ciabatta Roles, cut in half
- 3/4 cup Mayo
- 2-3 tablespoons Sriracha
- 1 teaspoon Garlic, minced
- 2 tablespoons Salt
- 2 tablespoons Cracked Black Pepper
- 2 cups Pickled Carrot & Daikon
- 1/2 cup Olive Oil
- 1/4 cup Hoisin Sauce

Direction

- Pickled Carrots and Daikon
- Place cut carrots and daikons in plastic mixing bowl with agave nectar and salt, toss to coat carrots and daikons
- Allow to sit for 20 minutes, remove contents into mason jar or container
- In pot add vinegar and water and cook on medium heat, until it starts to boil
- Once it has boiled, pour over carrots and daikon and allow to cool uncovered in fridge. Cover once done cooling. Will taste best after 24 hours of sitting, but you can use immediately

- 5 Spice Chicken Banh Mi
- Using a sharp knife, cut chicken breasts in half lengthwise. Season all four breasts generously with salt, pepper, 5 spice powder, olive oil- Set aside until ready to grill
- In a small mixing bowl, add mayo, sriracha, and minced garlic. Stir until combined. Taste to see if you need more sriracha to your liking, set aside
- On cut side of ciabatta rolls brush olive oil
- Clean and Preheat grill for 5-8 minutes
- Add Chicken Allow to cook for 3 minutes, flip and cook alternate side for 3 minutes
- Lower heat on grill, flip chicken again and drizzle 1 tbsp. of hoisin sauce over each chicken. Allow to cook until chicken reaches 160 degrees in the thickest part of the chicken, remove from grill and allow to rest
- Add ciabatta rolls to the grill on low heat and grill the oil side down until you have grill marks- Turn off grill
- To Assemble your 5 Spice Chicken Banh Mi, Start by adding sliced cucumbers to the bottom layer of ciabatta, next layer with chicken, on top of your chicken, add pickled carrots and daikon, top with sliced jalapenos and cilantro leaves (5-6 per sandwich). On the top slice of bread, spread your sriracha aioli
- Enjoy

9. A Happy Chicken Salad Roll, Herby & Nutty!

Serving: Serves 8 | Prep: | Cook: | Ready in:

Ingredients

- 1 1/2 pounds Skinless, boneless chicken breast, cooked* & chopped (about 6 cups)
- 1/3 cup Chopped chives (I like to cut them with scissors) or scallions if you prefer
- 1/3 cup Chopped red onions
- 1 Large garlic clove, crushed
- 1/2 cup Light mayonnaise (I like the Hellman brand; says 1/2 the calories of regular mayo)
- 1/2 cup Fat free (preferably Greek) yogurt
- 2 teaspoons Dijon (or regular) mustard
- 1 tablespoon Juice of a lemon and zest of half of the lemon.
- 1/4 teaspoon Turmeric (good for you and gives nice yellowish tint)
- 1/4 teaspoon Smoked sweet paprika
- 1 tablespoon Fresh chopped tarragon (or, if you prefer, you can use a different herb like 1-2 tsp chopped fresh rosemary)
- 1/4 teaspoon Sriracha sauce for a very mild hint of spiciness (at least to me) or more to taste
- 1/3 to 1/2 cups Chopped smoked almonds (I use Blue Diamond brand, almonds smokehouse)
- * I like to boil the chicken in plain water, cool, and then chop.

Direction

- Combine all ingredients except the chicken, almonds, chives and tarragon. Taste and adjust seasoning to taste if necessary. Stir the chicken and almonds; then fold the chives and tarragon.
- Serve (about 1/3 cup each) the chicken salad on 8 toasted (or grilled) buttery hot dog rolls (I use Pepperidge Farm Top Sliced Hot Dog Buns), or use 16 slices of good quality whole grain bread to make 8 sandwiches). Or do what you want with it. If desired, sprinkle additional chives or scallions.

10. A Spring Riff On Shepherd's Pie

Serving: Serves 6 | Prep: | Cook: | Ready in:

Ingredients

- for the filling
- 1 tablespoon extra-virgin olive oil
- 1 pound ground turkey meat

- 1 medium onion, chopped
- 3 cloves garlic, minced
- 1/2 cup white mushrooms, chopped
- 1/4 cup fresh italian parsley, chopped
- 2 sprigs fresh thyme leaves
- 2 sprigs fresh marjoram leaves
- salt to taste
- freshly ground black pepper to taste
- 1 1/2 cups low sodium chicken broth
- 1 cup fresh carrot juice
- 12-18 small to medium white turnips, trimmed, peeled, cut into 1/2 inch pieces
- Greens from turnips, long stems removed, leaves coarsely chopped
- for the gravy and topping
- 4 sprigs fresh thyme leaves
- 1/2 teaspoon fresh tarragon, chopped
- 3 tablespoons unsalted butter
- 1/2 cup vermouth or other dry white wine
- Cornstarch roux made from 2 tablespoons cornstarch mixed in 3 tablespoons water
- 2 cups leftover mashed potatoes

Direction

- Preheat oven to 400 degrees. Prepare a 9 X 13 inch ceramic baking dish by greasing with olive oil. Set aside
- Heat olive oil in 10-12" skillet over medium high heat. Sauté onions until softened and lightly browned, 2 minutes.
- Add ground turkey and brown, using spoon to break up pieces. Continue to cook until evenly browned and no longer pink, about 4 minutes.
- Add garlic, mushrooms, thyme and marjoram, stirring to combine.
- Add parsley and season to taste with salt and pepper. Turn off heat.
- Meanwhile, bring chicken broth and carrot juice to boil in a small saucepan.
- Add turnips; turn down heat and cover to simmer. Cook until turnips are tender, about 10 minutes.
- Add chopped turnip greens and cook for 2 minutes.
- Using a slotted spoon, remove turnips and greens (setting broth/carrot juice mixture to the side) and fold into skillet with turkey mixture. Spoon into prepared baking dish.
- Add butter to broth/carrot juice mixture. Turn up heat to bring to a slow boil.
- Add vermouth, fresh thyme and tarragon, and slowly whisk in cornstarch roux to thicken. Season to taste with salt and pepper.
- Spoon broth/carrot gravy over turkey/turnip mixture. Top with leftover mashed potatoes.
- Cover with foil and cook in preheated oven for 20-25 minutes until bubbly. Remove foil during last 5 minutes of cooking. (Prepared pie can be made 1 day ahead, skipping the mashed potato step, and refrigerated. Top pie with potatoes before immediately before cooking. Follow heating directions above).

11. Add Exotic Flavor To The Table Taiwanese Style Sesame Oil Chicken Rice

Serving: Serves 4 | Prep: | Cook: | Ready in:

Ingredients

- 75 grams ginger
- 2 pounds chicken (dark meat is better)
- 1/2 cup Asian-style Sesame oil
- 1/2 cup Cooking rice wine
- 2 cups Rice

Direction

- First, find Asian-style Sesame oil and a bottle of cooking rice wine. Asian-style Sesame oil usually looks dark and has a strong flavor because it is made with black seeds (Semen Sesami Nigrum). Instead of using of sherry wine or Vermouth as in Western-style cooking, people in East Asia use rice wine. Please note that some rice wines contain salt; if you buy a rice wine containing salt, be sure to cut back on the amount of additional salt that you add. My experience is Asian-style Sesame oil can be easily found in most stores. Rice wine is usually only found in Asian markets. If you cannot find the cooking rice wine I use, you can use "AJI-MIRIN" which can be easily found in most stores. However, since AJI-MIRIN is a sweet rice wine, the flavor is slightly different and you will have to add salt in your dish and reduce the amount of sweet rice wine you use to prevent it from becoming too sweet. I usually use half traditional rice wine and half AJI-MIRIN and my mom only uses rice wine in her recipe.

- Heat the cast iron on the stove. When the cast iron is hot, add the sesame oil and ginger (thin slices). Let the ginger cook in the hot oil for a while until you can smell the flavor and see the edge of the ginger slices begin to brown.
- Add the chicken legs to the pot and stir-fry them 3-5 minutes.
- Add rice wine to the pot and cook for one minute.
- We will use the same pot to cook the rice, so remove the chicken and liquid from the pot and add the rice to the pot. When using cast iron to cook rice, the ratio for Rice :Water should be 1:1, but since the sesame oil and rice wine are still in the pot, we need to subtract them from the amount of water we need to add. For 2 cups of rice, we only need to add 1 and 1/4 cups of water.
- Add the 2 cups rice and 1 and 1/4 cups water to the pot and then put chicken (and all the liquid) back top of the rice. Don't stir them -the chicken should be on top of the rice. Cover the pot and use the cast iron to cook the rice as usual (use medium heat to cook it until you see steam, then reduce to low heat and cook for 20 more minutes)
- When you feel the rice is well-done, open the lid and stir. Now you have amazing Taiwanese style Sesame oil Chicken Rice.
- If you don't use cast iron, you can stir fry the chicken in a regular pot and use any equipment to cook the rice. The procedure and rule for water is similar.

12. Adobo Hot Wings

Serving: Serves 4 to 6 | Prep: | Cook: | Ready in:

Ingredients

- For the glaze
- 2 tablespoons butter
- 4 cloves of garlic, minced
- 1 to 2 habanero chili peppers, minced
- 1/2 cup apple cider vinegar
- 1/4 cup dark soy sauce
- 2 tablespoons (heaping) brown sugar
- 3/4 to 1 teaspoons coarsely ground black pepper
- For the wings
- 2 pounds chicken wings, tips removed
- 2 tablespoons butter, melted
- 2 tablespoons peanut, corn, olive, canola or vegetable oil
- 1 teaspoon (heaping) granulated garlic powder
- 1 teaspoon kosher or sea salt
- 3/4 teaspoon freshly ground black pepper

Direction

- Heat a small pot over medium-high heat and add 2 tablespoons butter. Once melted, add the garlic and habaneros. Stir and sauté until the garlic is lightly golden and fragrant, 1 to 2 minutes.
- Slowly add the apple cider vinegar, soy sauce, brown sugar and 3/4 to 1 teaspoon black pepper to the pot. Bring the sauce to a boil, reduce heat, and let simmer for 10 to 15 minutes until sauce is reduced and thickens a bit. Set aside.
- Preheat oven to 400 degrees. Very lightly oil a large rimmed baking sheet. Dry chicken wings with paper towels and place in large bowl. In a cup, mix together melted butter, peanut oil, garlic powder, salt and 3/4 teaspoon black pepper. Pour over wings in bowl, mix, and massage seasoning mixture onto the wings to

coat. Lay wings out, not touching, on prepared baking sheet.
- Bake wings for 45 to 55 minutes until toasty brown and cooked through. Place cooked wings in a large bowl, drizzle with adobo glaze, gently toss to coat evenly and serve up with some blue cheese dressing and frosty beer. HA-CHA-CHA!

13. Air Fryer|Garlic Chicken Legs

Serving: Serves 3 | Prep: 0hours5mins | Cook: 0hours20mins | Ready in:

Ingredients

- Oil 2 tbsp
- Chicken legs 6
- Lemon juice 1 tsp
- Garlic powder 1tbsp
- Paprika 2 tsp
- Salt 1/2 tsp
- Dried oregano 1 tsp
- Black pepper 1 tsp
- Jaggery powder 1 tsp

Direction

- Start by adding oil and lemon juice in a bowl. Next add garlic powder and dried oregano
- Add pepper. Add the mixture to the chicken legs. Add jaggery powder to the chicken legs and set it aside for at least 30 min. Preheat the air fryer. After preheat set the air fryer to chicken setting. Place the chicken legs inside air fryer and close it. After 20-25 min, take out the chicken legs. Serve hot and enjoy

14. All Day Duck Gumbo

Serving: Serves a crowd | Prep: | Cook: |Ready in:

Ingredients

- 1 - 5 pounds duck
- 1 whole bulb garlic
- Kosher salt and sweet smoked paprika
- 1 pound pork andouille sausage (3 links)
- 1 cup chopped onion - fairly small chop
- 1 cup chopped celery - same size as the onion
- 1 cup chopped green bell pepper - same size as the onion and celery
- 1/4 cup minced garlic (I know this sounds like a lot but trust me)
- 4 cups low salt chicken broth
- 1 brown beer (I use Abita Amber)
- 1/2 cup vegetable oil
- 1/2 cup all purpose flour
- 1 teaspoon kosher salt
- 1/2 - 1 teaspoons cayenne pepper (a full teaspoon makes it pretty spicy)
- 3 whole bay leaf
- 1 teaspoon dried thyme
- 1 teaspoon smoked sweet paprika
- 1 tablespoon red wine vinegar
- 1 tablespoon gumbo file
- green onions, for garnish
- EQUIPMENT - roasting pan preferably with a rack, and a heavy gumbo pot - I use my Le Cruset dutch oven

Direction

- Start in the morning! Put the oven on 250, and arrange the racks so there is room for the duck on top and a baking dish below. Remove the neck and giblets from the duck, rinse him and pat him dry. Cut the top off the bulb of garlic. Salt the duck inside then put the garlic inside. Prick him all over with a sharp fork - pierce the skin but not the meat. Sprinkle him all over with salt and paprika, tuck his wings behind his back (I got a one armed duck so he only had one tucked). Spray the rack of your roasting pan or wipe it with oil, and put the duck on breast side down. Throw the neck in the pan too. Put him in the oven.
- Put the flour in a baking dish - I just use a 9x13 black metal one. I also do 4 cups at a time, you will use 1/2 cup for the gumbo and the rest can go in a jar in the pantry for future rouxs

and gravies. Put the flour in the oven too. For 3 30 minute intervals pull out the flour and stir it, and re-poke the duck skin with a fork. After the third time (you are an hour and a half in now) flip the duck over and repeat - 3 more 30 minute intervals with flour stirring and skin poking at the end of each one.
- NOW - turn the oven up to 350. The duck is going to roast for another 30 minutes until it is nice and brown. Then pull him out and set him aside to cool. Put the andouille links on a cookie sheet (I spritz with no stick) and into the oven. After about 10 or 15 minutes flip them - they should be browning and spattering. Give them a little poke with the fork too to let out some of the fat. Stir the flour and cook 10 or 15 more minutes, Pull the andouille out, and stir the flour. Put the duck and andouille on a big cutting board where you can process them and let them cool all the way. Chop the veggies while you wait and stir that flour every 10 or 15 minutes until it is a nice toasty brown. You won't think it's dark enough but when you add it to the oil in a while it will be.
- Chop the veggies. Time for music - suggested listening - The Subdudes (of course), Mingo Fishtrap, The Gourds, The Neville Brothers, Rockin' Dopsie.
- Open the beer and let it sit for a bit. Cut the sausage up into bite size discs. Break down the duck - this is what I do - first, pull off the breast skin which will still be a little soft - SAVE IT. Then I get a stock pot and literally pull the meat off with my hands and rip it up and throw the bones in the stock pot (duck and grilled steak bone stock is awesome). I pick what I can off the neck and add that to the duck pile and throw the neck bones in the stock pot. It's all completely barbarian. But it's fun.
- Wash your hands. Put vegetable oil and 1/2 c toasted flour in the gumbo pot on medium heat. Stir until it's hot - see how dark it got? Once it's hot add the onions and stir for a 2-3 minutes. Add the celery, peppers and garlic and cook for a few more minutes. Add the broth and the beer. It's going to look odd and lumpy - never fear it will smooth out as it simmers and you stir. Bring it to a simmer, then add the spices EXCEPT the gumbo file - that goes in last. Also, start with 1/2 tsp of cayenne and then taste it in about 15 minutes for heat. You can always add more.
- Add the duck and the sausage and the vinegar. Let the pot simmer away - now is a good time to clean the kitchen a bit. You could probably use a beer or a glass of wine or a giant iced tea. Cook the rice, too. Chop up the green onion. The gumbo is best if you can give it an hour to simmer on low, so do other stuff. Taste it now and then to see if it needs salt or cayenne.
- You are almost done! Now for a little lagniappe - get the duck skin and cut it up into small pieces. Fry it in a heavy skillet on medium heat until it is very brown and crispy. Drain it on to paper towels ... try not to eat it all right then. Now, right before serving, turn the heat up a bit and stir in the gumbo file.
- Time to EAT - rice goes in the bowl first, then gumbo. Top it off with green onion and duck cracklings, and enjoy. It has been a long day, right?

15. All In One Salad

Serving: Serves 2 as a main course | Prep: | Cook: |Ready in:

Ingredients

- Five to six 1/2-inch slices baguette
- 1 garlic clove, peeled
- 1 tablespoon olive oil
- 3 cups watercress (broken into small stems)
- 1 cup thinly sliced celery
- 2 cups cubed cooked lamb and chicken, and thinly sliced salumi (I'd do 1 cup lamb, 1/2 cup each chicken and salumi)
- 2 tablespoons sour cream
- 1 tablespoon heavy cream or mayonnaise

- 2 tablespoons prepared horseradish
- 1 tablespoon lemon juice
- Grated zest of 1 tangerine
- Salt and freshly ground black pepper

Direction

- Heat the oven to 400 degrees. Make the croutons: rub the baguette slices with the garlic clove, then cut the slices into 1/2-inch cubes. Measure out 2 cups. (Eat the rest while you prepare the salad.) Spread on a baking sheet and toss with the olive oil. Toast the croutons in the oven until golden, tossing once, 5 to 10 minutes. Let cool.
- In a large salad bowl, combine the watercress, celery, meats and croutons.
- In a small bowl, whisk together the sour cream, heavy cream, horseradish, lemon juice and tangerine zest. Season to taste with salt and pepper (and feel free to add more lemon juice and horseradish as desired).
- Pour the dressing over the watercress and meats and toss until lightly dressed. Taste and adjust seasoning. Let sit for 15 minutes before serving.

16. Alpine Turkey Burgers

Serving: Serves 4 | Prep: | Cook: | Ready in:

Ingredients

- 4 teaspoons olive oil, divided
- 1 1/2 cups finely sliced onion
- pinch of sugar
- 1 cup chopped mushrooms
- 1 pound ground turkey (93% lean)
- 1/2 teaspoon Worcestershire
- 1/4 teaspoon dried thyme
- 1 teaspoon salt
- 1 teaspoon Dijon mustard
- 1/2 teaspoon freshly cracked black pepper
- pinch of nutmeg
- 3/4 cup shredded Gruyere or Swiss cheese

Direction

- Heat 2 teaspoons of the olive oil over medium low heat in a large skillet. Add the onions and pinch of sugar and cook for about 20 minutes, stirring occasionally, until the onions are caramelized. Add in the mushrooms and cook for another 6 or so minutes or until the mushrooms are tender. Remove from heat and let cool slightly.
- Put the ground turkey in a bowl and add the Worcestershire, Dijon, thyme, salt, pepper and nutmeg. Add the onion/mushroom mixture and mix well. Add in the Swiss and mix thoroughly. Form into 4 patties. Raise the heat under the skillet to the medium and add the remaining 2 teaspoons of olive oil. Cook the patties about 7-8 minutes per side or until done to your liking.

17. Apple Chicken Salad With Hazelnut Curry Vinaigrette

Serving: Serves 4 | Prep: | Cook: | Ready in:

Ingredients

- Salad
- 8 cups baby spinach
- 2 honey crisp apples, chopped
- 1 cup grapes, sliced in half
- 8 ounces cooked chicken breasts, sliced
- Vinaigrette
- 1/4 cup hazelnut oil
- 2 tablespoons red wine vinegar
- 1 teaspoon curry powder
- 1 teaspoon dijon mustard
- 1/4 teaspoon salt
- pinch of sugar

Direction

- Wisk dressing ingredients together and set aside.

- Divide salad ingredients equally among four plates and drizzle 1-2 Tbsp. of vinaigrette on each salad.
- Note: apples should be rubbed in a bit of lemon juice to prevent browning if salad will not be served immediately.

18. Artichoke Turkey Panini With Basil Pesto Aioli

Serving: Serves 4-6 | Prep: | Cook: | Ready in:

Ingredients

- Basil Aioli
- 1 bunch basil leaves (1.5-2 cups)
- 4 cloves roasted garlic
- 1/2 cup parmeseano-reggiano cheese, finely grated
- 2 tablespoons lemon juice and zest
- 1/4 cup pine nuts
- salt and pepper to taste
- 1/2 cup olive oil
- 1/2 cup canola oil
- 1 egg yolk (2 if small)
- Artichoke-Turkey Panini Sandwiches
- 2 grilled artichokes, halved
- 4 cloves roasted garlic
- 2 tablespoons truffle oil or olive oil
- 12 ounces fresh turkey breast
- 12 pieces provolone cheese
- 6 multi grain, seeded ciabatta rolls

Direction

- Make basil pesto aioli. If possible, allow to refrigerate overnight for flavors to develop. I like to use roasted garlic as it is a sweeter, more rounded flavor, and it is less likely to give that "garlic burp". You can substitute walnuts for the pine nuts, but use the best olive oil and parmesan that you can afford. Follow Amanda's recommendations--if you just took the egg out of the fridge--go read a couple of chapters, take a catnap, etc... dinner will be worth the wait.
- If you haven't grilled artichokes before, cut in half, remove choke. Cut into quarters. Dymnyno and aargersi both have good recipes posted. If you make their recipe first, just toss on a couple of extra for this recipe. You want a nice char which is why I cut into quarters.
- After artichokes have cooled, make a rough chop of the artichokes. Add a little oil to help bind together. This can be made a day ahead. If you like a finer chop, you can use the food processor and pulse to desired consistency.
- Layer ciabatta bread with artichoke spread on the bottom, turkey slices and provolone and on top piece of bread spread the basil pesto aioli. Toast on panini grill until cheese is melted.

19. Asha Gomez's Kerala Fried Chicken

Serving: Serves 8 | Prep: 24hours0mins | Cook: 0hours30mins | Ready in:

Ingredients

- 2 cups buttermilk
- 10 garlic cloves
- 6 whole serrano peppers, seeded if desired
- 1 bunch fresh cilantro (about 1 cup)
- 1 bunch fresh mint (about 1/2 cup)
- 2 tablespoons plus 1 teaspoon kosher salt
- 8 boneless, skinless chicken thighs (about 3 pounds)
- Canola oil, for frying
- 4 cups unbleached all-purpose flour
- 2 tablespoons coconut oil, melted
- 2 stems fresh curry leaves, for garnish

Direction

- In a blender, combine the buttermilk, garlic, peppers, cilantro, mint, and 2 tablespoons of the salt and purée until smooth. Place the

chicken in a large container with lid, and pour the buttermilk marinade over the chicken. Toss the chicken in the marinade, making sure it is well coated. Cover and refrigerate for at least 18 hours and up to 24 hours.
- When ready to fry the chicken, fill a large cast-iron skillet with 1 inch of oil and heat gently over medium heat until the oil reaches 350°F. Place a cooling rack over a rimmed baking sheet and set aside. Combine the flour and 1 teaspoon of salt in a shallow dish and set aside.
- While the oil is heating, remove the chicken from the marinade and gently shake off the excess marinade. Dredge each piece of chicken in the flour, coating thoroughly.
- Place the chicken in the hot oil, taking care not to crowd the pieces. Cook the chicken until it is deep golden brown and cooked through, about 4 minutes on each side, or until a meat thermometer reads 165°F. Drain the chicken on the cooling rack and drizzle with the melted coconut oil.
- Dip the curry leaves in the hot frying oil until crisp, about 10 to 15 seconds. Set on the cooling rack.

20. Asian Sesame Chicken & Broccoli

Serving: Serves 4 | Prep: | Cook: |Ready in:

Ingredients

- 1 pound chicken breast, cut into 1 inch pieces
- 3 1/2 cups fresh, pre-cut broccoli, can also buy frozen and thaw in advance
- 1 1/2 tablespoons extra virgin olive oil or coconut oil
- 3 tablespoons white rice vinegar
- 1 1/2 tablespoons sesame seeds
- 1 tablespoon garlic powder (I really like garlic)
- 1/2 teaspoon red pepper chili flakes
- 1/2 teaspoon ginger
- 1/4 teaspoon paprika
- salt/pepper to taste

Direction

- Warm oil in a large sauté or stir fry pan on the stovetop
- Add broccoli to pan, stirring frequently cook ~7 minutes until broccoli begins to soften
- Add to pan cut chicken, seasonings & white rice vinegar
- Cook ~10 minutes turning frequently until chicken is cooked through
- Serve & top with sriracha hot sauce (optional)

21. Asian Spiced Chicken Livers With Lemon Grass And Ramps

Serving: Serves 6-8 | Prep: | Cook: |Ready in:

Ingredients

- • 1 pound freshest chicken livers (organic)
- • ½ cup good quality soy sauce
- • ½ cup water
- • ¼ cup dry sherry wine
- • 1 tablespoon sugar (I used honey)
- • ½ star anise
- • 1 small stick cinnamon (about 1-inch)
- • 1 ½ -inch slice fresh ginger (crushed)
- • 2 sprigs lemon grass (cut in 1-inch pieces, and crushed)
- • 1 bunch of Ramps or young garlic
- • ¼ teaspoon dry red pepper flakes
- 1 tablespoon vegetable oil

Direction

- Place livers in a pan, cover with water, and bring just to boiling; rinse and drain. In a sauce pan combine soy sauce, water, Sherry, sugar or honey, and oil. Add star anise, cinnamon, ginger, lemon grass or young garlic and red pepper flakes. Bring to a boil, reduce

to simmer, add chicken levers, and reduce to simmer. Cover and cook on the lowest flame for 15 minutes.
- Remove from heat and cool. Chill for at least 1-2 hours. To serve, drain, discard all spices, and reduce the sauce until lightly thickened. Serve the sauce separately, or pour over the livers.

- Add the chicken, broth, and water and bring to a boil. Simmer for about 20 minutes. Stir in the rice, salt, and pepper, and simmer, covered for about 25 more minutes, until the rice is done and the chicken is tender.
- Stir in the frozen peas and cook for an additional 5-10 minutes. Serve in bowls with baguette bread and butter on the side.

22. Asopao De Pollo (Chicken Stew)

Serving: Serves 4-6 | Prep: | Cook: | Ready in:

Ingredients

- For the Sofrito
- 1 onion, diced
- 1 sweet pepper, diced
- 2 garlic cloves, chopped
- 1 handful cilantro, washed and chopped
- 1 ajicito dulce
- For the Asopao
- 8 chicken thighs and drumsticks
- Adobo
- 3 tablespoons olive oil
- Sofrito recipe
- 1 cup tomato sauce
- 3/4 cup alcaparrado
- 4 cups chicken stock
- 2 cups water
- 2 cups short or medium-grain rice
- 2 teaspoons salt
- 1 teaspoon pepper
- 2 cups frozen green peas

Direction

- Combine the onion, garlic, sweet pepper, hot pepper and cilantro in the blender with a few tablespoons of water. Blend until pureed.
- Sprinkle the chicken on both sides with adobo. Set aside.
- Heat the oil in a large soup pot. Add the sofrito, tomato sauce, and alcapparado. Simmer together for five minutes.

23. Autumnal Zuppa

Serving: Serves 6 | Prep: | Cook: | Ready in:

Ingredients

- 1 tablespoon olive oil
- 1/2 diced yellow (or white) large onion
- 1 pound ground turkey
- 1 tablespoon fennel seed
- 1 teaspoon red pepper flakes
- 1/2 teaspoon garlic powder
- 1 tablespoon vegetable base (I use "Better than Bullion")
- 1/2 cup water
- 1 teaspoon kosher salt
- 5-6 grinds of freshly ground pepper
- 1 huge or 3 medium sweet potatoes skinned and cubed
- 2 white potatoes cubed (optional)
- 3-4 cups well washed curly kale (or any kale like green) stems removed and diced
- 2 quarts good quality chicken broth
- Salt and ground pepper to taste

Direction

- Drizzle olive oil in a medium sauté pan and add diced onion and diced greens stems. Cook on medium high until translucent. Add ground turkey and brown until no pink remains. Add fennel seed, red pepper flakes, garlic powder and vegetable base and stir well for 2 minutes lightly toasting the seasoning. Add 1/2 cup water and reduce until turkey mixture is just dry (slightly moist is cool too,

you don't want to burn it). Add salt and pepper. This mixture should be slightly salty to the taste and highly seasoned.
- While meat is browning, combine sweet potatoes, white potatoes, kale, and chicken stock in a large soup pot. Turn on medium high and watch for it to boil, when the bubbles are apparent turn it down. Gently add completed turkey meat mixture to the soup pot and turn it down further to a gentle simmer. The soup is done with then potatoes are fork tender, about 30 to 40 minutes. Salt and pepper to taste. This is good straight from the pot but it is magnificent the next day, when the flavors marry and bloom while chilling in the fridge. Serve with good crusty bread and a sprinkle of parmesan cheese if you desire.

24. BBQ Chicken Bacon Ranch Salad

Serving: Serves 4 | Prep: | Cook: | Ready in:

Ingredients

- Salad
- 2 Heads of romaine lettuce
- 3 Large boneless, skinless chicken breasts
- 5-6 Slices applewood smoked bacon
- 1/2 onion, thinly sliced
- 1 cup halved cherry tomatoes
- 1/4 cup BBQ sauce
- 3/4 cup Shredded cheddar cheese
- 1/2 avocado (totally optional)
- Easy Homemade Ranch
- 1 cup Mayonnaise
- 1 cup milk
- 1 packet ranch dressing seasoning (I used Hidden Valley Ranch)

Direction

- Make the Ranch Dressing first, or ahead of time. Follow package instructions- simply mix mayo, milk, and ranch seasoning in a bowl and whisk together
- Preheat the oven to 375*F. Spray a rimmed baking dish with cooking oil. Thinly slice the onions and put them in the dish. Then put the three chicken breasts on top of the onions.
- Pour the BBQ sauce over the chicken. Bake for 30 minutes.
- While the chicken in cooking, make the bacon according to package instructions. Fry in a frypan or wide saucepan until crispy, 7-15 minutes over medium heat depending on thickness. When done, put on a plate with a paper towel to dry. Crumble with your fingers when cool, or use a knife to help.
- After 30 minutes, check the chicken for doneness. I usually slice into the thickest part of the breast and if there is any pink in the middle, then it needs to cook for longer. Add the cheese, and put back in the over for another 5-15 minutes, depending on doneness. If you have a meat thermometer, you can use that- make sure the internal temp of the chicken reaches 165*F.
- It's done when the chicken is fully cooked and the cheese is gooey. Let cool in the pan for about 10-15 minutes. Meanwhile, assemble the beds of salad greens and cherry tomatoes.
- Chop the chicken into bite sized pieces. Add a little of the sauce and onions from the pan, and if you like things super tangy, you can add a little more BBQ sauce to the chopped chicken here.
- Top each serving of salad with chicken, sprinkle with crumbled bacon, and drizzle with Ranch. If you have avocado, add a few slices. Enjoy your amazing BBQ Chicken Bacon Ranch Salad!

25. BBQ Whiskey Chicken Thighs

Serving: Makes 8 chicken thighs | Prep: 0hours5mins | Cook: 0hours15mins | Ready in:

Ingredients

- 8 Boneless skinless chicken thighs
- 1 1/2 cups Your favorite bbq sauce
- 1/3 cup Whiskey

Direction

- Add chicken thighs to a bowl
- In a separate bowl mix together BBQ sauce and whiskey
- Add BBQ/whiskey mixture to chicken thighs and stir to coat.
- Grill chicken thighs over medium to high flame for about 15 minutes, flipping half way through.

26. BBQ Pulled Chicken Lettuce Wraps

Serving: Serves 4 | Prep: | Cook: | Ready in:

Ingredients

- 1 pound boneless, skinless chicken breasts or boneless, skinless chicken thighs
- 1/2 cup to 3/4 cup barbecue sauce
- 1 cup packaged shredded carrots or 2 medium carrots, shredded
- 2 tablespoons chopped fresh cilantro
- 8 Bibb or romaine lettuce leaves

Direction

- Place the chicken in a medium saucepan and add enough water to cover. Bring to a boil. Reduce the heat to low, cover, and simmer until the chicken is cooked through, 15 to 20 minutes.
- Transfer the chicken to a cutting board and let cool, slightly. Discard the water in the pan and wipe dry with paper towels. Use two forks to shred the chicken. Return the chicken to the pan and stir in the barbecue sauce. Cook over medium heat until heated through, about 2 minutes.

- In a small bowl, combine the carrots, cilantro, and lime juice. Serve the BBQ chicken and some of the shredded carrot mixture in the lettuce leaves.

27. Baby Potatoes In Cheese Sauce

Serving: Serves 4 | Prep: | Cook: | Ready in:

Ingredients

- 500 grams baby potatoes
- 1/2 tablespoon chicken bullion
- 1 teaspoon minced white onion
- 1 pinch salt
- 1 tablespoon chopped parsley
- 1/2 cup milk
- 1/4 cup grated cheddar
- 1 cup water

Direction

- Wash baby potatoes and cut in half.
- Boil potatoes in water with the chicken bouillon until cooked.
- Lower heat then add milk, cheese, onions and parsley.
- Mix until sauce thickens and add a pinch off salt.

28. Baby Spinach, Arugula, And Fruit Salad With Balsamic Dressing

Serving: Serves 4 to 40 | Prep: | Cook: | Ready in:

Ingredients

- Salad Ingredients
- Baby Spinach
- Arugula

- Mixture of Nuts & Berries: (I buy this at Costco) Cranberries, dried cherries, pistachios, walnuts, almonds
- Fuji apple, diced medium (1 apple for 3-4 people)
- Fresh blueberries, and/or blackberries, raspberries, Peaches, any fresh fruit
- Grilled chicken, sliced, 1 boneless breast per person
- Goat cheese, 2 ounces per person
- Dressing
- Equal amounts of extra virgin olive oil and balsamic vinegar. Add pepper to taste. My favorites combos are: Persian Lime Olive Oil with Blueberry Balsamic OR Persian Lime Olive Oil with White Peach Balsamic

Direction

- Mix equal amounts of the olive oil and balsamic together in a jar and shake well. Add pepper to taste, shake again.
- Toss spinach and arugula together, add the nuts and berries, apple, and fresh fruit. Toss with dressing.
- Place salad greens on a dinner plate and top with slices of grilled chicken and the goat cheese.

29. Bacon Blueberry Dog Biscuit

Serving: Makes 30 biscuits | Prep: 0hours30mins | Cook: 2hours0mins | Ready in:

Ingredients

- 2 1/2 cups old-fashioned oats
- 3/4 cup Bow Hill Organic Heirloom Blueberry Powder
- 1/2 cup flax seeds, ground
- 2 tablespoons bacon fat, olive oil or flax seed oil
- 1/2 cup applesauce or 2 eggs
- 1/2 cup chicken or vegetable stock

Direction

- Heat oven to 325°F.
- Grind the flax seed in a coffee grinder (or buy pre-ground).
- Set aside ½ cup of oat flour. Combine 1 ½ cups oat flour and remaining ½ cup of whole oats, blueberry powder, and flax meal.
- Stir in the bacon fat, eggs, and chicken stock until a sturdy dough forms.
- Generously sprinkle half the leftover oat flour on a counter top and use another fourth of it for the rolling pin (reapplying as needed). Roll the dough ½" thick and cut into your desired shapes.
- Place on a baking sheet lined with parchment paper or a Silpat (or nothing at all). After placing on the baking sheet, brush each shape with chicken stock or water.
- Bake 1 hour. Turn oven off and leave the biscuits in the oven with the door closed for another hour to completely dry out.
- Store in an airtight container until Fido has finished them off!

30. Bacon Wrapped, Spatchcocked Turkey In 80 Minutes

Serving: Serves 12 | Prep: 0hours0mins | Cook: 0hours0mins | Ready in:

Ingredients

- 4 Cloves garlic, peeled
- 1 handful Mixed fresh herbs (sage, rosemary, thyme, parsley, oregano)
- 3 pounds Thick cut bacon
- 12-14 pounds Turkey, spatchcocked
- Pepper
- 3 Carrots, peeled and cut into 3" pieces
- 2 Leeks, cleaned and cut into 3" pieces
- 2 Apples, unpeeled and cut into 8 slices
- 3/4 - 1 cups Chicken stock

Direction

- Heat oven to 400 degrees. Put the garlic in a food processor and whirl to finely chop. Add herbs and pulse to chop. Add 1/2 pound of bacon and butter and pulse until you have a smooth bacon herb butter.
- Prepare turkey by running your hands between the skin and the flesh to separate the skin from the flesh. Separate the skin for as much of the turkey as possible, including the breasts and the drumsticks. Rub the bacon, herb butter all over the turkey and in between the skin and the flesh, giving the turkey a good bacon-butter massage. Lay three strips of bacon between the breast and the skin. Season with pepper.
- Spread the vegetables and the apples over a large rimmed sheet pan and lay the turkey skin-side up on the pan. Starting with the neck-side of the turkey, begin weaving a turkey jacket by laying one long strip horizontally across the width of the turkey and then weaving a strip vertically. Alternate between horizontal and vertical strips, until the body of the turkey is covered in a woven jacket. Then continue weaving the jacket to include both drum sticks and the wings. Trim any excess lengths of bacon.
- Pour the stock into the bottom of the pan. Carefully put the pan in the oven and roast for about 80 minutes, frequently checking to see the bacon is not over cooking. If the bacon starts to become too dark, remove from the oven and cover with a sheet of foil and return it to the oven to continue roasting. The turkey is done when the internal temperature reaches 155 degrees. Remove from the oven and allow to rest for 30 minutes before slicing. The internal temperature will rise to 160 to 165 degrees while the turkey rests. Always use a thermometer to safely and consistently determine when your turkey is done.

31. Baid Mutajjan – Middle Eastern Fried Hard Boiled Eggs

Serving: Serves 4 | Prep: | Cook: | Ready in:

Ingredients

- 5   fresh eggs
- 3 tablespoons   vegetable oil
- 3 tablespoons   sumac
- 2 tablespoons   sesame seeds
- to season   salt
- to garnish   coriander leaves

Direction

- 1. Hard boil the eggs, remove shell and cut into halves. Season lightly with salt.
- 2. Dry roast the sesame seeds till light golden; make sure not to burn.
- 3. Coarsely grind the sumac and sesame seeds in a mortar and pestle and keep aside.
- 4. In a flat pan, heat oil (on medium heat) and place the eggs yolk side down. A bit of splutter is expected. (You can fry the eggs whole too without cutting into halves but ensure that you prick a couple of holes with a fork to avoid the eggs from exploding.)
- 5. After a minute or two, turn the eggs over and fry another minute. Remove from flame.
- 6. Roll or dust the eggs with the sumac-sesame seed blend. Garnish with chopped coriander leaves just before serving.

32. Baked Meat Cannelloni Cannelloni Di Carne Al Forno

Serving: Serves 8 | Prep: | Cook: | Ready in:

Ingredients

- Meat filling for the cannelloni
- 7 ounces   minced veal
- 7 ounces   minced pork
- 4 ounces   chicken breat minced

- 4 ounces Italian sausage without the casing and crumbled
- 3.5 ounces Parmesan grated
- 2 slices of Prosciutto, chopped very finely
- 1 whole egg
- 1/4 cup white wine
- nutmeg
- salt
- pepper freshly ground
- 5 tablespoons Extra Virgin Olive Oil
- For the Tomato Sauce
- 24 ounces bottle of tomato passata - see explanation at the bottom of the recipe
- 2 garlic cloves, green inner part removed and chopped very finely
- 1 medium red onion chopped very finely
- 5 tablespoons Extra Virgin Olive Oil
- 8 oven-ready lasagne noodles
- 1/3 cup parmesan for topping cannellonis
- Bechamel Sauce
- 4 cups milk
- 3 ounces all purpose flour
- 3 ounces butter cut in small pieces
- salt
- white pepper freshly ground
- 1 dash nutmeg

Direction

- Chop the Prosciutto finely and set aside.
- In a wide pan, over medium heat, add the 5 tablespoons of olive oil. Start by adding the crumbled sausage meat, stir well and let start get some color. Add the veal a bit at a time and stir. Let start to brown. Then add the pork, a little at a time and continue browning. Finally add the chicken. The procedure is a little slow because you want to brown the meat and if you put all the meat in one go it starts to lose its water and you end up with boiled rubbery meat instead of fried meat.
- Keep stirring the meat until golden brown all through, add the white wine, stir, let the alcohol evaporate, season with salt, freshly ground pepper and some nutmeg. Put the meat in a colander over a bowl and allow to cool. All the excess fat and liquid will fall through the colander.
- When cool, put the fried meat in a bowl, add the chopped prosciutto, the egg lightly beaten and the parmesan cheese. Mix everything very well to blend all the ingredients.
- For the Béchamel Sauce: Warm up the milk.
- In a medium saucepan, melt the cut up butter until it starts to get a little blond. Add the flour all at once and stir continuously over low heat until well blended.
- Slowly add the warm milk, stirring constantly (I actually prefer to use a whisk, I think it helps blending better). When it's all incorporated, continue cooking for 15 minutes over low heat. You need to cook the béchamel sauce for this amount of time to cook the flour and minimize the taste of raw flour.
- Season with salt, freshly ground white pepper, a nice dash of freshly grated nutmeg and let cool. The béchamel should remain soft, not thick.
- For the Tomato sauce: In a pan over medium heat add 5 tablespoons of olive oil, the 2 chopped garlics and the onion chopped very finely. Stir until the onion is translucent, add the passata, stir, add a pinch of salt and reduce the heat to low. Allow to simmer for about 15 to 20 minutes until you have a thick tomato sauce.
- For the cannelloni (see note at the bottom if you have dry pasta cannelloni): Bring a large pot of salted water to boil and add 1 tablespoon of olive oil. On the side have a big bowl of cold salted water with 1 tablespoon of olive oil.
- Prepare on your work surface 2 clean kitchen tea towels (linen or cotton - not terry cloth) to drain the cooked lasagna sheets.
- Add 2 or 3 pasta sheets a time and cook about 2 minutes. Remove each lasagna square out with a slotted spoon and dip it in a bowl with salted cold water. When cold, drain and set them on the clean kitchen tea towel, making sure they don't overlap so they don't stick to each other.

- Preheat oven to 350°F with rack in the middle. Prepare a 13- by 9- by 2-inch ceramic baking dish.
- Divide the meat filling on the lasagna rectangles in a line on the short side of the pasta rectangle, then roll up to close filling.
- Add half the béchamel sauce to the tomato sauce and stir well to mix.
- Cover the bottom of the baking dish with a good layer of tomato béchamel mixture. Align the rolled cannelloni's, seam side down, to baking dish, starting. On one of the ends. Finish putting all the cannelloni in the dish and cover completely with the tomato béchamel sauce.
- Sprinkle generously with parmesan on top, and finish with a few tablespoons of the remainder béchamel over the tomato sauce.
- Bake in the oven for 30 minutes. Turn off the oven, half open the door and leave the cannelloni to rest and the sauce will thicken a little.
- Serve hot.
- Note: in Italy people use cannelloni which are large tubes of dry pasta. Because there is a lot of sauce you don't have to pre-cook them and they also absorb some liquid from the tomato sauce, which is why you need this much tomato sauce. I don't know if in the U.S you can find these large pasta tubes. If you can, use them by all means, it's much easier than making them out of lasagna. You just fill them with a small spoon or preferably with a piping bag, until the whole tube is filled with meat, then put them on the tomato sauce, cover with tomato sauce, some béchamel and bake for 30 minutes.
- Tomato Passata: In Italy we have 2 different kinds of tomato sauce - one is Passata and the other is Pomarola. The Passata is fresh tomatoes, peeled and passed through a vegetable mill so you have in fact raw tomato juice. You can make it by processing canned peeled tomatoes with the liquid that comes in the tin - as easy as that! The Pomarola, or tomato sauce, is made with passata as a base, but is cooked with olive oil, onions, garlic, bay leaf, thyme, basil and sometimes some celery, salt and pepper. It is then cooked for about 45 minutes to reduce and obtain a thicker sauce that is already finished.

33. Baked Pasta With Chicken Sausage

Serving: Serves 8 | Prep: | Cook: | Ready in:

Ingredients

- 1 tablespoon olive oil
- 3/4 pound fresh sweet Italian sausage (I use chicken, but feel free to use pork)
- 1/2 onion, diced
- Kosher salt
- 1 fat clove garlic, peeled and smashed
- Handful basil leaves
- 4 cups chopped tomatoes (fresh or canned)
- 1 cup heavy cream
- 1/2 cup grated Parmesan
- 1/4 cup ricotta cheese
- 1 cup grated mozzarella
- 1 pound short pasta (I like penne or conchiglie)
- 2 tablespoons cold unsalted butter, cubed

Direction

- Heat the olive oil over medium-high heat in a medium heavy saucepan until shimmering. Remove the sausage from the casings and add it to the pan, breaking it up into small pieces with a wooden spoon. Brown the sausage well, stirring a couple times, about 5 minutes.
- Create a hole in the middle of the pan and add the onion and a pinch of salt. Cook until softened, stirring occasionally, for about 5 minutes. Add the garlic and cook for another minute. Add the tomatoes and the basil and stir well to combine. Bring the mixture to a simmer and cook until the sauce thickens and the flavors meld, at least 30 minutes. Taste and

add salt if necessary. Remove the basil leaves and set the sauce aside.
- Heat the oven to 500 °F and butter a 2-quart baking dish. Bring a large pot of salted water to a boil.
- In a mixing bowl, combine the sausage sauce with the rest of the ingredients, except the pasta and butter. Add 1/2 teaspoon salt and stir well.
- Drop the pasta into the boiling water and cook for 4 minutes. Drain well and add to the mixing bowl, tossing gently to combine everything.
- Spread the pasta evenly into the baking dish. Dot evenly with the butter, and bake until bubbly and brown, 7 to 10 minutes. Cool for a few minutes before serving.

34. Baked Salt And Pepper Wings

Serving: Serves about 15, depending on pack size | Prep: | Cook: | Ready in:

Ingredients

- 2 packets chicken wings
- 2 cups all-purpose flour
- 1 tablespoon ground black pepper
- 1 tablespoon ground white pepper
- 1 tablespoon ground Szechuan pepper
- 1 tablespoon sea salt
- 1 red bell pepper
- 3 spring onions
- 1 long red chili

Direction

- Prepare the chicken wings by trimming the tips and removing excess skin and fat.
- Tip the flour into a box with an air-tight lid, and add the salt and pepper. Stir well to mix.
- Put the chicken wings into the box, and put the lid on. Give the box a good shake, rattle and/or roll to thoroughly coat the wings with the seasoned flour. There will seem to be a lot of excess; this is OK.
- Refrigerate the wings overnight.
- When you're ready to cook, heat the oven to 400F/200C. Take the box out of the fridge and give another shake to loosen things up. Take the wings out and layer on a wire rack with a tray underneath. You'll find that the wings have stuck together and that the flour coating is now more of a thick batter - this is perfect, but be sure to separate them before cooking.
- Put the wings in the oven for 25 minutes. Turn them over once, halfway through the cooking time.
- While the wings are cooking, thinly slice the bell pepper, diagonally slice the spring onion and slice the chili into rings, removing or leaving the seeds as you prefer.
- When the wings are ready, put them in a serving bowl and toss with the bell pepper, spring onion and chili.

35. Baked Pineapple Fried Rice With Cashew Nuts

Serving: Serves 4 | Prep: | Cook: | Ready in:

Ingredients

- 1 pineapple
- 2 cups leftover, refrigerated cooked jasmine rice
- 1 egg
- 2 tablespoons raisins
- 1/4 cup toasted unsalted cashew nuts
- 1/4 cup shrimp
- 1/2 cup diced chicken thighs
- 1 cup diced carrots and peas
- 2 garlic cloves, coarsely chopped
- 1 tablespoon soya sauce
- 1/2 tablespoon sugar
- 2 tablespoons fish sauce
- 2 tablespoons coconut milk
- 2 tablespoons oil

- white pepper to taste
- cliantro leaves and chopped green onion for granish

Direction

- Preheat an oven to 375 F.
- Cut the pineapple in half lengthwise and hallow out the fruit so that the shell can be used as a container. Put the pineapple shell into the oven for about 5 minutes to dry out the moist. Meanwhile, coarsely cube 1 cup of the pineapple fruit. Set the shell and the fruit aside.
- Heat the wok or the skillet in medium high heat, add 1 tablespoon of oil, stir fry the garlic for about 30 seconds until the garlic is light golden brown. Increase the heat to high, sauté the shrimp and chicken until both are cooked through. Set aside.
- Crack the egg in a bowl, briefly mix the yolk and the white with a folk, add a pinch of salt and pepper. Heat the skillet in medium high heat, add 1 tablespoon of oil, pour the egg into the skillet without stirring, cook until set about 30 seconds. Add the diced carrot, peas and the cooked rice. Break up any clumps of rice. Add the cooked shrimps, chickens, cashew nuts, raisins, chopped pineapples, soya sauce, sugar, fish sauce, coconut milk, stir fry until evenly seasoned.
- Cover the pineapple leaves with foil (so that they are not burn when bake). Transfer the rice mixture to the pineapple shell and baked until hot, about 10 minutes. Garnish with cilantro leaves and chopped green onion.

36. Balsamic Chicken Sandwich With Peach Jam And Brandied Onions

Serving: Serves 4 | Prep: | Cook: | Ready in:

Ingredients

- For the chicken and brandied onions:
- 1 pound boneless free-range chicken breast, cut into strips
- 1 cup balsamic vinaigrette
- Sea salt, to taste
- Freshly cracked pepper, to taste
- Olive oil
- 1 red onion, thinly sliced
- 1 tablespoon brandy
- 1 loaf of bread from the bakery (I used French bread), sliced
- Peach jam (see below)
- Your favorite mayonnaise (or a vegan substitute)
- 1 head of lettuce (Boston, green, or red leaf would work)
- For the peach jam:
- 1 peach, peeled and chopped
- 2 tablespoons organic sugar
- 1 teaspoon brandy
- 1 pinch sea salt

Direction

- For the chicken and brandied onions:
- Marinate the chicken for at least one hour and up to 12. When you're ready to cook, preheat a grill or a grill pan over medium-high heat. Drizzle the grill with a little olive oil and cook chicken strips for 4 minutes per side. Remove and set aside.
- Meanwhile, in a small pan, heat a glug of olive oil over medium heat and add the onion slices. Season with salt and pepper and cook for 6 to 7 minutes, stirring often.
- Add the brandy and continue to cook until the alcohol is absorbed, about 2 to 3 minutes. Remove from the heat and set aside.
- Lay out the slices of bread. Spread the jam on one side and the mayonnaise on the other. On top of the jam, add the chicken, onion, then the lettuce. Voilà!
- For the peach jam:
- Add the ingredients to a pan set over high heat. Bring to a boil, then reduce heat to medium and continue to cook for about 7

minutes. Using a potato masher, smash the peaches until the big lumps are gone.
- Turn off heat and transfer to a jar to cool. The jam will keep for up to 3 weeks in the refrigerator (if you don't eat it all first!).

37. Basil Chicken

Serving: Serves 4 | Prep: | Cook: |Ready in:

Ingredients

- 4 breasts of chicken, boneless & skinless
- 2 cups mozzarella cheese, shredded
- 4-5 sprigs fresh basil, chopped (per breast)
- several pats garlic butter (per breast)
- salt to taste
- pepper to taste

Direction

- Butterfly your breasts
- Add basil, cheese, garlic butter, salt & pepper to inside of breasts
- Close breasts back together and secure by threading a wooden skewer through it
- Grill breasts until done
- Add a little more cheese & basil to the tops and melt

38. Beer Can Chicken

Serving: Serves 2 (with leftovers) to 4 | Prep: | Cook: |Ready in:

Ingredients

- 1 3 1/2 lb. chicken
- 1 lemon, halved (preferably Meyer)
- 2 sprigs of rosemary
- Kosher Salt
- water
- 1 tablespoon lavender
- 1 tablespoon peppercorns
- 1 tablespoon lavender
- 1 can of beer

Direction

- Make a brine by dissolving salt in 2 quarts cold water in large container. I find the easiest way to do this is add the salt to the container and about 1 inch of hot water, dissolve the salt by stirring briskly and then add the cold water.
- Lower the chicken into the salted water and brine, refrigerated for at least 1 hour and up to 4 hours. Remove chicken from brine and rinse inside and out with cold water.
- Turn all burners on gas grill and pre-heat until hot as can be. If using charcoal - and, yes, I know that is better - light the coals.
- Grind the peppercorns, lavender and fennel in a spice grinder and massage spice rub all over chicken, inside and out. Lift up skin over breast and rub spice rub directly onto meat. Stick the rosemary sprigs, crunched up, into the cavity.
- Open beer can and pour out (or drink) about 1/3 cup. With church key can opener, punch two more large holes in top of can (for a total of three). Slide chicken over can so that drumsticks reach down to bottom of can and chicken stands upright. Take one half of the lemon and cover the hole on top, pulling excess skin over the lemon if possible.
- Place chicken and beer can on the part of grill closest to front and balance the bird using the drumsticks as a tripod. Turn off first burner. Close lid and bring heat back to 350 degrees. Fiddle with grill controls so that you keep the bird at 350 degrees. I have three burners and it works with the first off, the middle on low-medium and the back one high. If you are using the better alternative - charcoal - I am afraid you are on your own.
- After 30 minutes rotate bird 180 degrees using wads of paper towels to help you. Roast bird about 60 minutes for a 3 1/2 lb. bird or until instant-read thermometer inserted into

thickest part of thigh registers 170 to 175 degrees. Allow to rest for 15 minutes tented with foil. Remove carefully from the beer can - a job sometimes best done over the sink - and serve.

39. Best Ever Turkey Chili

Serving: Serves 4 | Prep: | Cook: | Ready in:

Ingredients

- Olive oil
- 2 tablespoons tomato paste
- 1 medium to large onion, chopped
- 5 cloves garlic, minced
- 1/2 red bell pepper, chopped
- 1 teaspoon chili powder
- 1/2 teaspoon hot paprika
- 1/2 teaspoon dried coriander
- 1/4 teaspoon oregano
- Dash of cinnamon
- 1 pound ground turkey breast
- 1 cup dark beer, such as Leffe Brown
- one 28-ounce can diced tomatoes
- one 15 1/2-ounce can kidney beans, drained
- 1/2 teaspoon hot sauce or chile paste
- Salt and pepper
- Sour cream, chopped chives, cilantro, and/or shredded cheese, for topping

Direction

- Heat a bit of olive oil in a large pot over medium heat. Add the tomato paste, onion, garlic, and red pepper, then cook, stirring occasionally, until softened. Add the chili powder, hot paprika, coriander, oregano, and cinnamon; stir and allow to cook until aromatic, 1 minute.
- Add the ground turkey and cook, breaking it up with a spoon, until lightly browned. Pour in the beer and allow to cool down slightly.
- Add the tomatoes, beans, and hot sauce or chili paste.

- Allow the chili to simmer, uncovered, until thickened, about 40 minutes. Season with salt and pepper to taste. Top with sour cream, chopped chives, cilantro, and/or shredded cheese.

40. Best Stuffed Peppers

Serving: Makes 8 | Prep: 0hours10mins | Cook: 1hours0mins | Ready in:

Ingredients

- 4 large bell peppers, gutted and halved
- 1 tablespoon canola oil
- 1 teaspoon onion powder
- 1 teaspoon garlic powder
- 1 teaspoon kosher or sea salt
- 1 teaspoon ground black pepper
- 1 pound ground meat (turkey, chicken, or beef)
- 1 pound sweet longanisa sausage (can use honey garlic, or any sweet sausage, as a substitute)
- 2 cloves of garlic, minced
- 1 cup diced mushrooms, drained
- 1 cup mushrooms, diced
- 1 cup tomato sauce
- 1 cup Minute Rice
- 1 cup mozzarella cheese, shredded
- 1/4 cup parmesan cheese, grated
- Fresh parsley for garnish

Direction

- Heat grill on high heat.
- Place halved peppers on grill and grill until slightly charred with grill marks - approx. 5 minutes a side.
- Remove from grill and place on a plate. Set aside.
- In a large skillet, heat cooking oil.
- Add minced garlic and sauté until fragrant; make sure not to brown the garlic.

- Add the ground beef (or chicken/turkey) and the sausage. (If the sausage was in casing, make sure you squeeze it out of its casing).
- Add the onion powder, garlic powder, sea salt and ground black pepper.
- Stir well until meat is cooked.
- Add mushrooms, diced tomatoes, tomato sauce, and Minute Rice.
- Bring the heat to high until mixture reaches a simmer, and then bring the heat to low. Allow to simmer for approx. 5 minutes.
- Remove from heat and add 1 cup of shredded mozzarella cheese. Mix well and set aside.
- Pre-heat oven to 375F.
- With a tablespoon, carefully scoop the meat mixture into the peppers.
- Pack the peppers as much as you can and press down on the mixture to secure.
- Sprinkle each pepper with the remaining shredded mozzarella.
- Finish off by sprinkling each pepper with shredded parmesan.
- Place the peppers in the oven for approx. 15 minutes or until the mozzarella cheese melts and bubbles.
- Turn the broiler on to high heat and place the peppers under the broiler for approx. 2 minutes, or until cheese browns slightly.
- Garnish with fresh flat leaf parsley and serve.

41. Bev's Chicken (or Pork Or Beef) Or Vegetarian Tortilla Casserole

Serving: Makes 13 x 9 baking dish | Prep: | Cook: | Ready in:

Ingredients

- 15 ounces can of black beans
- 15 ounces can of refried beans
- 7 ounces can of Ortega chilies
- 2 cups Shredded Monterey Jack cheese
- 1 medium onion, diced
- 2 cups shredded cooked meat (pork, chicken or beef}
- white corn chips

Direction

- Preheat oven to 350° F
- Spray a 9"x13" pan with vegetable oil
- Place a layer of corn chips in the bottom of the pan.
- Mix black beans and refried beans together in a separate bowl
- Pour ½ of the bean mixture on top of the chips.
- Spread meat over the beans
- Spread ½ of chilies over the meat.
- Place another layer of chips over the chilies.
- Pour remaining ½ of beans over the second layer of chips and put the remaining chilies over that.
- Top with cheese and chopped onions.
- Bake uncovered at 350° for 30 minutes or until warmed through.

42. Bibimpap

Serving: Serves 2-4 | Prep: | Cook: | Ready in:

Ingredients

- 1 cup basmati rice, cooked
- 2 eggs, done any way you like
- 1 cup roughly chopped/shredded chicken (I used leftovers from the Sweet Chili Chicken Wings recipe)
- 2 carrots, peeled, sliced, and blanched
- 1 English Cucumber, sliced
- 20 or so Brussels spouts, quartered and blanched
- 2 tablespoons Asian sesame dressing

Direction

- This is pretty much a prep and put together kind of meal. I heated up a teaspoon of olive oil and lightly sautéed the shredded chicken.

Since it was already seasoned from the previous day's wing recipe, it took on this smoky flavor after cooking it in the pan. It was quite delicious.

- After blanching the vegetables, I separately sautéed each in the same pan for about 1-2 minutes each, just to kind of get a semi-browning on them.
- This is supposed to go in a large bowl, but I thought it would look better on a large plate, so just place each vegetable, chicken, and rice, along the edge of the plate, kind of in a circular fashion (you can see why I was supposed to use a bowl) and place the fried egg in the middle. Top the rice with a little bit of Asian sesame dressing and dig in!

43. Big Mama's Fried Chicken

Serving: Serves 8 | Prep: 0hours0mins | Cook: 0hours0mins | Ready in:

Ingredients

- 8 pieces chicken
- 3 large eggs, beaten
- 1 teaspoon hot sauce
- 1 teaspoon Worcestershire
- 2 1/2 cups all-purpose flour
- 3 tablespoons seasoned salt
- 3 tablespoons cornstarch
- 2 teaspoons paprika
- 1/2 teaspoon cayenne pepper
- 2 teaspoons black pepper
- 1/2 teaspoon garlic powder
- 1 tablespoon onion powder

Direction

- In a medium sized bowl, whisk together eggs, hot sauce and Worcestershire and set aside.
- Next add flour, cornstarch, seasoned salt, paprika, cayenne pepper, black pepper, garlic powder and onion powder to a paper bag and shake to mix well.
- Dip each piece of chicken into egg wash coating both sides then dip into seasoned flour thoroughly coating each piece. Then add piece to baking sheet to rest.
- Finish coating all chicken and let sit for 10-15 minutes until coating has set.
- While coating sets, add 1-1/2 inches of oil to a cast iron skillet or heavy bottom skillet and heat over medium high heat. Also turn on oven to 275 degrees.
- This is my test for knowing when the oil is ready: Big Mama always tossed a tiny bit of flour in the oil and if it began to fry and sizzle, the oil was ready.
- Fry four pieces at a time on each side starting with dark meat since it takes longer. Make sure you don't overcrowd the pan. After each side has turned slightly golden, put the top on the skillet to steam the inside of the chicken ensuring doneness. After a couple of minutes, remove the top and continue to fry until the crust is crispy again and completely golden brown.
- Remove chicken from oil and place on paper towels or rack to drain. Place chicken on a baking sheet covered with parchment and add to warmed oven while finishing the other chicken pieces.
- Fry the remaining chicken pieces and drain and add to oven. Add the remaining chicken to the oven.
- Serve chicken when ready.

44. Bikini Bolognese

Serving: Serves 2 | Prep: | Cook: | Ready in:

Ingredients

- 2 1/2 large zucchinis, peeled and spiralized
- 1/2 pound ground turkey, lean
- 2 tablespoons olive oil
- 1/2 red onion
- 1/2 celery stick, diced
- 1/2 whole carrot, diced

- 1 teaspoon red hot pepper flakes
- 2 garlic cloves, minced
- 14 ounces can of crushed tomatoes
- 3/4 tablespoon tomato paste
- 1/4 cup chicken broth
- 1/3 cup chopped basil
- 1 tablespoon oregano flakes
- 1/4 cup shaved parmesan cheese, for garnish

Direction

- Add your carrots and celery to a food processor and pulse until chopped finely. There can still be chunks, just no big ones. The end mixture should be somewhere in between chunky and pureed.
- Put a large skillet over medium heat and add in the olive oil and season with salt and pepper. Once oil heats, add in garlic and cook for 30 seconds. Add in red pepper flakes, cook for 30 seconds and then add in the onions. Cook onions for 1-2 minutes or until they begin to soften. Add in carrot/celery mixture and cook for 1 minute.
- Push the veggie mixture to the side and add in the ground turkey, crumbling as you add. Crumble with a spatula or wooden spoon. Add a pinch of the oregano flakes. Cook turkey until the meat is no longer pink.
- Combine the veggies with the turkey and season with another pinch of oregano flakes. Add in the chicken broth and cook until reduced (water evaporates).
- Add in the crushed tomatoes, tomato paste and season generously with salt and pepper. Add in the remaining oregano flakes. Bring to a boil and then lower heat and let simmer for 15 minutes.
- After 15 minutes, add in the zucchini pasta and mix thoroughly to combine. Plate onto dishes and garnish with Parmesan cheese. Feel free to eat this while wearing a bikini!

45. Bison And Chicken Sausage Chili

Serving: Serves 5 | Prep: | Cook: | Ready in:

Ingredients

- 1.5 pounds ground bison
- .5 pounds mild Italian chicken or turkey sausage (about 2 links)
- 1 tablespoon olive oil
- 1 medium onion, chopped
- 2 bell peppers (orange and/or yellow), roughly chopped
- 4 cloves garlic, minced
- 56 ounces (2-28 oz. cans) whole tomatoes with juice, roughly chopped
- 14.5 ounces (1 can) black beans, drained and rinsed
- 14.5 ounces (1 can) kidney beans, drained and rinsed
- 8 ounces tomato sauce
- 1 tablespoon tomato paste
- 1 tablespoon chili powder
- 2 teaspoons garlic powder
- 2 teaspoons onion powder
- 1 bay leaf
- salt and freshly ground black pepper, to taste

Direction

- Heat 1 T of olive oil over medium heat.
- Add chopped onion and cook for 5 minutes, until it is just becoming translucent.
- Add chopped bell peppers and cook for 2 minutes, then add garlic.
- When garlic becomes fragrant, but not brown (1 minute or so), add ground bison.
- Remove the chicken sausage from its casings and add the chicken as well. Discard casings.
- Add half of chili powder (about 2 tsp.) and pinches of salt and pepper. Stir frequently.
- When meat is no longer pink (8-10 minutes), reduce heat to low and add the chopped tomatoes with their juice.
- When incorporated, add the rinsed and drained beans.

- Add tomato sauce (you can use less, if you prefer, but the bison will soak it up) and the remaining seasonings: 2 tsp of chili powder, garlic and onion powders.
- Add bay leaf.
- Simmer chili on the stove, still on low heat, stirring occasionally, for 45-60 minutes. This allows the flavors to merry and the excess liquid to burn off.
- Remove the bay leaf and serve with light sour cream and a little cheddar cheese if you can't help yourself!

46. Blue Hubbard Squash Chili

Serving: Serves 6 | Prep: | Cook: |Ready in:

Ingredients

- 5 cups Blue Hubbard squash, peeled & diced
- 1 cup sweet onion, diced
- 1 poblano, diced
- 2 hatch chiles, diced
- 1 garlic clove, minced
- 6 cups chicken stock (preferably homemade)
- 2 medium tomatoes, diced
- 1 can great northern beans, drained and rinsed
- 1 cooked chicken breast, diced
- 1 teaspoon pasilla chile powder
- 1 tablespoon ancho chile powder
- 1 teaspoon paprika
- 1/2 teaspoon smoked paprika
- 1/2 teaspoon pepper
- Salt, to taste

Direction

- Spray heavy bottomed Dutch oven with cooking spray, then add diced onions, peppers, garlic, and squash to pan.
- Sauté vegetables until soft, about 5-7 minutes.
- Add chicken stock, tomatoes, beans, diced chicken, and herbs.
- Bring to boil, then reduce to a simmer for about 30 minutes.
- Season with salt & pepper to taste.

47. Blueberry Sweet Tea–Brined Chicken Thighs From Todd Richards

Serving: Serves 4 | Prep: 0hours0mins | Cook: 0hours0mins |Ready in:

Ingredients

- 8 bone-in, skin-on chicken thighs
- Blueberry Sweet Tea Brine (recipe below)
- 2 tablespoons blended olive oil
- 1 tablespoon kosher salt
- 1 teaspoon coarsely ground black pepper
- BLUEBERRY SWEET TEA BRINE
- Blueberry Sweet Tea (recipe below)
- 1 cup kosher salt
- 1 tablespoon black peppercorns
- 1/4 teaspoon red pepper flakes
- 4 garlic cloves
- 4 star anise pods
- 4 bay leaves
- 2 large thyme sprigs
- 2 medium-size oranges, cut into quarters
- 1 large lemon cut into quarters
- BLUEBERRY SWEET TEA
- 2 quarts (8 cups) water
- 12 orange pekoe black tea bags
- Blueberry Simple Syrup (recipe below)
- BLUEBERRY SIMPLE SYRUP
- 1 cup granulated sugar
- 1 tablespoon lemon zest (from 1 lemon)
- 6 black peppercorns
- 1 star anise pod
- 2 cups (16 ounces) water
- 1 cup fresh blueberries

Direction

- Combine the chicken thighs and Blueberry Sweet Tea Brine (recipe below) in a large bowl and refrigerate 4 hours or up to overnight.
- Heat broiler with oven rack 6 inches from heat.
- Remove the chicken from the brine, and pat dry with paper towels. Let stand at room temperature 1 hour. Rub with the oil, and sprinkle with the salt and pepper.
- Line a rimmed baking sheet with aluminum foil, and top with a wire rack. Place chicken, skin side up, on rack, and broil until skin is golden brown and crisp, about 15 minutes. Turn chicken over, and broil until chicken starts to pull away from the bone, about 10 minutes. Let stand for 10 minutes.
- BLUEBERRY SWEET TEA BRINE: Add the salt, black peppercorns, red pepper flakes, garlic, star anise, bay leaves, thyme sprigs, and orange and lemon quarters to the Blueberry Sweet Tea (recipe below), squeezing the citrus juice into the pan as you add them. Return to medium-high and bring to a simmer. Remove from the heat, and let stand for 1 hour. Remove the solids, and store in an airtight container in the refrigerator for up to 5 days.
- BLUEBERRY SWEET TEA: Bring 2 quarts of water to a boil in a medium saucepan over high heat. Add the tea bags, and remove from the heat. Cover and let stand 7 minutes. Stir in the Blueberry Simple Syrup (recipe below), and cool complete, about 20 minutes.
- BLUEBERRY SIMPLE SYRUP: Bring the sugar, lemon zest, peppercorns, star anise, and 2 cups water to a boil in a saucepan over medium. Add the blueberries and reduce the heat to low. Cover and simmer for about 8 minutes. Remove from heat, and let stand 30 minutes. Mash the blueberries in the syrup using a potato masher or the back of a slotted spoon. Pour the syrup through a fine-mesh strainer into a bowl; discard solids. Store in an airtight container in the refrigerator up to 2 weeks.

48. Braised Mediterranean Cinnamon Chicken

Serving: Serves 4 | Prep: | Cook: | Ready in:

Ingredients

- 4 pieces Chicken Thighs, bone in and skin on
- 1 tablespoon Olive Oil
- 1.5 teaspoons Ground Cinnamon
- 1.5 teaspoons Ground Cumin
- 1.5 teaspoons Salt
- 1 Sprinkle of Ground Pepper
- 1 Can of Diced Roasted Tomatoes
- .5 Yellow Onion, sliced thin
- 2 tablespoons Minced Sweet Cherry Peppers in brine (the kind in the jars found where the Olives are)
- 1 tablespoon Minced Garlic
- 2 cups Sliced Mushrooms
- .25 cups Balsamic Vinegar
- .75 cups Red Wine
- Chicken Stock
- .5 teaspoons Red Pepper Chili Flakes (optional)

Direction

- Pat dry your chicken thighs and leave the "fatty bits" on :) Heat your olive oil on Medium-High in an oven safe pan. Preheat your oven to 375 degrees.
- Sprinkle the chicken thighs with the salt, pepper, cinnamon, and cumin on both sides. When the oil is hot, place the chicken thighs skin down and get a nice brown crust going - this should take about 3-4 minutes. Turn the chicken and brown the bottom as well, for another 3-4 minutes.
- Remove the chicken to a plate and set aside for later. In the same pan, add your sliced onions and sauté until golden brown. Then add your garlic and minced sweet peppers and sauté for 5 minutes. Add the mushrooms and sauté for about 7-8 minutes, until most of the water is gone and they are almost cooked through. Mix everything together well.

- Add the red wine, mix well, and let reduce for 3-4 minutes. Then add the balsamic, mix well and let reduce for another 3-4 minutes. Finally add the canned tomatoes and mix everything together nicely. Even out the mixture, and place the chicken thighs skin side up in the pan. Don't crowd them too much!
- Add enough chicken stock to the pan to raise the liquid level, but don't cover that beautiful crisped chicken skin! Just up to the skin will be wonderful, and you'll get the benefits of braising without soggy, crispy, operatic fatty bits :) Place the pan (open) on the middle rack in the oven, and bake for 45 minutes.
- When finished, remove the chicken pieces and set on a platter. Put the pan back on the stove burner and medium high and reduce the leftover stock for about 5 minutes, adding the red chili flakes and half a teaspoon of salt to taste. Spoon the wonderfulness on top of the chicken and serve!
- Note: The leftover sauce is to die for. I love mixing it in with pasta, scrambled eggs, or sautéing it with some spicy sausage the next day.

49. Breaded Turkey Meatballs

Serving: Makes 13 meatballs | Prep: | Cook: | Ready in:

Ingredients

- For the Meatball Mix:
- 1/4 Onion - Chopped
- 1/2 Carrot - Finely Chopped
- 1 Garlic Clove - Finely Chopped
- 3 tablespoons Olive Oil
- 9.1 ounces Ground Turkey (260 grams)
- 1/2 teaspoon Garlic Powder
- 1 teaspoon Dried Oregano
- 3 tablespoons Bread Crumbs
- 1/2 teaspoon Ground Cumin
- 1 Egg
- 1/2 cup Vegetable Oil (For Frying)
- For the Bread Crumbs Coating:
- 1/2 cup Bread Crumbs
- 1 tablespoon Sesame Seeds

Direction

- On a frying pan, preheat the olive oil over medium heat and add in the chopped onion, chopped carrot. Sauté while stirring for about 3 minutes. Add the chopped garlic and stir for another 30 seconds. Remove from heat.
- Place the fried onion mix in a medium bowl and add all the other meatballs ingredients, except for the frying vegetable oil. Mix all together until form and even mix.
- For the coating, place 1/2 cup bread crumbs and 1 tablespoon sesame seeds in a small bowl and mix.
- Using your hands, form ping pong size balls from the turkey mix. Flatten the balls just a bit and dip in the coating (bread crumbs) mix until fully coated on both sides. Form coated balls from the whole mix and set aside in a plate.
- Over medium heat , preheat the 1/2 cup vegetable oil in a frying pan (depending on the size of your pan, the oil should be about 1/4 inch or 1/2 cm deep.
- Fry the coated meatballs until brown. About 3-4 minutes on each side.

50. Breakfast Salad

Serving: Serves 2 | Prep: | Cook: | Ready in:

Ingredients

- 4 Eggs
- i bunches Kale , spinach or lettuce of your choice
- 1 Avocado
- 6 ounces Turkey bacon cooked & crumbled
- 1/2 Sliced cucumber
- 2 ounces Crumbled feta or Goat cheese
- Handful Shredded carrot

Direction

- Simply toss all your vegetables together. You may add or subtract to your preference. Cook turkey bacon or sub shredded chicken or turkey leftovers. Scramble eggs in nonstick pan with just a coating of Olive oil brand of your choice. Be sure and season eggs. I love Trader Joes lemon pepper seasoning.
- Arrange scrambled eggs on salad portioning two plates. Top with sliced avocado, turkey & crumbled cheese. A squeeze of fresh lemon juice with 2 tablespoons olive oil is fine for dressing.
- The great thing about this salad us you can add or subtract to your liking. Fresh herbs, scallions etc... I like to add a dollop of siracha hot sauce!

51. Broccoli Chicken Alfredo Skillet

Serving: Serves 6 | Prep: | Cook: |Ready in:

Ingredients

- 1 pound whole wheat penne
- 1 pound boneless, skinless chicken breast
- 1 pound blanched,broccoli florets or defrosted frozen works great as well.
- 1/2 cup heavy cream
- 2 tablespoons butter
- 1/2 teaspoon each: Smoked paprika, garlic salt, black pepper (spice blend)
- 1 cup grated parmesan cheese, you can do an assortment, I used romano in mine as well.
- drizzle or two of olive oil

Direction

- Get your pasta water going, salt it. Season chicken breast on both sides with spice blend.
- Heat a large skillet to medium high, add olive oil, add chicken turn after about five minutes, cook other side for four minutes or so (depends on thickness). Once cooked place chicken on a plate to rest.
- Cook pasta in boiling water for 10 minutes, during the last 2 minutes toss the broccoli in to reheat. Drain.
- In the chicken skillet add butter, cream, cheese and whisk over medium low, add pasta back to pan and toss with sauce, chop chicken up and add back to pan with any reserved juice that accumulated while it was resting.
- Top with a bit more parm and done. It's kinda healthy, well I guess nourishing is a good term as it covers all your nutritional bases. It does have cream….and butter…but it's still healthier than the versions you eat at restaurants.

52. Buffalo Chicken Frittata (or Egg Cups)

Serving: Serves 6 | Prep: | Cook: |Ready in:

Ingredients

- Ingredients for Chicken
- 1/2 pound boneless chicken breast, cut into cubes
- 1/2 teaspoon sea salt
- 1/4 freshly ground pepper
- 2 tablespoons buffalo wing sauce
- 2 teaspoons olive oil
- Ingredients for Egg Mixture
- 8 large eggs
- 2 tablespoons water
- 1 tablespoon and 1 teaspoon buffalo wing sauce
- 1/2 teaspoon sea salt
- 1/4 teaspoon freshly ground pepper
- 2-3 scallions, sliced
- 2 tablespoons gorgonzola, optional
- Olive oil or cooking spray

Direction

- In a medium bowl add cubed chicken, salt, pepper and wing sauce. Coat chicken well.
- In a 10 inch non-stick oven safe sauté pan set over medium heat. Once heated add in chicken and let cook for about 7 minutes; turning often. Take off heat and let cool. Once cooked, shred.
- In a medium bowl add the eggs and whisk. Continue whisking and add in the remaining ingredients. Add in chicken.
- Clean and wipe down the same pan and set temperature to medium heat. Once heated add in olive oil or coat with cooking spray.
- Preheat broiler
- Add the entire egg and chicken mixture into the pan and let cook until the bottom starts to brown (about 3 minutes). Take a rubber spatula and run between the pan and frittata and loosen up a little from the pan.
- Add to the oven and broil for 3 minutes or until the top begins to brown. (NOTE**Do not walk away from the oven. You want to keep an eye on the broiler).
- Take out of the oven (using mits) and let cool for a minutes then using the same rubber spatula loosen and move to a board to cut and serve!

53. Buffalo Chicken Grilled Cheese Sandwiches

Serving: Makes 4-6 | Prep: 0hours5mins | Cook: 0hours15mins | Ready in:

Ingredients

- 4 chicken breasts
- 6 tablespoons butter, divided
- 1/2 cup Frank's red hot sauce
- 1/2 teaspoon salt
- 1/4 teaspoon black pepper
- 2 pieces sliced cheddar cheese per sandwich
- 1/4-1/3 cups shredded mozzarella cheese per sandwich
- 1-2 tablespoons crumbled blue cheese
- 8-12 pieces of sliced bread (Italian, Frech, Ciabatta)
- Ranch dressing for dipping

Direction

- Heat a skillet over medium heat, melt 2 tbsp. of butter, and add the chicken.
- Season with salt and pepper, and cook for about 4 minutes on each side until it's cooked completely.
- Transfer to a plate, and shred the chicken using two forks.
- Add 2 tbsp. of butter to the same pan, then add the chicken back and the Frank's.
- Mix well, and cook for a minute until heated through.
- To assemble the sandwiches, start with 2 slices of bread, butter one side of the first piece and place butter side down in a frying pan.
- Place the cheddar cheese on the bread, then the mozzarella, then the blue cheese.
- Spoon the chicken over the cheeses, then top with the other piece of bread, butter side facing up.
- Grill over medium heat until golden on both sides, and all cheese is melted.
- Dip sandwiches in ranch dressing.

54. Buffalo Chicken Sausage Salad

Serving: Serves 1 qt. | Prep: | Cook: | Ready in:

Ingredients

- 1 packet Dietz & Waston Buffalo Style Chicken Sausages, sauteed or grilled, and cooled, and cut into 1/4 inch rounds
- 2 cups celery, very thinly sliced
- 1 cup sour cream
- 1/4 cup buttermilk
- 1/3 cup Maytag blue cheese, crumbled
- kosher salt and fresh ground pepper

- 1/4 teaspoon cayenne, optional the sausages are pretty hot
- 1 tablespoon minced chives, plus a teaspoon for garnish

Direction

- In a large mixing bowl whisk the buttermilk and sour cream. Season with salt, pepper and the optional cayenne if using. Add the rest of the ingredients and mix thoroughly. Taste and adjust the seasoning. Garnish with chives and serve.

55. Buffalo Chicken Soup

Serving: Serves 3-4 | Prep: | Cook: | Ready in:

Ingredients

- 2 large chicken breasts, cut into chunks
- 1/4 cup whole wheat flour
- salt and pepper to taste
- 2 tablespoons unsalted butter, divided
- 1 onion, diced
- 2 carrots, peeled and sliced
- 2 stalks of celery, sliced
- 4 cups chicken broth
- 1/4 to 1 cups Frank's Red Hot Sauce
- 1 cup shell pasta
- blue cheese, for topping

Direction

- In a medium bowl, add flour, salt, and pepper. Dredge the chicken chunks and set aside.
- In a Dutch oven over medium heat, melt 1 tablespoon of butter. Add the chicken and cook until browned on all sides. Remove the chicken and set aside again.
- Add remaining tablespoon of butter to pot and add vegetables. Cook until soft and translucent, about 10 to 15 minutes, stirring occasionally.

- Add back in the chicken, chicken stock, hot sauce, and shells. Cook until noodles becomes soft. The longer you let it sit, the spicier it will get!
- Top with blue cheese and dig on in!

56. Buffalo, Blue Cheese Chicken Burgers

Serving: Serves 3 | Prep: | Cook: | Ready in:

Ingredients

- 1 pound Ground Chicken or Turkey
- 5 ounces Crumbled Blue Cheese
- 3 Carrots, peeled and finely diced, shound be between a 1/4 cup and 1/2 cup
- 3 Celery Stalks, finely diced, sould between 1/4 cup and 1/2 cup, I prefer the light colored heart stalks with the leaves
- 1 Egg
- High quality Buffalo Suace
- dash Liquid Smoke
- bread crumbs Home-made, I add by the handful, about 1- 1.5 cups plus some for coating burgers
- 3 High Quality Hamburger Buns
- 1-2 tablespoons Vegetable Oil

Direction

- Preheat oven to 400F degrees.
- Dice the carrots and soften slightly by placing them in a microwave bowl and adding a little water, cover and steam the carrots under high power. I have also used left over carrot puree from my infant food that the lid refused to eat, works but not as good for the texture of the burger
- Once the carrots have cooled enough to handle mix them in a larger bowl with the chicken, celery, blue cheese, Egg, and Buffalo Sauce (Add to taste, more the spicier) Add a couple of dashes of Liquid Smoke. If you want to

- really spice it up add a couple dashes of hot sauce like habanero or Louisiana hot sauce.
- Add breadcrumbs to by the handful until the chicken mixture can hold and form a burger. Mix breadcrumbs in well.
- Warm a large cast-iron or other large oven proof skillet over medium high heat.
- Put remaining breadcrumbs in a shallow bowl, and press the burgers into the breadcrumbs turnover and repeat.
- Place the burgers in the hot skillet with a little oil and brown, 1-2 minutes until a nice color forms. Flip the burgers when brown and place in the oven until done, internal temp should be 165F. (I tend to remove at 155-160, cover and let rise for five minutes until 165.)
- Place burgers on buns, spread a little more buffalo sauce on the burgers and serve with the dressing on the side so each person can choose the amount of dressing they want.

57. Burmese Chicken Salad

Serving: Serves 2 | Prep: | Cook: |Ready in:

Ingredients

- 200 grams cooked chicken (poached or roasted)
- 1/2 cup chopped cilantro leaves
- 2 hot chiles, like jalapeños, deseeded and thinly sliced
- 2 fresh shallots, thinly sliced
- 3 teaspoons lime juice
- 2 teaspoons fish sauce
- 1 teaspoon vegetable oil
- 2 tablespoons fried shallots
- Salt and pepper, to taste

Direction

- Shred the chicken meat using hands or forks.
- Place the chicken and all of the other ingredients in a mixing bowl and gently toss. Season to taste, keeping in mind that the fish sauce itself is rather salty.

58. Butter Chicken

Serving: Serves 4 | Prep: | Cook: |Ready in:

Ingredients

- 4 chicken breasts
- 1 tablespoon olive oil
- 1 teaspoon salt
- 1/2 teaspoon pepper
- 1 teaspoon Mrs. Dash onion & herb
- 1/2 teaspoon rosemary
- 1 teaspoon Weber roasted garlic & herb
- 2-3 garlic cloves, minced
- 2 teaspoons Worcestershire sauce
- 1 stick butter, cut in large slices
- 1/4 cup fresh cilantro, finely chopped

Direction

- Heat a nonstick frying pan (cast iron is best), and make sure it's hot so the chicken will sear nicely.
- Add olive oil and chicken, sprinkle with salt, pepper, and seasonings.
- Cook about 4 minutes, then flip the chicken over.
- Add garlic, Worcestershire, and butter.
- Cook another 4-5 minutes until chicken is cooked through.
- Sprinkle with fresh cilantro and spoon butter sauce over chicken when plated.

59. CHA! Hoisin Glazed Roasted Chicken Wings

Serving: Makes 48-50 | Prep: | Cook: |Ready in:

Ingredients

- Wings
- 4 pounds Chicken Wings
- 1 cup CHA! By Texas Pete
- 1 piece Butter
- Salt and Pepper
- Glaze
- 1/4 cup CHA! by Texas Pete
- 3/4 cup Hoisin Sauce
- 1 bunch Scallions, sliced thin for garnish

Direction

- Marinate the chicken wings in the CHA! By Texas Pete® for 24 hours.
- Preheat the oven to 400 degrees Fahrenheit.
- After 24 hours, place the chicken wings in a large mixing bowl.
- Melt the stick of butter and pour over the chicken wings. Season with salt and pepper and mix well.
- Place the chicken wings on as many baking trays as needed, keeping space between each chicken wing and not over-crowding the pans.
- . Roast the chicken wings in the oven for approximately 45 minutes or until golden brown, crispy, fork tender and fully cooked to an internal temperature of 165 degrees. Flip them once halfway through the cooking process so they crisp evenly on both sides.
- Depending upon the size of the wings, you may need to cook them for over an hour.
- While the wings are cooking, prepare the glaze and slice the scallions.
- Mix the ¼ cup of CHA! by Texas Pete® with the ¾ cup of Hoisin sauce and mix well.
- When the chicken wings are finished cooking, carefully place them into a large mixing bowl and toss them with the spicy CHA! Hoisin glaze.
- Arrange the chicken wings on a serving platter, garnish with the sliced scallions and serve.

60. CHA!Cho's

Serving: Serves 2-4 | Prep: | Cook: |Ready in:

Ingredients

- 1 Rotisserie Chicken
- 1/2 cup CHA! by Texas Pete
- 2 cups Shredded Cheddar Cheese
- 1 bag- Green Mountain Gringo Corn Chips
- 1 jar-Green Mountain Gringo Hot Salsa
- 2 ounces Sour Cream

Direction

- Preheat the oven to 375 degrees Fahrenheit.
- Pull and shred all the meat from the rotisserie chicken and place the meat in a mixing bowl.
- Arrange the spicy shredded chicken over the tortilla strips.
- Sprinkle all of the shredded cheddar cheese over the chicken and tortilla strips.
- Place the nachos in the oven to bake for approximately 10-15 minutes or until golden brown, toasted and all of the cheese is melted.
- Garnish the nachos with the Texas Pete® Hot Salsa and sour cream and serve immediately.

61. Cajun Honey Grilled Chicken

Serving: Serves 8 | Prep: | Cook: |Ready in:

Ingredients

- 1 teaspoon dried oregano
- 1 teaspoon paprika
- 1 teaspoon cayenne pepper
- 1 teaspoon freshly cracked black pepper
- 1/2 teaspoon KOSHER SALT
- 8 boneless, skinless chicken breasts (5 oz. each)
- 1 tablespoon olive oil
- 1 teaspoon honey

Direction

- Prepare grill for medium-high direct heat. Stir together first 5 ingredients in a small bowl. In a large bowl, toss chicken, olive oil and honey. Sprinkle with spices and let stand 30 minutes at room temperature.
- Place chicken breasts on grill and cook, 5 to 6 minutes per side or until fully cooked.

62. Cajun Spiced Chicken And Fettuccine

Serving: Serves 4 | Prep: | Cook: |Ready in:

Ingredients

- 1 red bell pepper sliced thin
- 1 yellow bell pepper sliced thin
- 1 red onion sliced thin
- 4 cloves of garlic diced
- 1 tablespoon paprika
- 1 teaspoon garlic powder
- 1/2 teaspoon Cajun seasoning
- 1/2 teaspoon red cayenne pepper
- 1 pinch of thyme, oregano, smoked paprika and dried, ground chipotle
- 1 tablespoon olive oil
- 2 large boneless, skinless chicken breasts
- 2 cups heavy whipping cream
- 1 pound dried fettuccine - preferably flavored (spicy) cooked, drained

Direction

- Slice vegetables, set aside.
- Combine all spices in a small dish.
- Wash and pat dry chicken.
- Rub chicken all over with spices (you may have some leftover).
- Heat a large, heavy skillet over medium high heat.
- Add olive oil to the pan.
- Add chicken and cook on medium high heat on one side for about 7 minutes. Flip chicken, reduce heat slightly, cover and cook until chicken is cooked through (internal temperature should be 165°F). Remove and set chicken aside.
- In same pan, add vegetables and cook until very tender.
- Add cream to vegetables and heat through.
- Add cooked pasta and stir to combine and heat through.
- Transfer pasta and vegetables to bowl. Slice chicken and serve on top of pasta.

63. Calabrian Style Chicken

Serving: Serves 4 | Prep: | Cook: |Ready in:

Ingredients

- 8 boneless and skinless chicken thighs
- 6 tablespoons olive oil
- 1 small red onion, diced
- 5-10 stems of parsley, leaves only, chopped
- 2 sprigs rosemary
- 2 teaspoons salt
- 1 teaspoon oregano
- 3/4 cup white wine (or chicken stock)
- 2-3 garlic cloves, thinly sliced
- 2 fresh or dry bay leaves
- 5-6 basil leaves, thinly sliced
- 16 green olives

Direction

- Thoroughly wash the chicken in cold water and set aside in a large skillet.
- To the skillet, add the oil, onion, parsley, rosemary, salt and oregano.
- Open the gas to medium and bring to a slight sizzle allowing the chicken to get some color on both sides. Lower the heat if the chicken is browning too quickly.
- Add the wine or chicken stock and bring chicken to a low simmer.
- You don't want to brown your garlic or it will become bitter, so add it now that you have added the wine.

- Cook the chicken uncovered for about 25 minutes on medium-low heat, if it looks like it's getting too dry quickly, add about ¼ cut of water.
- About 25 minutes into the cooking, add the bay leaves, basil and olives and cook for an additional 10 minutes.
- Remove bay leaves before serving

64. Can't Believe Its Not Beef!

Serving: Makes 6 patties | Prep: | Cook: |Ready in:

Ingredients

- 1 pound Whole Foods Turkey Burger
- 10 ounces Package of Frozen Chopped Spinach, thawed and drained
- 1/2 cup Portabella Mushroom, chopped
- 2 cloves garlic, minced
- 1/4 cup finely chopped red onion
- 1 teaspoon Salt
- 1 teaspoon Pepper
- 1 tablespoon Whole Foods Barbeque Sauce

Direction

- Pre heat grill to 300 degrees.
- Combine all ingredients in a medium bowl and mix well.
- Form mixture into patties and grill 8 minutes on each side.
- Do not flip each side more than once. This way it gives the turkey burger a chance to cook all the way through.
- When browned on each side, burger is done.

65. Caprese Chicken Breasts

Serving: Serves 4 | Prep: | Cook: |Ready in:

Ingredients

- 4 Boneless, Skinless Chicken Breast Halves
- 2 Roma Tomatoes
- 8 Slices Pancetta
- 4 Slices Mozzarella (I used Part-Skim)
- 1 bunch Basil
- 2 teaspoons Olive Oil (Or cooking spray)
- Toothpicks
- Salt and Pepper

Direction

- Preheat oven to 425 degrees and oil a cookie sheet or baking pan with the olive oil (or spray it with cooking spray).
- Cut a large pocket in each chicken breast. Salt and pepper the outside.
- Slice tomatoes thinly, long ways. Cut each slice in half, long ways. Slice mozzarella no thicker than 1/4 inch.
- Slice mozzarella to fit in chicken breasts.
- Stuff one slice pancetta, 1 slices mozzarella, 3-5 basil leaves, and 2 pieces of tomato inside the pocket of each breast. Secure the pockets with toothpicks.
- Place one leaf of basil on top of each stuffed breast. Place one slice of pancetta on top of the basil.
- Bake on pan for 25-30 minutes.

66. Cardamom Carrot Meatball Soup

Serving: Serves 6 for dinner | Prep: | Cook: |Ready in:

Ingredients

- Carrot Soup Base
- 2 pounds carrots
- 2 tablespoons olive oil
- 2 leeks
- 1-2 teaspoons salt (depending on your preferences)
- 1 teaspoon ground black pepper
- 3 cloves garlic
- 7-8 cups water

- 1/8 teaspoon cayenne pepper
- 1/8 teaspoon cardamom
- 1/4 cup uncooked white rice
- 1 tablespoon apple cider vinegar
- 1/2 to 3/4 cups white wine
- Turkey Meatballs
- 1 pound ground lean turkey meat
- 3/4 to 1 cups shredded carrot
- 1 finely diced onion
- 2 finely minced cloves of garlic
- 1 tablespoon minced fresh herbs (I used sage and thyme, but parsley works too)
- 1/2 teaspoon cardamom
- 1 teaspoon salt
- 1/2 teaspoon ground black pepper
- 1/3 cup dry bread crumbs
- 1/3 cup old fashioned oats
- 1 egg

Direction

- Carrot Soup Base
- Peel the 2 lbs of carrots. Save one or two carrots for the meatballs. Dice the rest into 1/2" wide rounds. Heat a large pot over medium-high heat and add the olive oil. When the oil has heated a bit, add the carrots and stir to coat in oil. Brown the carrots a bit (to add flavor) while you prep the leeks.
- To prepare the leeks, cut off the dark green tops and discard. Slice the leeks in half, lengthwise, and rinse thoroughly under cold running water to remove all the dirt and sand. Slice the cleaned leeks and add to the pot with the carrots.
- Peel the garlic cloves and smash slightly to open them up. No need to dice - just toss them in the pot. Add the salt and pepper and continue to cook the veggies until the leeks are nice and tender and the carrots have begun to soften on the outside, approx. 10 minutes.
- Add the water and the 1/4 c uncooked white rice, along with the cardamom and cayenne pepper. Stir and simmer the soup on medium-low heat for 20-25 minutes until the carrots and the rice are completely cooked. This gives you time to prep the meatballs.
- Once the soup base is ready, remove it from the heat and break out your immersion blender. If you don't have one, you can do the soup in batches in a regular blender. Blend the soup until it's completely smooth. Add the white wine and apple cider vinegar. Taste the soup at this point and correct seasoning if needed. Put the soup back on the heat and bring it to a simmer on low heat (not too high or you will have exploding hot soup splatters). Add the turkey meatballs and cook on low for 15-20 minutes or until the meatballs are completely cooked. A meat thermometer inserted in the center of a meatball should read 165F. Serve into bowls and enjoy! For a fancy touch, you can garnish with a sprig or two of fresh herbs.
- Turkey Meatballs
- Peel 1-2 carrots and shred using a box grater. Mix the carrots and all the dry ingredients (not the eggs or the ground turkey) in a bowl until well-blended.
- Add the egg and the ground turkey and mix well with your hands or a fork until everything is evenly incorporated.
- Shape the mixture into golf-ball-sized meatballs and set aside.
- When the carrot soup has been blended, add the meatballs to the soup and simmer on low for 15-20 minutes or until the inside of a meatball registers 165F on a meat thermometer.

67. Chai Spiced Chicken, Barley, And Chickpea Stew

Serving: Serves 4 to 6 | Prep: | Cook: |Ready in:

Ingredients

- 4 tablespoons olive oil, divided
- 4 skinless, boneless chicken thighs
- Kosher salt, to taste
- 1 tablespoon minced ginger

- 3 large garlic cloves, minced
- Leaves from 2 teabags Chai spice black tea, emptied
- 2 teaspoons ground cumin
- 3/4 teaspoon crushed red pepper flakes
- 2 finely chopped roasted red bell peppers (can be from a jar)
- one (15-ounce) can good quality tomato sauce + 1cup water
- 5 1/2 cups homemade chicken stock or store-bought low sodium chicken broth, divided
- 1/2 cup quick-cook pearl barley
- two (15-ounce) cans organic chickpeas, rinsed well and drained
- 2 tablespoons fresh lemon juice
- 3 tablespoons coarsely chopped cilantro or flat-leaf parsley
- Plain yogurt and flatbread, for serving

Direction

- Heat 2 tablespoon oil in a medium pot over medium-high heat. Season chicken with salt; add to pot and cook, turning once, until browned, about 8 to 10 minutes. Transfer to a plate. Reduce heat to low and let oil cool a little. Add the ginger and garlic. Sauté until the ginger and garlic just start to brown.
- Add cumin, red pepper flakes, and the tea leaves; sauté for 30 seconds. Stir in the roasted red bell peppers and tomato sauce. Rinse the tomato sauce can with 1 cup water and add it to the saucepan. Bring to a boil, then reduce the heat and simmer, uncovered, until thickened, about 15 minutes.
- Return reserved chicken with any accumulated juices and 4 cups of chicken stock to the pot. Scrape up any browned bits. Bring to a boil; reduce heat to medium-low and simmer, uncovered, occasionally stirring, until chicken is tender, about 25 minutes.
- Combine 1/2 cup barley and 1 1/2 cups chicken stock in a 2-quart saucepan with a lid. Bring to a boil over high heat, reduce to low heat, cover, and simmer for 10 minutes. Remove from heat and let stand covered for 5 minutes.
- When the chicken is cooked, transfer to a plate. Add barley and chickpeas to the pot; bring to a simmer and cook for 10 more minutes. Using 2 forks, shred chicken and add to stew. Stir in remaining 2 tablespoons of oil and 2 tablespoons of lemon juice and simmer for a couple more minutes. Taste and season with salt and more lemon juice, if needed.
- To serve: Ladle hot stew into bowls; garnish with cilantro or parsley. Place a serving dish with plain yogurt and a plate with flat bread on your table.

68. Chcken Dupiaza

Serving: Serves 2-4 | Prep: | Cook: |Ready in:

Ingredients

- 3 chicken thighs, skinned, de-boned, and cut into thin slices or cubes
- 1 & 1/2 cups chicken stock
- 2 teaspoons grated ginger
- 4 garlic cloves
- 2 teaspoons tumeric
- 4 teaspoons curry powder
- 1 teaspoon chili powder
- 2 teaspoons garam masala
- 4 onions, chopped
- 2 sticks celery, chopped
- 2 carrots, peeled and chopped
- 1/2 to 1 cups plain yogurt
- 2 tablespoons tomato paste
- 2 teaspoons unsalted butter

Direction

- In a medium sauce pan, add enough water to fill it halfway and bring to a boil. Add half of the chopped onions and cook until soft. About 10-15 minutes or so. Drain the onions and puree until semi-smooth. This will be your onion paste, but you can set it aside for right now.

- In a large skillet, under medium high heat, add the butter and melt. Once melted, add in the remaining onions, celery, and carrots. Reduce heat to medium-low and cook until vegetables are soft and starting to turn brown in color, about 10-15 minutes.
- Meanwhile, you can make your curry paste. In a food processor, add ginger, garlic, curry powder, garam masala, turmeric, and about 1-2 tablespoons of water. Pulse to get a nice paste-like consistency. You may add more water if it is still too thick. Add paste to saucepan with vegetables and stir for about 2-3 minutes.
- Add in chicken and coat well with mixture.
- In a medium bowl, mix yogurt, tomato paste, onion paste, and chicken stock. Mix until tomato paste is dissolved. Then add mixture to pan with vegetables and chicken. Mix well and simmer for about 15 minutes and chicken is cooked all the way through.
- I served this with some red rice and it was phenomenal. You could sense the onion flavor, but it wasn't too much. The curry really mellowed the onion out. It was definitely sensationally delicious and great the next day! Enjoy!

69. Cheater's Chicken Schnitzel

Serving: Serves 2 | Prep: 1hours0mins | Cook: 0hours15mins | Ready in:

Ingredients

- Mayo marinade
- 3/4 cup mayonnaise
- 3 tablespoons Dijon mustard
- 3/4 teaspoon kosher salt
- Chicken schnitzel
- 1 1/2 cups peanut or vegetable oil, adjusted as needed for frying
- 2 (3/4-pound) chicken breasts
- 2 cups panko breadcrumbs
- 4 pinches kosher salt, divided

Direction

- Combine the marinade ingredients in a large plastic bag or bowl. Squeeze the bag or stir with a spoon to mix.
- Halve the chicken breasts horizontally. Pound each half to 1/4-inch thickness. You could do this between two pieces of plastic or parchment or, my favorite, in a plastic bag (splatter-free!). You could use a meat mallet or heavy skillet or, my favorite, a rolling pin.
- Add the prepped chicken to the marinade. If it's a bag, seal. If it's a bowl, cover. Refrigerate for at least 1 hour or up to 1 day.
- When you're ready to fry, add enough oil to a large cast-iron skillet to reach just shy of 1/2-inch in depth. Set over medium-high heat.
- Spread out the panko on a plate. Remove each chicken piece from the marinade and swipe away any excess. (No need to be obsessive but it should look mostly mayo-free, otherwise it won't crisp properly.) Dredge each chicken piece in the panko, pressing firmly to completely coat.
- The oil should be about 365° F. If you don't have a thermometer, you can test its readiness by dropping a crumb in the oil. It should immediately sizzle—not sink (too cold), nor burn (too hot).
- Fry in batches, taking care not to overcrowd, which would lead to steaming over browning. Cook for 3 to 4 minutes per side until deeply browned. Transfer to a paper towel–lined plate to drain. Repeat with the remaining chicken.
- Serve immediately.

70. Cheesy Stuffing

Serving: Serves 4-6 | Prep: | Cook: | Ready in:

Ingredients

- 1.5 cups multi grain bread-cut into 1/2 inch cubes

- 2 ounces olive oil
- 3/4 cup mushrooms-quartered
- 1 teaspoon cayenne pepper
- 1/4 cup onion-small dice
- 3 ounces olive oil
- 1/2 cup eggplant-cut into 1/2 inch pieces
- 1/2 cup carrots-cut into 1/2 inch pieces
- 1 clove garlic-minced
- 1 egg-whisked
- 1/2 cup ricotta cheese
- 1/2 cup grated Parmesan cheese
- butter/cooking spray for coating baking dish
- 3/4 cup chicken stock
- salt to taste
- pepper to taste

Direction

- Place bread cubes on baking tray and toast on 400F until just browned; reserve.
- On high heat, brown mushrooms in olive oil; add cayenne pepper, season, and reserve.
- Sweat onion on medium heat in olive oil; add eggplant, and carrots until soft, finish with garlic, season, and reserve.
- In a bowl, combine bread cubes, mushrooms, eggplant/carrot mixture, egg, ricotta cheese, and half of the Parmesan cheese-mix well.
- Butter/spray a baking dish and transfer stuffing mixture.
- Pour chicken stock on top of stuffing; top off with remaining Parmesan cheese.
- Bake at 400F until top is golden brown (~17-22 min); see serving suggestions above.

71. Cherry Poppy Seed Chicken Salad

Serving: Serves 4-6 | Prep: | Cook: | Ready in:

Ingredients

- 10-12 ounces chicken breast meat
- 1 tablespoon vegetable or canola oil
- 2 ribs celery, chopped finely
- 1 cup sweet cherries, pitted and quartered
- 1/4 cup chopped walnuts
- 1/3 cup mayonnaise
- 1.5 teaspoons poppy seeds
- salt and pepper to taste

Direction

- Heat the oil in a skillet over medium heat for 1-2 minutes. Cook chicken until meat is no longer pink, about 5-7 minutes per side. Chop the cooked chicken into small pieces (no bigger than 1/2-inch cubes). Place in the refrigerator to cool for 5-10 minutes.
- While the chicken is cooling, place the remaining ingredients in a mixing bowl and stir to combine. Season with salt and pepper to taste.
- Once cooled, add chopped chicken. Serve as a side dish or in sandwiches.

72. Cherry Tomato Hot Browns

Serving: Serves 10 people | Prep: | Cook: | Ready in:

Ingredients

- 1 pint cherry tomatoes
- 3 tablespoons chopped garlic
- 2 tablespoons chopped basil
- 1 handful chopped parsley
- 2 tablespoons Olive oil
- Salt and Pepper to taste
- 2 cups chopped turkey breast
- 2 tablespoons flour
- 2 tablespoons butter
- 2 cups whole milk
- 1 cup grated gruyere cheese
- 1 cup grated white cheddar cheese
- 1 sweet onion
- 1 packet puff pastry
- 6 pieces thick cut smoked bacon
- 2 tablespoons honey

Direction

- Chop basil, garlic, parsley and mix will 2 tabs Olive oil plus salt and pepper. Cut pint of cherry tomatoes in half, and toss with oil mixture. Please tomato mixture on baking sheet and roast at 425 until tomatoes start to caramelize (around 7-8 minutes). Take out of oven and set aside. While oven is hot place bacon on sheet pan and bake till done.
- Chop some leftover chicken or turkey into bite sized pieces.
- Mix flour and butter in pan until slightly golden. Slowly whisk in heated milk and bring to boil. When sauce has thickened, whisk in cheeses and remove from heat. Set sauce aside.
- Chop sweet onion in half, then slice. Place onion slices in pan will olive oil and cook on low heat for roughly 10-12 minutes to caramelize the onion. Place aside to cool.
- Thaw the package of puff pastry if frozen. Cut into circular pieces that will fit into cupcake baking sheet. Place circles in baking sheet bake at 350 for 5-6 minutes until slightly golden. Remove from oven and fill with pieces of turkey, then top with onion mixture, then top with the roasted tomatoes, then drizzle on cheese, and back in the oven for 5-6 additional minutes. When ready to eat, toss on chopped bacon, and drizzle with honey.

73. Chestnut, Pork And Nut Stuffing My Family's Traditional Recipe

Serving: Serves 8 | Prep: | Cook: | Ready in:

Ingredients

- Braised Meat
- 14 ounces pork loin
- 1 onion
- 6 chicken gizzards, clean
- 2 celery stalks
- 5 sage leaves
- 2 bay leaves
- 3 garlics, green inside part removed and chopped
- 1 sprig fresh rosemary
- 2 carrots
- 1/4 cup Extra Virgin Olive Oil
- 1/2 cup vegetable stock - hot
- 1/8 cup white wine
- salt
- 6 black peppercorns
- Stuffing
- 5 chicken livers clean and cut up in small pieces
- 3 tablespoons butter
- 2 big blond onions thinly sliced
- 1/8 cup cognac
- 3 fresh Italian sausages remove the casing
- 7 Italian rustic bread slices, crusts removed
- 1/4 cup milk
- 2 egg yolks
- 12 black olives in water, pitted and diced
- 2 tablespoons fresh parsley chopped finely
- 1/3 cup chopped shelled pistachios
- 1/3 cup pecans, chopped
- 2/3 cup boiled and skinned chestnuts, chopped
- 1/2 lemon - juice
- Sechuan pepper
- Salt
- 1/2 cup breadcrumbs

Direction

- Clean the gizzards of all the skin attached and cut up in pieces. Cut the pork loin in medium sized cubes.
- Braising the meat: Chop the onion, celery and cut the carrots in big pieces. Put all the vegetables in a sauté pan with 1/4 cup olive oil, the sage leaves, the rosemary sprig, the bay leaf and the peppercorns.
- When the olive oil starts to sizzle add the gizzards and the pork, brown the meat, stirring once or twice. When brown all over add the white wine, allow the alcohol to evaporate and then add the vegetable stock.

- Stir, cover, lower the heat to the minimum and let it braise for 20 minutes, stirring once in a while. Uncover and allow to cool.
- Livers: Slice the onions and sweat them in the butter over medium heat for about 15 minutes. Add the chicken livers, brown them. Allow to cool in a bowl.
- In the same frying pan, no need to wash it, add a drizzle of olive oil and fry the sausage meat crumbling it with the back of a wooden spoon. Remove and add to the bowl with the liver.
- While the meats are cooling, chop up with a knife the pistachios, the pecans and the chestnuts (don't use a processor because they will be either too small or part big and part small). Set aside. Chop the olives in pieces and set aside.
- Cut up the bread in medium pieces, add the milk and allow to soak. The bread has to be at least a day old and depending on the type of bread and how humid the dough is, you may need more or less milk. The bread should soak up the milk completely and neither be floating in milk or have any dry parts.
- Remove the pork and gizzards from the pan and put in a food processor. Discard the vegetables. Pulse 7 or 8 times, you want the meat to be grainy and not pureed. Add the liver with the onions and the sausage and pulse 4 or 5 more times. Don't overdo it. Take the meats out of the food processor and put in a big bowl.
- In the food processor (no need to wash it) add the soaked bread, squeezing out any excess milk, add the 2 egg yolks, 2/3 of the boiled chestnuts and puree well. If the mixture is too dry add a little extra milk.
- Add the bread and chestnut puree to the bowl with all the meats, add the parsley, nuts and remaining chestnuts and mix with your hands very well to combine all the ingredients together. Season with salt and Sichuan pepper (it adds a little lemon taste) and some lemon juice. Taste and rectify the seasoning to your liking.
- Make a ball with the stuffing and on a countertop roll it into a log form on breadcrumbs. As the meats are crumbly and not pureed, keep pressing the mixture together. Put the meat on an aluminum foil and roll the foil around, pressing together the mixture. Chill 6 hours or overnight
- Take the stuffing out to room temperature at least 1 hour and then cook it in a pre-heated oven at 350 degrees F in the turkey juices, basting the stuffing while it browns. Remember the stuffing is already cooked, it needs to warm up and get some flavour from the turkey.
- If you decide to make this stuffing for a meal, cook it with some olive oil and orange juice, it will taste very nice on its own.

74. Chicken "Stoup"

Serving: Serves 4 to 6 | Prep: | Cook: | Ready in:

Ingredients

- 2 lbs. chicken pieces, on the bone (dark meat is best, but you can use a mix if you'd like)
- 3 medium carrots, peeled
- 3 stalks celery
- 1 large sweet onion, peeled
- 2 cups homemade or good quality chicken stock
- Salt
- 2 tablespoons chopped fresh dill
- 1 lemon
- Freshly ground black pepper
- Crusty bread for serving

Direction

- Remove the fat from the chicken pieces, saving it if you like to make your own schmaltz or something. Put the chicken in a large soup pot. Cut one of the carrots into large chunks and add these to the pot with the chicken. Cut one stalk of celery and half the onion into similar sized chunks and add to the pot. Add the chicken stock and then enough water to submerge the chicken and vegetables. Add a generous pinch or two of salt. Bring to a boil over high heat and then lower the heat so that it simmers gently. During the first 5 minutes, skim any of the foam that accumulates on the surface with a shallow spoon. Cook the chicken for about 10 minutes, just until it's firm and opaque. Transfer to a plate, cover loosely with foil, and let the chicken cool for a few minutes while you continue to simmer the stock, partially covered.

- Remove the chicken from the bones and reserve the meat, returning the bones to the pot. Re-cover and simmer the stock for at least 45 minutes more. Remove the bones and the vegetables with a slotted spoon and discard, and then strain the stock through a fine mesh sieve into a clean pot.
- Cut the remaining carrots and celery into bite-sized chunks, and then do the same with the onion. Return the stock to a simmer and taste for seasoning, adding more salt if necessary. Add the carrots and onion to the pot and simmer for 5 minutes. Add the celery and cook for another 3 minutes, then stir in the dill, a good amount of lemon juice and several grindings of black pepper.
- When you're ready to serve the soup, tear or cut the chicken into bite-sized pieces and add it to the pot. Simmer for a minute or so, just until the chicken has a chance to reheat. (Be vigilant here -- this is the step that determines whether your chicken is tender or dry.) Taste once more for salt, and then serve immediately in shallow bowls with some good, crusty bread.

75. Chicken & Cabbage Salad With Sesame Seeds, Scallions & Almonds

Serving: Serves 6 to 8 | Prep: 0hours20mins | Cook: 0hours20mins | Ready in:

Ingredients

- 2 tablespoons plus 1 teaspoon kosher salt
- 1 whole chicken, about 3 lbs
- 1 head cabbage, about 2.5 lbs
- 1/2 cup neutral oil such as canola or grapeseed
- 1/4 cup white balsamic vinegar
- 1 tablespoon fresh lemon juice
- 2 tablespoons sesame oil
- 2 teaspoons sugar
- 1 cup sliced almonds
- 1/3 cup sesame seeds
- 6 scallions, thinly sliced

Direction

- Bring a large pot of water to a boil. Add 1 tablespoon kosher salt. Drop in the chicken and simmer for 15 minutes. Remove pan from heat, cover, and let sit for 15 minutes. Remove chicken, let cool briefly, then remove meat from bones, and pull or shred into pieces.
- Meanwhile, cut the cabbage into quarters through the core. Thinly slice it, discarding the core. Place in a large bowl and sprinkle with 1 tablespoon kosher salt. Using your hands, massage the salt into the cabbage. Let sit for 15 minutes. Fill bowl with cold water and jostle the cabbage with your hands. Drain into a large colander. Don't worry about drying the cabbage.
- Meanwhile, make the dressing: Whisk together the neutral oil, sesame oil, vinegar, lemon juice, sugar, and remaining teaspoon kosher salt.
- In a large bowl, place the cabbage, pulled meat, almonds, sesame seeds, and scallions. Add the dressing and toss to coat. Serve.

76. Chicken & Quinoa Stuffed Peppers

Serving: Serves 5 | Prep: | Cook: | Ready in:

Ingredients

- 5 Red Bell Peppers
- .5 tablespoons Coconut Oil
- 1 Onion
- 2 tablespoons Minced Garlic
- 1 pound Diced Chicken Breast
- 1 teaspoon Italian Seasoning
- .25 teaspoons Black Pepper
- .25 teaspoons Red Chili Flakes
- .25 cups Shredded Carrots
- 3 Campari Tomatoes
- 2 handfuls Chopped Baby Spinach
- .33 cups LowFat Cottage Cheese
- 1 cup Cooked Quinoa

Direction

- Pre-Heat Oven at 400 degrees
- Heat 1/2 TB Coconut Oil in a Sauté Pan on a medium flame. Add 1 small Onion, Diced and 2 TB Minced Garlic. Cook for 2-3 minutes.
- Then add 1 lb. Diced Chicken Breast, Italian Seasoning, Black Pepper & Red Pepper Flakes (optional).
- Stir occasionally and when Chicken is nearly cooked through, add 1/4 Cup Shredded Carrots, 3 Chopped Campari (or 2 Plum) Tomatoes. Sauté for about 4-5 more minutes.
- Turn heat off and Stir in 2 Handfuls of Chopped Baby Spinach, 1/3 Cup Low-fat Cottage Cheese & 1 Cup Cooked Quinoa.
- Cut off the tops of peppers, remove seeds and place in a deep pan. Fill Peppers with Chicken Mix and cover with foil. Bake for 20 minutes. Remove Foil and turn oven up to broil for about 5 minutes (to crisp up the top of the filling)

77. Chicken & Vegetable Ramen Noodles

Serving: Serves 6-8 | Prep: | Cook: | Ready in:

Ingredients

- Chicken
- 4 chicken breasts, cubed
- 1 tablespoon olive oil
- 1 teaspoon salt
- 1/2 teaspoon black pepper
- Broth
- 64 ounces organic chicken broth
- 3 organic carrots, shredded
- 1 bunch organic kale, torn
- 1 bunch organic green onions, sliced
- 2 teaspoons fresh ginger, or jarred
- 2 garlic cloves, minced
- 3 tablespoons soy sauce
- 1/4 teaspoon sesame oil
- 2 teaspoons salt
- 1/2 teaspoon black pepper
- 2 packages Chinese noodles
- Garnish with chopped fresh cilantro, bean sprouts, and Sriracha sauce

Direction

- Chicken
- Heat a large skillet over medium heat, and add olive oil and chicken.
- Season with salt and pepper, and cook for about 5-7 minutes, leaving chicken partially pink. Set aside.
- Broth
- In a large stockpot add chicken broth, carrots, green onions, garlic, ginger, soy sauce, sesame oil, salt and pepper; bring to a boil.
- Add the kale and cook on a low boil for about 5-7 minutes until kale is soft.
- Add chicken back and cook an additional 3 minutes.

- Place cooked noodles into a bowl, top with vegetable chicken broth, then garnishes of your choice.

78. Chicken Asparagus Penne Pasta

Serving: Serves 10-12 | Prep: | Cook: | Ready in:

Ingredients

- 1 pound Chicken Tenders
- 1 packet Zesty Italian Dressing Mix - Dry
- 14.5 ounces box of Dreamfield's Penne Pasta
- 2 tablespoons Extra Virgin Olive Oil
- 3 Garlic Cloves, minced
- 1 pound Asparagus, trimmed and chopped into 1" pieces
- 3 cups Cherry Tomatoes
- 1/2 cup fresh chopped Celery
- 1/2 cup finely chopped Onion
- 1/2 cup Chicken Stock
- 1/2 cup Pasta Water
- 2 tablespoons White Balsamic Vinegar
- 1 small can sliced Black Olives
- 1 small can sliced green olives (or sub capers)
- 2 cups fresh grated Parmigiano-Reggiano Cheese
- 4 tablespoons fresh chopped Basil
- 2 tablespoons fresh cracked Pepper

Direction

- Cook pasta according to directions. Reserve 1/2 cup pasta water for later.
- Grill chicken tenders in 1 Tbsp. olive oil and season with 1 Tbsp. of the Italian dressing mix. Save the rest of the dressing mix for later.
- Sauté garlic and asparagus pieces in 1 Tbsp. olive oil until asparagus is slightly tender. Add tomatoes and stir over medium high heat for 2 minutes. Add all sautéed ingredients to pasta.
- Add all other ingredients, except for 1/4 cup cheese and basil to pasta. Mix thoroughly. Salt to taste. When ready to serve, sprinkle with basil and remaining cheese. Serve warm or chill before serving. Your choice.

79. Chicken Avocado & Veggie Egg Rolls With Sweet & Sour Sauce

Serving: Makes 20 | Prep: 0hours15mins | Cook: 0hours30mins | Ready in:

Ingredients

- Egg Rolls
- 1 package egg roll wrappers
- 2 chicken breasts, cut in small pieces
- 3 cups green cabbage, finely chopped
- 1 large carrot, shredded
- 1/2 red pepper, diced
- 1/2 cup white onions, diced
- 1 avocado, chopped
- 1/2 teaspoon sesame oil
- 2 teaspoons olive oil, divided
- 1 teaspoon salt
- 1/2 teaspoon black pepper
- 24 ounces Grapeseed oil for frying
- Sweet & Sour Sauce
- 1/2 cup fresh squeezed orange juice
- 2 tablespoons brown rice vinegar
- 1/3 cup brown sugar
- 3 tablespoons ketchup
- 1 tablespoon soy sauce
- 1 tablespoon corn starch
- 1 tablespoon water

Direction

- Egg Rolls
- Heat a deep skillet over medium heat, and add sesame oil and 1 tsp olive oil, and chicken.
- Cook until the chicken is done, about 5 minutes. Transfer to a mixing bowl.
- In the same pan, add 1 tsp olive oil, and all of the veggies except the avocado.
- Cook for about 2 minutes, then add to the chicken.

- Add the avocado and mix well.
- Take an egg roll wrapper and place it with pointed end up (like a diamond).
- Place a heaping spoonful of the filling in the center of each wrapper, then roll both sides over tightly, then roll the bottom over the fillings, and brush water on the tip of the wrapper to seal it.
- Heat grapeseed oil in a heavy pot or deep fryer to 375*, then drop the egg rolls in batches leaving enough room to turn them.
- Turn when golden and crispy, and place on paper towels.
- Sweet & Sour Sauce
- Place all the sauce ingredients except corn starch and water in a small saucepan and bring to a boil over medium heat stirring often.
- Mix the corn starch and water in a small bowl. Once sauce comes to a boil, add the corn starch mixture and stir until it thickens. Remove from heat.

80. Chicken Bog

Serving: Serves a crowd | Prep: | Cook: | Ready in:

Ingredients

- 4 pounds bone-in, skin-on chicken thighs
- Kosher salt and pepper
- 2 tablespoons extra-virgin olive oil, peanut oil, or vegetable oil
- 3 bell peppers, diced (all red, or a mix of colors)
- 1 large (or 2 small) yellow onion, diced
- 4 celery ribs, trimmed and diced
- 1 tablespoon finely minced fresh thyme
- 1 tablespoon minced garlic
- 1 28-ounce can whole tomatoes, with liquid
- 4 tablespoons butter
- 4 tablespoons flour
- 1 pound kielbasa (could also add cooked ham, bacon, andouille, etc.), chopped into bite-sized pieces
- 2 cups chicken stock
- 2 bay leaves
- 1 tablespoon apple cider vinegar, plus more to taste
- 1/4 cup Dijon mustard
- Hot sauce, to taste
- For serving: 1/4 cup chopped fresh parsley; cooked long-grain white rice

Direction

- Dry chicken well. Season both sides with salt and pepper. Add oil to a Dutch oven over medium-high heat. Add the chicken thighs (skin-side down) and sear until golden on both sides, about 4 minutes per side. (Brown in batches if needed so they don't steam.) Remove chicken to a plate; set aside. Leave 2 to 3 tablespoons of fat in the pan; drain off any excess.
- To the pan, add the peppers, onion, celery, thyme, and cook, stirring occasionally, until vegetables are soft, about 10 minutes; season with pinch or two of salt and pepper. Add garlic and cook for another minute. Add tomatoes (cut into small chunks with kitchen shears right in the pan) and bring to a boil; adjust heat so mixture gently simmers.
- While you're sweating the vegetables, make the dark roux by melting the butter in a small skillet or saucepan over medium heat. Add flour and stir until smooth. Cook, stirring occasionally, until mixture turns a deep chestnut brown in color, about 10 minutes. Add the roux to the simmering tomatoes; cook about 5 minutes.
- Return the chicken thighs to the pan, and add kielbasa, stock, and bay leaves; simmer, stirring occasionally, for about 30 minutes, or until the chicken is fully cooked through.
- Remove chicken with tongs to a large plate; when cool enough to handle, remove skin and chicken from the bone; shred the meat; and return to the pan. Continue to simmer. (At this

point, the bog can gently simmer on the stove for several hours; add a little water or stock, if needed, if it starts to dry out.)
- When ready to serve, stir vinegar and mustard into stew. Taste, and adjust seasoning and acidity (I usually add at least 2 tablespoons of apple cider vinegar). Remove and discard bay leaves. Add hot sauce, to taste, and pass more when serving. Stir in parsley, and serve over white rice.

- Next, add the rest of the white wine and reduce by half. Next add the cream and chicken stock. Simmer until all reduced by half being sure to stir well. Season to taste with salt and any other desired spices.
- Finally add the chicken breasts back to the pan with the sauce reduce the heat to low and cover with lid. Simmer for several minutes
- Fluff sauce white fork and add any other desired seasonings. Serve with two long chive stems forming an X over the chicken and sauce to garnish.

81. Chicken Breast With Cream Of Herb Sauce

Serving: Serves 4 | Prep: | Cook: | Ready in:

Ingredients

- 4 pieces chicken breast
- 1 cup white wine
- 2 cups heavy whipping cream
- 2/3 cup fresh chopped chives
- 2 average shallots
- salt to taste
- 1 tablespoon flour or xanthan gum
- 2 teaspoons butter
- onion powder to taste
- 3 tablespoons fresh basil leaves
- 10 ounces chicken stock

Direction

- Season the chicken breasts with salt and onion powder. Pan sauté with the butter. About 2 minutes, flip and cook about 2 more minutes.
- Then remove the breasts from the pan and set on separate plate, and place in a 200 degree oven to keep warm.
- Next use some of the white wine to deglaze the pan. Being sure that all bits are well scrapped from the pan. Add minced shallots and flour or xa. gum and stir. Sauté for a minute then add the basil and chives. Sauté another 45 seconds.

82. Chicken Breasts & Thighs Pounded, Wrapped In Pancetta, Filled W/ A Cilantro, Feta, Mint Pesto And Covered In A Blood Orange Sauce

Serving: Serves 4 | Prep: | Cook: | Ready in:

Ingredients

- For the Chicken Breasts and/or Thighs:
- 2- 4 boneless breasts and/or thighs of chicken – pounded to about ½ inch thick
- 1 recipe Mint, Feta, Pine Nut, Cilantro Pesto (to follow)
- 1 recipe 3-day Blood Orange Reduction (to follow)
- 1 tablespoon olive oil
- about 3 slices pancetta (thinly sliced) per thigh or breast (aprox. 12 total if making 4 pieces)
- Additional kitchen tools: Kitchen twine/string
- For the Pesto: (can be made a day ahead)
- A handful of mint (a little under a cup)
- A large handful of cilantro (a very full cup)
- a little under ½ cup pine nuts (raw if possible)
- ¼ cup fresh lemon juice (from about one small lemon)
- ¼ cup Bulgarian feta (or any feta will work)
- your very best extra virgin olive oil

- ¼ teaspoon sea salt
- 5 turns course ground black pepper

Direction

- For the Chicken Breasts and/or Thighs:
- Preheat oven to 400 degrees.
- Lay chicken out on flat surface. Place about 1-2 tablespoons of Pesto in each pounded chicken breast or thigh. Roll up tight, like a burrito (some of the pesto make attempt to escape; just roll as tight as you can and know that you can patch it up with the pancetta and the string.) Cover each breast or thigh in pancetta, making sure to cover all ends, so there are no holes. Wrap tightly with kitchen string; first on long ends, then twice around middles, so all is secure.
- Heat saucepan over medium high heat. Place olive oil in pan. Add rolled breasts or thighs and sear until gold and uniform in color (you may have to adjust the heat a bit from medium to medium high as you cook). Making sure to get the small (horizontal) ends as well – you want the whole thing nicely golden and browned, no raw pancetta pieces!
- Place in casserole dish and bake for 15 minutes (for breasts) and 25 minutes for thighs. When cooked remove from oven and let rest for about five minutes.
- Place on serving platter or individual plates; slice on the diagonal; spoon sauce over top and eat to your hearts content!
- For the Pesto: (can be made a day ahead)
- Place all ingredients into food processor (or blender if you do not have). Drizzle a little olive oil in to moisten, then pulse a few times, and continue to drizzle olive oil in until reaches a smooth and fluid, but still very thick consistency. Check for salt and pepper and add more lemon juice if necessary; then blend on high until as smooth as possible.
- For the Blood Orange Reduction:(can be made up to three days ahead – it gets better with time...)Ingredients:9 large blood oranges - peeled and skinned 1 regular orange1 cup tangerine juice2 cups red wine½ cup orange liquor (we used Orange Curacao)¾ cup port
- Just throw everything into a large pot and cook down for about 5 hours or so, until thick and fragrant. Spoon over stuffed chicken or use for other (very interesting) things...

83. Chicken Breasts Over Fennel In Parchment

Serving: Serves 2 or as many as you wish. | Prep: | Cook: | Ready in:

Ingredients

- 2 Boneless Chicken Breasts
- 1 Fennel Blub, sliced thinly
- 4 Lemon slices
- 4 sprigs fresh thyme
- 1 tablespoon Olive Oil
- 1 teaspoon salt
- 1/4 teaspoon Pepper
- 2 17" long Sheets of Parchment Paper

Direction

- Slice Fennel and toss in olive oil with the chicken breasts and the rest of the ingredients.
- Fold Parchment paper in half and arrange chicken on top of fennel and top that with lemon and thyme sprigs.
- Bake in 400 degree preheated oven for 20 minutes.

84. Chicken Cordon Club

Serving: Serves 2 | Prep: | Cook: | Ready in:

Ingredients

- 2 Chicken, boneless breasts
- 1 ounce Swiss cheese, grated
- 1 slice of bacon, cooked and crumbled

- 2 tablespoons Dijon mustard
- 1/2 cup Panko bread crumbs
- 1 tablespoon Olive oil
- 1/2 cup white wine
- 1/2 cup chicken broth
- 1 tablespoon capers

Direction

- Pound chicken breasts to about 1/2 inch thickness.
- On one half of the chicken breast, place about 1/2 ounce grated cheese and half the bacon. Fold the other half over to cover the filling.
- Cover the top sides with mustard, then coat with Panko. Flip and do the same on the other side. Press the crumbs into the mustard. Save about 1 t. of mustard for the sauce.
- Heat oil in heat proof frying pan (cast iron) until shimmering. Carefully add the breasts and brown, about 3 minutes. Turn and brown the other side.
- Place pan in 350 degree oven for about 15 minutes, or until the chicken is throughly cooked.
- Remove from the oven. Place chicken on plate and cover loosely with foil. Over medium heat, add wine and stock to the pan and stir to dissolve any juices. Add reserved 1 t. mustard and the capers. Taste for salt and pepper. Stir until sauce reduces. Serve the breasts with sauce over half, the remainder on the plate.

85. Chicken Crepes With Ricotta, Parmesan And Spinach With Parmesan Bechamel

Serving: Makes 12-18 | Prep: 1hours0mins | Cook: 0hours30mins | Ready in:

Ingredients

- Crepes
- 4 eggs
- 3 tablespoons melted butter
- 2 cups milk
- 1 1/2 cups flour
- 1/2 teaspoon sugar
- Pinch salt
- Crepe Filling and Parmesan Bechamel
- 1 tablespoon olive oil
- 1/2 onion, chopped finely
- 1 garlic clove, crushed
- 1/2 bag fresh spinach, washed
- 1 cup ricotta cheese
- 2 cups chopped chicken (rotisserie or leftover)
- 1/2 cup parmesan cheese, finely grated
- 1/2 cup fontina cheese, grated
- 3 tablespoons fresh basil, chopped (or 1 1/2 TB dried)
- 2 teaspoons fresh thyme (or 1 tsp dried)
- 1/2 zest of 1/2 lemon
- 2 teaspoons kosher salt
- 1/2 teaspoon white pepper
- 1 egg, beaten
- 4 tablespoons flour
- 4 tablespoons butter
- 2 cups warm milk
- 1/2 cup parmesan cheese, grated
- 1/2 cup asiago or mozzarella cheese
- 1 teaspoon salt
- 1/8 teaspoon nutmeg
- 1/4 teaspoon cayenne pepper
- 1 tablespoon paprika

Direction

- Crepes
- Mix all ingredients together in a blender and process until smooth. Let sit for 1/2 hour, refrigerated.
- Melt a small knob of butter in medium size frying pan (non-stick is best). Add about 1/2 a ladle of batter and swirl quickly to coat. The crepes should be thin.
- Cook the crepe until bubbles appear on the top uncooked side. Lift carefully to check for browning, and if browned, gently flip. Cook the other side for 1-2 minutes only. Repeat until batter is done. Stack them on a plate as you cook them.
- Crepe Filling and Parmesan Béchamel

- In a large frying pan, add olive oil and chopped onion. Cook on medium heat until onion is softened. Add garlic and spinach. Cook until spinach is wilted. Set aside to cool.
- In a large bowl, combine ricotta cheese, chicken, cheeses, herbs, lemon zest, salt, and pepper. Add spinach mixture from frying pan. Combine with a spoon or clean hands. Taste for seasoning and add herbs, salt or pepper to taste. Add egg and combine again.
- Grease a large baking dish. Take a crepe (either store bought or homemade). Add 1 1/2 to 2 TB of filling in a log shape across the crepe, and roll tightly. Place in baking dish seam side down. Repeat until dish is full. Set aside and make the béchamel.
- Parmesan Béchamel: Melt butter in a medium saucepan. Add flour. Over medium heat, stir constantly with a whisk for 2-3 minutes until flour has cooked. Do not brown.
- Add milk gradually and whisk while sauce thickens. Lower heat to low. Stir in parmesan and asiago or mozzarella cheese, nutmeg, salt, and cayenne pepper. Remove from heat and taste to correct for seasoning.
- Pour sauce over the crepes. Sprinkle with paprika and additional parmesan cheese.
- Bake in a preheated 350 degree oven for 30 minutes or until sauce is bubbly and slightly browned.
- Variations: Add sautéed mushrooms to filling and/or sauce. Use ground chicken or veal in filling, or use spinach and asparagus. Use your favorite tomato sauce instead of béchamel. Don't cook the crepes without sauce, they will dry out.

86. Chicken Curry

Serving: Serves 3 | Prep: | Cook: | Ready in:

Ingredients

- 3 organic/free range chicken legs
- 2 yellow/orange peppers
- 1 thumb ginger
- 4 cloves garlic
- 3 onions
- 1 or 2 fresh chillies (depends how spicy)
- 2 teaspoons curry powder (homemade if possible)
- 1 teaspoon ground turmeric
- 1 teaspoon cinnamon
- 1 teaspoon ground cloves
- 400 milliliters chicken stock (home made if poss)
- 2-3 teaspoons raw organic honey
- 2 teaspoons coconut oil
- half cup organic double cream
- extra vegetables of your choice (optional - I like without too)

Direction

- Take your casserole pot and fry off chicken in coconut oil for 10 minutes until it browns. Take it out of the pot to one side and let it sit.
- Peel your onion, garlic, ginger and deseed your peppers and chili and blend them in a food processor with the curry powder and turmeric until a smooth paste.
- Put the paste into the chicken fat and coconut oil left in your pot and heat through for 5 minutes.
- Add all of the chicken stock and bring back to the boil then add your chicken legs back in and cover with the liquid
- Add your teaspoons of cinnamon, clove, honey and a good pinch of salt and pepper and simmer gently for 45 - 60 minutes (the liquid should darken and thicken - you can cook on high for 5-10 minutes to reduce liquid at the end)
- Towards the end take out the chicken and shred it off the bone being careful to get rid of gristle and skin and pop the tender meat back into the curry.
- Slowly add the cream to your desired consistency and taste - I find I don't need much to create and creamy texture.
- Put 1 cup rice to 1 1/2 cup of cold water in a pan, bring to the boil and simmer gently for

exactly 12 minutes, WITHOUT taking the lid off or stirring, for perfect fluffy rice. While the rice is cooking leave the curry off the heat covered to stew further.
- Serve with steamed vegetables - cauliflower and broccoli go well drizzled with a little olive oil, salt, pepper and lemon.
- Eat and enjoy. Delicious the next day for lunch.

87. Chicken Curry With Moringa

Serving: Serves 4 | Prep: | Cook: | Ready in:

Ingredients

- 1/4 cup onion strips
- 2 teaspoons ginger strips
- 2 teaspoons chopped garlic
- 1/4 cup coconut oil
- 1/2 pound chicken cut into strips
- 2-3 teaspoons yellow curry powder
- 2 teaspoons fish sauce
- 1-2 teaspoons sea salt
- 1/4 teaspoon white peper
- 1 cup heavy coconut milk divided in half
- 1 1/2 cups diced potatoes
- 1 cup diced carrots
- 1/2 cup water
- 1/4 cup red pepper cut into strips
- 1 cup fresh moringa leaves - green tea powder can be substituted
- 1/2 teaspoon cayenne pepper

Direction

- In a heavy, enamel-coated pot, sauté the onion, ginger, and garlic in coconut oil for 3-4 minutes.
- Add the chicken strips and cook another 5 minutes
- Add the curry powder and cook for 1 minute. Then add the fish sauce, salt, and pepper.
- Add 1/2 cup of the coconut milk and bring to a boil.
- Add the potatoes and carrots and boil for 15 minutes or until they are soft and cooked through, stirring frequently. Add 1/2 cup water if the curry is too thick.
- Add the red peppers and remaining coconut milk. Boil for 5 minutes.
- Remove from the heat and add the moringa and cayenne pepper (if using).

88. Chicken Flautas

Serving: Makes 6-8 servings | Prep: | Cook: | Ready in:

Ingredients

- Prep the Chicken:
- 3 tablespoons unsalted butter
- 1/4 cup organic unbleached flour
- 1 cup chicken stock (preferably homemade)
- 1 tablespoon chopped flat leaf parsley (or cilantro, if you prefer)
- 1 tablespoon fresh lemon juice
- 1 teaspoon grated onion
- Dash each of nutmeg and paprika
- fine sea salt and freshly ground pepper to taste
- 1 1/2 cups diced cooked chicken
- 12 flour tortillas
- Crème Fraîche or Sour Cream
- Avocado Sauce
- 2 ripe avocadoes (I prefer Hass)
- 1/2 teaspoon grated onion
- 1/2 cup sour cream or plain yogurt
- 1 teaspoon fresh lime juice
- 10 drops Tabasco sauce
- Pinch fine sea salt

Direction

- Prep the Chicken:
- Melt butter and blend in flour to make a light roux. (Be sure to cook the flour for a couple of minutes.) Add salt and stock. Cook, stirring until thick. Add parsley, lemon juice, onion, paprika, nutmeg and a dash of freshly ground pepper. Stir in chicken. Cool slightly.

- To Assemble Flautas, Place a heaping tablespoon of mixture on tortilla. Roll tightly, and fasten with a toothpick. Fry in deep hot fat for 1 or 2 minutes until tortilla is crisp and brown. Serve with a dollop of Crème Fraîche or sour cream and this sauce:
- Avocado Sauce
- Peel, seed and smash avocados. Add all the other ingredients. Mix until smooth. Spoon sauce over the cooked Flautas.
- Teacher's Tip: You could also make this dish with leftover Thanksgiving Turkey. No one would ever guess it was "leftovers."

89. Chicken Fricassee

Serving: Serves 6 to 8 | Prep: | Cook: | Ready in:

Ingredients

- 1 whole 3-pound chicken, cut into 10 pieces
- Kosher salt and freshly ground pepper
- 1 tablespoon expeller-pressed peanut oil
- 1 cup onion, small dice
- 1/2 cup red bell pepper, small dice
- 3 tablespoons fresh garlic, minced
- 1 tablespoon dried oregano
- 1 tablespoon dried thyme
- 1 tablespoon cumin, crushed
- 2 teaspoons paprika
- 2 bay leaves
- 16 ounces crushed tomatoes
- 2/3 cup green olives, halved
- 1/2 tablespoon capers, minced
- 2 tablespoons hot pepper of your liking, minced

Direction

- Season the chicken with salt and pepper.
- Place a large heavy bottomed pot over medium high heat. Add the peanut oil and swirl it around in the pan to coat the bottom. When the oil is hot add the chicken skin side down and brown it deeply on all sides. Adjust the heat as necessary to avoid scorching the oil.
- Once the chicken is caramelized remove it to a plate. Add the onions, pepper and garlic to the pan. Sweat the vegetables until they just become tender then add the dried spices. Stir the spices into the vegetables and let them toast until they become fragrant. Add the tomato and a cup of water. Season the sauce with a pinch of salt and a few grinds of pepper reminding yourself that the olives and capers are salty so don't season with a heavy hand. Taste and make adjustments.
- Add the chicken back to the broth and then bring the whole thing to a boil. Reduce the heat to a simmer. Cook until the chicken is just tender. If you plan to strip the meat from the bones remove it and place it on the same plate you used before. While it is cooling let the sauce reduce until it becomes unctuous.
- Cook your rice according to the instructions on the bag or box or however it works best for you.
- Add the pulled chicken (or chicken pieces) back to the reduced sauce. Add the olives, capers and any hot peppers you might want to add. Taste and add more salt if needed. Warm through and serve with rice.

90. Chicken Liver Pate With Bourbon, Honey, And Sage

Serving: Makes 2 cups or so | Prep: | Cook: | Ready in:

Ingredients

- 4 tablespoons butter
- 3 large shallots, sliced
- 1 pound chicken livers, trimmed
- 1 1/2 teaspoons kosher salt
- 1/4 teaspoon allspice
- 1/2 teaspoon freshly ground black pepper
- 1/4 cup loosely packed fresh sage leaves
- 1/4 bourbon

- 1 teaspoon honey, or to taste
- 2 tablespoons melted butter

Direction

- In a large sauté pan, heat the butter over medium-high heat until melted. Add the shallots and cook until translucent. Add the livers, sprinkle with salt, allspice, and pepper. Add sage leaves. Cook for about 2-3 minutes, turning livers occasionally. Add bourbon and increase heat to high. Cook until liquid in pan is almost, but not quite, evaporated.
- Remove liver mixture from heat and place in food processor bowl. Add honey. Pulse until smooth. Pack paté into 2 cup mold or individual ramekins. Pour melted butter over top. Cover and refrigerate for up to three days. Flavor improves as it sits.
- Serve with crusty bread.

91. Chicken Liver Paté

Serving: Serves 6-8 | Prep: | Cook: | Ready in:

Ingredients

- 1 pint chicken livers
- 1 tablespoon butter
- 1 cup milk (enough to cover livers)
- 1 medium onion, chopped
- 4 eggs
- 4 tablespoons chicken fat
- 1/8 cup cognac (optional)
- parsley

Direction

- Rinse livers, trim the sinewy bits, and then soak in milk in the fridge for a couple hours. Rinse, pat dry. Season with salt and pepper, then brown in butter until barely pink inside.
- Add cognac to pan and simmer until evaporated. Cool.
- Bring eggs to a boil, turn off heat, cover and let sit 6 minutes. Rinse under cold water, peel, set aside.
- Finely chop onions and slooowwwwwlllllly brown onions in chicken fat or butter (I have also used duck fat) with a pinch of salt until very, very brown. Almost black, they are so slowly and perfectly browned.
- My dad would now just put the livers and eggs through a meat grinder and stir in the fat and onions, season and be done. For me, the grainy texture was never appealing, so I put the livers, onions, 2 eggs, s&p into the Cuisinart and blended until smooth adding about 4 tablespoons of fat a pinch at a time until it was incorporated and velvety. I also stirred in some chopped parsley.
- Finally, separate the whites and yolks of the remaining eggs and push them through a sieve decorating the top of the paté like an egg.
- I served this with slices of grilled baguette brushed with oil but my dad served them with "tiny rye breads" or saltines which are equally good.

92. Chicken Liver Spread (née Pâté)

Serving: Makes 1 cup | Prep: | Cook: | Ready in:

Ingredients

- 7 ounces chicken livers
- 3 tablespoons unsalted butter
- 1 shallot, finely chopped
- 1 sprig rosemary
- 1 tablespoon capers, rinsed and dried
- 2 tablespoons dry vermouth
- 1 teaspoon red wine vinegar
- Coarse salt

Direction

- In a frying pan, melt the butter over medium-low heat. Add the shallot and the rosemary sprig and cook for about five minutes, until

the shallot has softened. (It should smell heavenly.)
- Meanwhile, dry the livers and season with salt and pepper. After the shallot has softened, add the livers to the pan and cook for about three minutes per side, or until they're just pink in the middle. Take the pan off the heat and transfer the livers and shallots to a food processor. (Discard the rosemary.) Add the capers to the liver and shallot mixture.
- Return the pan to the heat and add the vermouth. Bring the vermouth to a boil and deglaze the pan, scraping the brown bits off the bottom. When the vermouth has reduced by half, add 1/2 teaspoon coarse salt and the vinegar. Stir and then add to the food processor along with the livers.
- Pulse the food processor until you have a coarse paste. Taste for seasoning and serve.

93. Chicken Marsala

Serving: Serves 2 | Prep: 0hours25mins | Cook: 0hours45mins | Ready in:

Ingredients

- 8 ounces fresh button or cremini mushrooms, stems removed and sliced
- 2 tablespoons extra-virgin olive oil, divided
- 2 boneless, skinless chicken breasts
- Salt and pepper, to taste
- 1/2 cup plus 1 splash sweet Marsala wine, divided
- 3 garlic cloves, minced
- 1/2 cup heavy cream
- 1/2 cup chicken broth
- 2 tablespoons unsalted butter

Direction

- In a large skillet, sauté mushrooms in 1 tablespoon of the olive oil until lightly caramelized. Remove mushrooms from heat and set aside in a small bowl.
- Carefully slice each chicken breast horizontally, making four thinner pieces of chicken total. Lightly salt and pepper the chicken breasts.
- Heat remaining olive oil in the same skillet and brown chicken breasts on each side until almost done (They will continue to cook in the sauce in Step 6.). Remove from skillet and keep warm.
- Deglaze the pan with the 1/2 cup Marsala wine. Add the garlic. Continue to cook until wine is reduced to be thick and syrupy (au sec).
- Add cream and reduce slightly. Add the broth and continue to reduce slightly until sauce coats the back of a spoon.
- Nestle chicken breasts into the skillet, add the mushrooms and spoon sauce over top. Simmer, uncovered, until chicken is cooked through, about 5 minutes.
- Transfer the chicken to a serving platter and keep warm.
- Swirl butter into the sauce remaining in the skillet, season to taste with salt and pepper, and allow to reduce slightly. Add a splash of Marsala wine to the sauce and pour over the chicken. Serve immediately with a side of linguine or risotto, if desired.

94. Chicken Meatball Tikka Masala

Serving: Serves 4 | Prep: | Cook: | Ready in:

Ingredients

- For the meatballs
- 1 pound ground chicken thigh meat
- 2 shallots, minced
- 1/2 cup cilantro, minced
- 3/4 cup fresh white breadcrumbs
- 1 egg
- 1 tablespoon tomato paste
- 1 tablespoon ginger, minced
- 1 teaspoon salt

- For the masala sauce
- 1 1/2 tablespoons vegetable or other neutral oil
- 1 teaspoon mustard seeds
- 4 shallots, minced
- 4 cloves garlic, minced
- 2 tablespoons ginger, minced
- 1 teaspoon cumin
- 1 1/2 teaspoons coriander
- 1/4 teaspoon cayenne pepper
- 1/2 cup canned tomatoes
- 1 1/2 tablespoons tomato paste
- 1 teaspoon salt
- 1 teaspoon sugar
- 1 serrano chile, halved lengthwise
- 1/4 cup coconut milk
- 1/4 cup cilantro

Direction

- Preheat the oven to 400°F.
- In a large bowl, combine all the ingredients for the meatballs. Form into small golf-sized balls (you should get 24-26), and arrange them about 1 inch apart on a parchment-lined baking sheet.
- Bake for 15-20 minutes. Peak inside and make sure they're no longer pink before eating.
- Make the sauce: Combine the diced tomatoes and tomato paste in a mini food processor and process until smooth. Set aside.
- Heat the oil over high heat in a large cast iron pan until smoking. Add the mustard seeds and cover immediately, and wait till they stop popping (15 seconds). Turn the heat to medium-low and add the shallots, garlic, and ginger. Cook for 3-5 minutes, stirring nearly constantly, until the shallots are quite golden. Add the cumin, coriander, and cayenne, and cook for another minute or so, to toast the spices. Pour in the pureed tomato, and cook down for 3-4 minutes. It should be reduced to an almost paste-like consistency.
- Pour in the coconut milk, the salt and sugar, and about 1/4 cup of water. Bring to a boil.
- Simmer covered for 5-10 minutes, to let the flavors meld. Taste for salt and spiciness.
- Add the meatballs and the cilantro to the sauce. Toss well, heat the meatballs through, and serve.

95. Chicken Paillard With Lemon Salad

Serving: Serves 4 | Prep: | Cook: | Ready in:

Ingredients

- 2 teaspoons grated lemon peel
- 3 tablespoons lemon juice
- 2 teaspoons olive oil
- 1 garlic clove, crushed
- 1/2 teaspoon salt, divided
- 1/2 teaspoon pepper
- 4 cups arugula mixed green salad
- 4 boneless, skinless chicken breast halves
- Organic cooking spray
- 1 cup cherry tomatoes, halved

Direction

- Combine lemon rind, juice, oil, and garlic in a large bowl. Sprinkle with 1/4 teaspoon salt and 1/4 teaspoon pepper.
- When ready to serve add arugula and toss well, making sure to coat leaves evenly.
- Place each chicken breast half between 2 sheets of heavy-duty plastic wrap; pound each piece to 1/4-inch thickness using a meat mallet or small heavy skillet. Sprinkle both sides of chicken with remaining 1/4 teaspoon salt and remaining 1/4 teaspoon pepper. You can do this earlier in the day and cover and refrigerate if needed.
- Heat a grill pan or a large nonstick skillet over medium-high heat. Coat pan with cooking spray. Add chicken, and cook for 4 minutes on each side or until done. Remove chicken from pan, and keep warm.
- On a plate, place one chicken breast top with a heaping of salad and top with a handful of tomatoes.

96. Chicken Paprikash With Rhubarb, Cherry, And Red Pepper

Serving: Serves 4 | Prep: | Cook: | Ready in:

Ingredients

- 4 free range airchilled small chicken breasts, bone in and skin on
- 4 tablespoons flour mixed with 1 tbl of sweet smoked paprika for dredging chicken
- 1/4 teaspoon freshly ground black pepper
- oil for browning chicken (grapeseed or olive)
- 1 tablespoon Hungarian sweet smoked paprika (or plain sweet paprika is ok)
- 1/3 cup Rainier cherries, pitted, if available, black cherry tomatoes are an alternative
- 1 stalk of rhubarb chopped, with some of their stringiness removed
- 1/2 cup red bell pepper, sliced lengths, @ 1/4" wide
- 1 cup red onion loosely chopped
- 1 cup dry white wine
- 1 cup sour cream (or Greek yogurt)
- 3 tablespoons chopped flat leaf parsley
- kosher salt to taste
- additional paprika for garnish

Direction

- Dredge your prepared chicken breasts with flour seasoned with paprika and pepper (and a little salt).
- Heat a heavy pan with a small amount of oil. Stir in 1/2 tbsp. paprika.
- Add the floured chicken and brown thoroughly.
- Add the onions, red peppers, and rhubarb. Simmer for @ 5 minutes.
- Next add the cherries.
- Add the wine so the pan sizzles. Reduce. Add half the chopped parsley.
- Reduce to a simmer, cover and let cook until chicken is done (@30-40 minutes depending upon the size).
- Remove the chicken and stir in the sour cream. Stir in 1/2 tbsp. paprika. Return the chicken to the pan. Add a pinch of salt now. Make sure the sour cream has heated through (but don't boil it).
- Place the chicken over spaetzle. Smother it with the sauce. Garnish with chopped parsley and paprika.

97. Chicken Pot Pie Provencal

Serving: Serves 8 | Prep: | Cook: | Ready in:

Ingredients

- Jacques's Poached Chicken
- 4 pounds roasting chicken
- 6 carrots, ends trimmed, peeled
- 4 celery stalks, ends trimmed
- 1 leek, white and light green parts only
- 1 cup dry white wine
- 2 sprigs tarragon
- 3 sprigs thyme
- fronds from a large fennel bulb
- 10 ounces pearl onions, peeled
- 1 tablespoon kosher salt
- 12 black peppercorns
- Chicken Pot Pie Provencal (recipe will make two 9" round by 3" deep pies, each will serve 4-6 people) If making only one pot pie, freeze 1 pastry disc and half of the filling for later use.
- 3 cups plus 2 tablespoons all-purpose flour
- 2 sticks plus 5 tablespoons cold, unsalted butter, cut into 1" pieces.
- 2/3 cup ice water
- 1 teaspoon kosher salt
- reserved chicken
- reserved carrots
- reserved pearl onions
- 10 fingerling potatoes

- 1 large fennel bulb, quartered and roasted
- 10 ounces button mushrooms, thickly sliced and sauteed
- 1/2 pound haricot verts, topped and tailed, blanched, refreshed, and chopped
- 1 1/2 cups frozen green peas, thawed
- 1/4 cup diced oven roasted tomatoes (store bought)
- 1 tablespoon brown mustard seeds
- 1/4 cup vermouth
- 6 tablespoons butter
- 8 tablespoons flour
- 1 cup heavy cream
- 1 cup creme fraiche
- 4 tablespoons dijon mustard
- 1 tablespoon finely chopped tarragon
- 2 teaspoons finely chopped thyme
- 1 egg, whisked for egg wash
- salt and pepper

Direction

- Jacques's Poached Chicken
- Place chicken in a large stockpot.
- Tie whole carrots, leek, celery, and fennel fronds into a bundle and add to the pot with the chicken. Tie tarragon and thyme together and add to the pot. Toss in the peppercorns and the pearl onions, white wine, and 1 tablespoon of salt. Fill with water to just cover the chicken, put over a high heat and bring to a boil.
- Once boiling, lower the heat to maintain a gentle boil for 20 minutes. Raise the heat back to high, to again achieve a rapid boil, turn off the heat, cover and let sit for 1 hour.
- Remove chicken from the pot and set aside to cool. Remove the bundle of vegetables, discard the fennel fronds and leek, and cut the carrots and celery on the bias into bite-sized pieces, reserve.
- Skin the chicken and pull all the meat from the bones, tearing into bite-sized pieces, reserve.
- Strain the cooking liquid through a fine meshed strainer into a clean saucepan, skim any fat from the top and set over medium high heat to reduce to 4 cups of concentrated stock, reserve.
- Chicken Pot Pie Provencal (recipe will make two 9" round by 3" deep pies, each will serve 4-6 people) If making only one pot pie, freeze 1 pastry disc and half of the filling for later use.
- For the pastry crust - Place the flour into a bowl of a food processor, toss the butter on top, and pulse in short bursts until the butter is reduced to pea sized pieces. Add the salt to the water and stir to dissolve. Pour the water through the feed tube of the processor and pulse until the dough just starts to come together in a ball, you should still see some small butter chunks in the mix.
- Dump the dough out onto a well-floured work surface, and divide it into two equal sized balls. Press each ball into a disc about an inch thick, wrap in plastic wrap and refrigerate for at least a couple of hours, or overnight.
- For the pot pie filling - Pre-heat the oven to 400. Quarter the fennel bulb, and cut out the wedge shaped core. Toss with a little olive oil, salt and pepper, and place on a baking sheet. Roast in the oven for about 20-25 minutes, until nicely caramelized. Remove from the oven, roughly chop and reserve.
- Place the fingerlings in a pan of cold water to cover. Place over high heat and bring to a boil. Lower the heat to a gentle boil and cook until just cooked through, about 10-12 minutes. Drain, place on a cutting board, and cut into coins. Toss in a bowl with a touch EVOO and reserve.
- Sauté mushrooms in a little olive oil with salt and pepper, until caramelized. Add mustard seeds and vermouth, and cook until all the liquid has evaporated, reserve.
- Make a roux by melting the butter over medium heat in a medium saucepan, add the flour, and whisk constantly for 2-3 minutes. Remove from the heat and add the 4 cups of reduced stock, whisk until smooth. Put back on the heat, add the cream and crème fraiche, and cook, whisking, until the sauce thickens to coat the back of a spoon. Whisk in the

mustard and season with salt and pepper to taste. Add the minced tarragon and thyme, remove from heat to cool slightly.
- Put all filling ingredients (potatoes, tomatoes, onions, carrots, fennel, celery, haricot verts, mushrooms, and chicken) into a large mixing bowl, add the mustard velouté and mix well. Check for seasoning, reserve.
- Whisk the egg in a small bowl.
- Pour the filling to within 1/2" of the top of a 3" deep, 8-9" round soufflé dish (or other such ramekin or earthenware vessel)
- Roll the pastry dough on a well-floured surface to about 1/8" thickness.
- Brush egg wash onto the rim of the ramekin and about halfway down the outside of the dish to hold the crust in place while baking.
- Place the rolled pastry on top of the pie, allowing about 2" to drape over the edges. Press into place to adhere to the dish, cut away any excess.
- Brush the entire crust with egg wash, and cut 8 small vent slits in the top. Put the pie on a sheet tray and place in the 400 oven for 30-35 minutes, until the crust is nicely browned, and the contents are seen bubbling through the vent holes. Remove from the oven and serve with a simple green salad.

98. Chicken Prosciutto Roll Ups

Serving: Serves 4 | Prep: | Cook: |Ready in:

Ingredients

- 2 pounds Chicken breasts, sliced thin and pounded
- 1/2 pound Prosciutto
- 1/2 pound Fresh Mozzarella
- 1/3 cup Sun dried tomatoes in oil
- Salt, to taste
- Pepper, to taste

Direction

- Preheat oven to 350 degrees. In between Saran Wrap, place each piece of chicken breast (will make 4 roll-ups) until thin. Take 3 slices of Prosciutto, 2 slices of mozzarella and three pieces of sundries tomatoes on each piece of chicken. Add a little salt and pepper to taste. Roll up each chicken breast and the trick is to wrap them with butcher's twine instead of toothpicks so they don't fall apart! Bake on an uncoated baking sheet for 40 minutes.
- Let cool for ten minutes and slice each to desired thickness.
- Enjoy!

99. Chicken Salad With Wild Rice And Oranges

Serving: Serves 4 to 6 | Prep: 1hours20mins | Cook: 0hours40mins | Ready in:

Ingredients

- 1/3 cup Mayonnaise
- 2 tablespoons Frozen Orange Juice Concentrate, Thawed
- 3 cups Cubed Cooked Chicken (From Rotisserie Chicken)
- 1/2 cup Pecans, toasted and coarsely chopped
- 1/2 cup Dried Cranberries
- 1 Orange, segments removed and chopped
- 1 Celery rib, cut into small dice
- 1/2 teaspoon Salt
- 1/4 teaspoon Pepper
- 1/3 cup Wild Rice
- 1 cup Water
- Lettuce leaves and Orange segments for serving

Direction

- Whisk together mayonnaise and orange juice concentrate in a large bowl. Add chicken, nuts, cranberries, orange, celery, salt and pepper and mix well. Chill, covered, at least 1 hour.

- Rinse rice in a fine sieve under running cold water, then drain. Bring water to a boil in a heavy saucepan and stir in rice. Simmer, covered, until rice is tender, about 40 to 50 minutes. Drain rice and cool, then stir into chicken salad and serve over greens.

100. Chicken Skillet With Sweet Potatoes & Wild Rice

Serving: Serves 8 | Prep: | Cook: | Ready in:

Ingredients

- 1 tablespoon olive oil
- 1 onion, chopped
- 3 carrots, sliced
- 1 pound boneless skinless chicken breast, cut into 1-inch cubes
- 1 teaspoon salt
- 1 teaspoon pepper
- 4 cloves garlic, minced
- 1 18.5-ounce can chicken & wild rice soup
- 2 cups chicken stock as needed (more may be required depending on the rice you use)
- 1 cup brown & wild rice blend, uncooked (or your preferred rice variety)
- 2 tablespoons fresh thyme, chopped
- 1 teaspoon ground mustard
- 1 large sweet potato, cut into 1-inch cubes
- 14 ounces broccoli (1 head rinsed and chopped into small florets)
- 6 ounces cheddar cheese, shredded

Direction

- Heat one tablespoon olive oil over medium-high heat in a large (12-inch) oven-proof skillet. Add onion and carrot, then sauté for 3 minutes.
- Add chicken, salt, and pepper, and continue cooking over high heat for 5 minutes.
- Add minced garlic and cook for one more minute.
- Add Progresso Reduced Sodium Savory Chicken & Wild Rice Soup, chicken stock and bring to a simmer. Add wild rice, cover, and cook for 25 minutes.
- Add thyme, ground mustard, and sweet potatoes. Cover and cook for another 10 minutes or until rice is cooked to the doneness you prefer. If the mixture seems to be dry add a little extra chicken stock or water to loosen it up. (Different rice requires different cook times so check the package instructions and modify accordingly.)
- Stir in broccoli, cover and cook another 4 minutes.
- Remove cover and stir in 2 ounces of cheddar cheese, then sprinkle the remaining cheddar on top. Broil for 2-3 minutes or until cheese has melted (keep a close eye on it while broiling).

101. Chicken Sophia

Serving: Serves 2 | Prep: | Cook: | Ready in:

Ingredients

- 2 chicken breast, 6 oz. each
- 2 Alaskan king crab legs, picked of their meat
- 6 to 8 asparagus spears, top 3 inches only, blanched in heavily salted water until crunchy tender
- 2 egg yolks
- 1 teaspoon Dijon mustard
- 1 tablespoon fresh lemon juice
- 2 teaspoons fresh tarragon, minced
- 1 stick, unsalted butter, melted and kept warm
- kosher salt and fresh ground pepper

Direction

- Pull a 24 inch long piece of plastic wrap out of the container and then fold it in half so you have approximately a 12 by 12 inch square. Working with one chicken breast at a time

- place it off center on the wrap and then fold the wrap over the top. Pound the breast until it is about 1/4 to 1/2 inch thick. Repeat with the other breast. Cut the plastic wrap in half.
- Place each breast, what would have been skin side down, onto the plastic wrap. Rub a little butter across the center of each breast. Season each with pepper. Taste the crab if it is salty don't salt the chicken, your call on the salt here. In a straight line make a mound of crab meat down the center.
- Roll the chicken breast up in the plastic wrap taking care not to roll the plastic into the chicken. Now take two pieces of foil and place each roulade on a piece of foil. Roll the roulades in the foil and twist the ends of the foil tightening up the chicken roulade into a tight firm cylinder.
- Lace a large pot of water over high heat.
- While the water is coming to a boil place the yolks, lemon juice, mustard, tarragon, a teaspoon of water, salt and pepper into a heat proof mixing bowl. Whisk to combine.
- Place the bowl over low heat and continually whisk until the mixture starts to thicken and follow you whisk by leaving ribbon trails. Remove from the heat and place the bowl on a damp towel. The towel is to keep the bowl from moving. Adding a drizzle whisk the butter into the eggs. Really only do this at a drizzle and make sure the oil is emulsifying with the yolks before you add more. Slowly keep adding the butter while whisking until all but the last tablespoon, which is water, is combined. Keep the béarnaise in a warm spot but not over any flame.
- If the large pot is boiling, remove a cup of water and then add the chicken roulades and then reduce the heat to low. Simmer the roulades for 10 to 12 minutes. Remove them from the heat and let them rest.
- Place the asparagus tips into the reserved hot water to warm them.
- Remove the chicken from its wrapper and slice. Plate it and serve topped with béarnaise.

102. Chicken Soup Pipian

Serving: Serves 4 | Prep: | Cook: |Ready in:

Ingredients

- Pipian
- 2 jalapenos, stemmed and quartered, seeded and ribbed for less heat
- 2 small or 1 1/2 medium onions, peeled and trimmed at the root, quartered
- 4 cloves garlic, peeled
- 1 lime, halved
- 1 pound tomatillos, husked, rinsed and halved
- 1 1/2 cups pepitas (raw shelled pumpkin seeds)
- 1/4 cup sesame seeds (white/raw)
- 1/2 teaspoon ground cumin
- 1 cup cilantro leaves (save the stems for your stock)
- Soup base
- 1 whole chicken, cut into 10 parts (do not buy precut parts or you won't get the backbone to flavor the broth! You can ask the butcher to break down the chicken for you, if you prefer.)
- 8 cups water
- Springs from a bunch of cilantro, tied in a bunch with butcher's twine. I also save my cilantro sprigs regularly and put them in a zip top baggie in the freezer, so I add more if I have it to further flavor the stock
- 1 bay leaf
- 1 cinnamon stick
- 2 teaspoons salt
- cubed queso blanco (or cotija, queso Oaxaca), chopped avocado, chopped fresh cilantro, radish slices, and more pepitas, for topping and serving

Direction

- To make the Pipian, preheat the oven to 450F. Place the jalapenos through tomatillos in a large (16") cast iron skillet; alternatively you can use a baking tray. Dry roast in the oven for

15 minutes, flipping halfway through. Meanwhile, toast the pepitas about 5 minutes in a dry pan and remove to a food processor. Toast the sesame seeds 2 minutes and remove to the food processor. Process until ground. Place all of the roasted vegetables, except the limes, in the processor. Squeeze in the juice of the roasted limes, and add the cumin and cilantro leaves. Process all together until you have a thick sauce. You can add up to 2 Tbsp. vegetable oil if the sauce is too thick to blend. Salt to taste.

- To make the soup: in a large Dutch oven or stockpot, cover the chicken with the water. Add the bay leaf, cinnamon stick, salt and parcel of cilantro sprigs. Bring to a boil, then reduce to a simmer and cook for 30 minutes. Remove the chicken to a plate, discarding the backbone, and allow to cool enough to remove the skin and pull the meat from the bone. Shred or roughly chop the meat and stir in the pipian sauce. Remove the cilantro, bay and cinnamon stick from the stock. Strain the stock then return to the pot and bring back to a simmer to keep warm.
- To serve, place a generous amount of shredded pipian chicken in the base of a soup bowl and ladle over the broth. Top with sliced radish, cilantro, cubed queso blanco, cubed avocado, and extra pepitas.

103. Chicken Souvlaki Naan Plate

Serving: Serves 2 | Prep: | Cook: | Ready in:

Ingredients

- Chicken Souvlaki
- 2 pieces garlic naan, approx 8" diameter
- 1 large boneless chicken breast, cut in 1" cubes
- 1 red bell pepper, cut in 1" squares
- 1/2 red onion, cut in 1" squares
- 1 baby cucumber, cut into spears
- 1 vine ripened tomato, hulled and diced
- 4 sprigs romaine lettuce, chopped
- 8 pieces sliced banana peppers (optional)
- 1 dash sriracha (optional)
- 1 ounce feta, cubed (optional)
- 1/4 cup olive oil
- 1/4 cup soy sauce, low sodium
- 1/8 cup lemon juice
- 8 tablespoons tzatziki
- Awesome Dill Tzatziki (for 4 pitas)
- 1 cup plain greek yogurt
- 2 medium cucumbers, skinned and seeded
- 3 garlic cloves, chopped
- 2 teaspoons dry dill
- 1/2 teaspoon salt
- 1/2 teaspoon ground black pepper
- 2 tablespoons lemon juice

Direction

- Prepare the marinade of olive oil, soy sauce, and lemon juice, and soak chicken for 30-60 minutes at room temperature.
- While chicken is marinating, prepare the awesome dill tzatziki. Pulverize cucumber in food processor and strain excess water. Combine the remaining cucumber pulp and other awesome dill tzatziki ingredients in a bowl. Save some for next time or for other recipes.
- Skewer the chicken, alternating with red bell pepper and red onion. Grill the kebabs on medium-high heat for 5 minutes, rotate and grill for another 5 minutes.
- Wrap naan in aluminum foil and place on grill with kebabs for 5 minutes.
- Plate with the naan at the base, lettuce, deconstructed kebabs, cucumber, tomato. Top with optional ingredients and 4 tbsp. of tzatziki per souvlaki.

104. Chicken Stew

Serving: Serves 4 | Prep: 0hours10mins | Cook: 1hours0mins | Ready in:

Ingredients

- 1 pound chicken cut in pieces
- 4 carrots
- 1 onion
- 1 leek
- 1 green pepper
- kosher salt
- Freshly ground black pepper
- Extra Virgin Olive Oil
- 1 cup white wine
- Chicken broth

Direction

- In a large pot over medium heat, add oil. Add cut carrots and leek and season with salt and pepper. Cook, stirring often, until vegetables are tender, about 5 minutes.
- Then add chicken and white wine. Bring mixture to a simmer and cook until the chicken is no longer pink. Add broth until cover the chicken and cook for 45 minutes.
- Serve.

105. Chicken Thigh Surprise

Serving: Serves 4 | Prep: | Cook: | Ready in:

Ingredients

- 6 Chicken thighs
- 3/4 pound Chopped butternut squash
- 3/4 pound Brussel sprouts
- 1 cup Low sodium chicken broth
- 1/2 cup Onion chopped
- 1/2 cup Green peppers chopped
- 1/2 cup Celery chopped
- 1/2 cup Carrots chopped
- 2 Cloves of minced garlic
- 1 tablespoon Black Pepper
- 1 tablespoon Kosher Salt
- 1 tablespoon Turmeric
- 1 tablespoon Herbs de Provence
- 1 tablespoon Curry powder
- 1 tablespoon Smoked paprika
- 1 tablespoon Garlic powder
- 2 tablespoons Olive oil
- 2 tablespoons Brown or Dijon mustard
- 1 cup Water

Direction

- Preheat oven at 350 degrees Season chicken thighs with a tablespoon of the above seasonings and mix to distribute evenly.
- Add olive oil to cast iron skillet; allow pan to heat.
- Place seasoned chicken thighs to pan skin side down. Flipping after 3 mins.
- Once both sides are brown remove chicken from pan and let rest.
- Reduce heat and deglaze by adding the mustard and chicken stock by stirring the little bits from the pot (my favorite part).
- Add chopped veggies. Allow to cook for five minutes. Add pinch of salt and pepper. While they are cooking take Brussels sprouts chop into quarters. Afterwards take the butternut squash and cut into the same size as the sprouts.
- Stir veggies that are sautéing and add sprouts and squash. Allow all to cook for five minutes. Reseason with a pinch of ALL seasonings used for the chicken.
- Add back chicken thighs and add remaining water.
- Remove from oven and serve.

106. Chicken Thighs Smothered In Gravy

Serving: Serves 5 | Prep: | Cook: | Ready in:

Ingredients

- 2 & 1/2 tablespoons canola oil
- 5 skinless chicken thighs
- salt and freshly ground pepper
- 1 thick slice bacon, cut crosswise in thin strips
- 1 & 1/2 tablespoons flour
- 1 onion, thinly sliced
- 1 garlic clove, thinly sliced
- 1 tomato, peeled, seeded, & chopped
- 1 teaspoon tomato paste
- 1 cup milk
- 1/2 cup chicken broth
- 2 sprigs parsley, plus 2 teaspoons, chopped

Direction

- Preheat oven to 375 F. In an ovenproof skillet, heat 1 tablespoon of the oil under medium to high heat. Season the chicken with salt and pepper and add it to the skillet. Cook until browned all over, about 8 to 10 minutes, flipping once in between. When chicken is browned, transfer it to a plate and set aside.
- Add the bacon to the skillet and cook until fat is rendered, about 2 minutes. Drain off the fat and add remaining oil to skillet. Stir in flour until incorporated. Add the onion and garlic. Cook until soft and translucent, about 3 to 5 minutes. Add the tomato and tomato paste and cook until tomato is somewhat soft, about 5 more minutes. Add the milk and broth and bring mixture to a boil. Stir until it begins to slightly thicken, about 3 to 5 minutes. Return the chicken and any juices to skillet. Stir in parsley sprigs as well.
- Cover the skillet and braise the chicken in the oven for about 20 minutes, or until cooked all the way through. You can't really go wrong with chicken thighs because as long as you don't burn it (which is practically impossible in a braising situation), then you can't dry it out, or cook it "too long".
- Carefully take skillet out of oven with an oven mitt and remove chicken and place on a platter. Then, STILL wearing oven mitt, (I say this because I damn near burnt myself by grabbing onto the skillet handle without one), place skillet under moderate heat and stir mixture until smooth, about 2 to 4 minutes. Stir in the remaining chopped parsley and spoon the gravy onto the chicken.

107. Chicken Tikka Masala

Serving: Serves 4 | Prep: | Cook: |Ready in:

Ingredients

- For chicken marination
- 2.2 pounds chicken breast
- 5 tablespoons yogurt
- 2 tablespoons chicken tikka masala powder
- 1/2 tablespoon turmeric powder
- 1/2 tablespoon dried fenugreek leaves
- 2 tablespoons ghee
- 1 tablespoon lemon juice
- 1/4 teaspoon saffron food colour
- 1/2 tablespoon Salt
- For gravy
- 1 big onion
- 2 tomatoes
- 2 green chilies
- 1 tablespoon ginger garlic paste
- 1/2 teaspoon cumin seeds
- 1 teaspoon Coriander powder
- 1 teaspoon Turmeric powder
- 1 teaspoon Red chili powder
- 1 teaspoon chicken tikka masala powder
- 1/2 teaspoon sugar
- 1/4 cup cream
- 1 handful Coriander leaves
- 1 teaspoon salt

Direction

- Cut chicken breast in medium sized kebab pieces. Transfer chicken pieces in a bowl and mix all the ingredients mentioned for marinating with yogurt.
- We need thick yogurt for this. Just keep the yogurt in a strainer for some time, this will

drain off excess water and you will get thick creamy yogurt. Let chicken marinate for couple of hours.
- Pre heat the oven at 200'C or 390 F. Put chicken pieces on a skewer, if not, simply put it in oven dish and place it in oven for 10-15 minutes. With this chicken tikkas are ready for the gravy.
- For making gravy for chicken tikka masala, heat oil in a pan. When oil is hot add cumin seeds. When cumin seeds start to splutter, add finely chopped onion and split green chili. Let it cook till onions are slight golden brown in color.
- Add finely chopped tomatoes at this point. You can also make a paste of the tomatoes in blender and add if you like it that way.
- In a small bowl, add coriander, red chili, turmeric and chicken tikka masala powder with little water and transfer this paste in the pan.
- Let it cook for 2-3 minutes or till masala gets cooked, you will know masala is cooked when oil starts separating from masala. Add sugar and salt.
- When masala is fully cooked add cream. You can also substitute cream with yogurt if you like. Slowly add yogurt in masala.
- Add little water to make the gravy of the desired consistency. Wait for 3-4 minutes then add chicken tikka to it.
- After a boil, garnish with chopped coriander. With this chicken tikka masala is ready. Serve with naan or rice.

108. Chicken Tsukune

Serving: Serves 14 skewers | Prep: 0hours40mins | Cook: 0hours15mins | Ready in:

Ingredients

- 14 5-inch flat bamboo skewers
- 10 shiso or perilla leaves
- 4 green onions/scallions
- 1 pound ground chicken
- 1 tablespoon sesame oil (and more for coating your hands)
- 1 tablespoon miso (I use awase miso, which is a combination of red and white miso)
- kosher salt
- 1/2 cup yakitori tare (recipe below)
- shichimi togarashi (Japanese seven spice) (optional, for spicy taste)
- Yakitori Sauce (Tare)
- 1/2 cup soy sauce
- 1/2 cup mirin
- 1/4 cup sake
- 1/4 cup water
- 2 teaspoons brown sugar, packed
- 1 scallion, green part only

Direction

- Gather all the ingredients.
- Soak the bamboo skewers in water for 30 minutes.
- Pile and roll up the shiso leaves, then cut into thin julienne slices. Cut the scallion into thin slices.
- Heat a nonstick frying pan over medium heat. When it's hot, add ⅓ of ground chicken and break it up into small pieces using a wooden spatula. Cook until no longer pink and transfer to a plate to let it cool.
- Combine the cooked chicken and uncooked chicken in a large bowl and mix well with rubber spatula.
- Add sesame oil and miso and mix well.
- Add the scallions and shiso leaves and combine well with silicone spatula.
- Now with your hand, knead 30 times clockwise. Then knead counterclockwise 30 times. The meat will become more pale in color and sticky. This part is very important for the meat to stay on stick so please do not skip this step.
- Grease the grill rack with brush. I use a roasting pan and rack as it can support the skewers very well while the excess oil drips down to the bottom of roasting pan when cooking.

- Lightly coat your hands with sesame oil to prevent the meat from sticking. Scoop a handful of the chicken mixture (1 ½ scoop for my hand using an OXO cookie scoop) and form into a round patty.
- Toss the meat to left and right hands to release the air pockets and gently squeeze to form the meat into a long oval patty, about 3-4 inches in length. Insert the skewer on the prepared wire rack.
- Lightly sprinkle salt over the chicken skewers.
- Put aluminum foil around the skewers to prevent them from burning.
- Preheat the oven to High Broil (550F) for 5 minutes. Boil in the middle rack, for 6 minutes. Then flip the skewers over and broil more for 4 minutes.
- When both sides are cooked, brush the yakitori sauce on the meat and broil for another 30 seconds. Transfer the skewers to a serving plate and brush the extra sauce on the meat. Serve with shichimi togarashi.
- Yakitori Sauce (Tare)
- In a small saucepan, add the soy sauce, mirin, sake, water, brown sugar, and the green part of 1 scallion, and bring it to a boil over high heat.
- Once boiling, reduce the heat to low and simmer, uncovered, until the liquid is reduced by half. It will take about 30 minutes. The sauce will be thicker and glossy.
- Let it cool to room temperature before using.

109. Chicken Under A Brick With Pickled Peppers

Serving: Serves 2 to 4 | Prep: | Cook: | Ready in:

Ingredients

- 2 chicken thighs and drumsticks, still attached
- Kosher salt
- 2 tablespoons olive oil
- 3 sprigs marjoram, thyme, or rosemary
- 2 sprigs sage
- 1 garlic clove, smashed, skin left on
- 1/4 cup rose or white wine
- 1/2 lemon
- 5 peppadew or other small pickled, slightly spicy peppers, thinly sliced

Direction

- An hour before cooking, season the chicken on all sides with salt. Place in the refrigerator for 1 hour.
- Pat the chicken dry. Place a medium cast iron skillet over medium high heat. When a drop of water sizzles in the pan, add the oil. Then the herbs, garlic clove, and chicken pieces, skin-side down.
- Use a pastry brush to brush the top of the chicken with oil. Lay a piece of foil on top of the chicken, then weigh it down with a large, heavy sauté pan. Let the chicken cook for 20 to 30 minutes, checking every couple of minutes to make sure it's browning steadily and evenly. You want the chicken to cook through just as the skin turns a nice hazelnut brown. When the chicken reaches this color, carefully turn the pieces over, making sure you don't tear the lovely crisp skin you've just worked so hard on. Crisp the other side just until the chicken is cooked through, 2 to 5 minutes.
- Remove the chicken to a plate. Add 1/2 cup water to the pan and bring to a boil. Scrape up any sticky bits. Discard the herbs. Pour this mixture into the sauté pan you used as a weight. Add the rose. Bring to a boil and reduce by half (or more, if desired). Season to taste with lemon juice and salt. Stir in the peppers. Spoon the sauce onto a serving dish (or into the cast-iron skillet) and top with the chicken.

110. Chicken Veggie Soup

Serving: Serves one full crock pot | Prep: | Cook: | Ready in:

Ingredients

- for the chicken
- 2 pounds boneless chicken breast
- 2 tablespoons Mrs Dash original
- 2 tablespoons minced garlic
- olive oil
- for the soup
- 1 leek, cleaned and separated
- 6 celery stalks, cleaned
- 2 cups bean sprouts
- 2 cups carrots, peeled
- 2 cups broccolli florettes
- 2 tablespoons minced garlic
- 1 quart chicken broth, low-sodium
- olive oil

Direction

- Cut the chicken breast into 1 -2" cubes. You can cook the chicken before cutting it, but it's more flavorful when cut first.
- Pour some olive oil into a skillet on medium heat and add garlic and Mrs. Dash.
- Add chicken pieces and stir to mix chicken, seasoning and garlic well.
- Cook chicken in covered skillet, tossing frequently to ensure even cooking and to distribute seasonings.
- Be careful not to overcook chicken! It will still be cooking in the crock pot, so just barely finish the chicken in the skillet. If it's overcooked, it will be tough and dry in the soup.
- When chicken is done, remove from skillet and place in bowl, along with any juices that may be in the pan.
- Prepare all vegetables by washing, trimming off any brown or root ends, and chopping coarsely. You do not need to chop the bean sprouts. Keep each vegetable separate after chopping, so they can be layered into the crock pot.
- Pour olive oil into skillet and add garlic. Add leek pieces and toss until oil and seasonings are distributed. It will look like a lot, but the leeks will cook down.
- Cover skillet and cook until barely tender, tossing frequently. Remove from skillet to a bowl.
- Return skillet to stove and use a little more olive oil, then pour in the bean sprouts. Again, cook until barely tender, tossing frequently.
- In a large crock pot, place the uncooked carrots in the bottom of the pot.
- Then, add the uncooked broccoli.
- Add celery to the pot next.
- Add chicken pieces and juices.
- Add cooked leeks, then cooked bean sprouts.
- Crock pot should be close to full. Pour in the quart of chicken broth.
- Cover crock pot and turn on low setting. Let cook for 2 - 3 hours.
- Once soup has cooled, it can be frozen in reheatable containers or stored in the fridge. This is especially easy if the ceramic pot in your crock is removable.

111. Chicken Vermicelli Soup

Serving: Serves 4 | Prep: | Cook: | Ready in:

Ingredients

- 2 chicken breasts sliced into strips
- 2 tablespoons any flavourless vegetable oil such as canola or sunflower
- 1 large onion finely chopped
- 2 potatoes quartered
- 2 carrots cut into large quarters
- 4-5 cups chicken stock
- 1 1 inch piece of cinnamon
- 1 teaspoon chilli flakes
- 1 pinch saffron strands soaked in 2 teaspoons of warm water

- Juice of half lemon
- 1 tablespoon chopped, fresh parsley
- 150 grams thin, rice vermicelli
- flour for dusting the chicken
- salt
- 1/2 teaspoon freshly ground black pepper
- 2 eggs, separated

Direction

- Heat oil in a thick casserole dish and fry the onions till slightly soft. Add the chicken pieces dusted with flour and quickly brown (not too much or the onions will burn).
- Throw in the carrots and potatoes, cook for a couple of minutes and pour in the stock, cinnamon stick, chili flakes and salt. Bring to a boil, lower heat, cover and simmer till vegetables are tender but not mushy.
- In a small bowl, beat the egg yolks with the lemon juice and mix in the herbs and the soaked saffron with the water (cooled or else the eggs will be cooked).
- Add the vermicelli to the soup and cook for a further 7-8 minutes till they are done. Mix in the chicken followed by the egg mixture. It's important to keep the heat low or take the pan off the heat while stirring the eggs in. Once mixed, return to low heat, simmer for 2 minutes, add the pepper and serve piping hot.

112. Chicken Yellow Curry

Serving: Serves 4 | Prep: | Cook: |Ready in:

Ingredients

- 1 pound chicken thighs or tenderloins
- 14 ounces can of diced tomatoes
- 14 ounces can of light coconut milk
- 1/2 large onion, diced
- 1-2 carrots, diced
- 1-2 tablespoons fresh ginger, minced
- 1-2 tablespoons yellow curry powder (depending on heat preference)
- 1/2 teaspoon ground coriander
- 2-3 tablespoons olive oil
- 1 tablespoon fish sauce
- salt and pepper to taste
- cilantro, chili peppers, lime, and green onion as garnish

Direction

- In a Dutch oven style pot, heat 2 tablespoons of olive oil over medium heat. When heated, throw in the onion, carrots, and ginger. After 5 minutes or so, add in the garlic. Give it a good stir and add in more oil if the mixture gets too dry. Then, add in the curry powder, coriander, salt and pepper. Get those veggies coated in the spices.
- Next, add in the diced tomatoes. Give the mixture a good stir and then move the heat to a low simmer. Cover the pot and let the tomato mixture simmer, simmer, simmer for about 45 minutes, stirring fairly regularly.
- At this point, the chicken can get started. Preheat the oven to 400°F. Salt and pepper the thighs or tenderloins. Next, place a sauté pan over medium heat with a bit of olive oil. When hot, brown the chicken for a minute on each side. Then place the pan in the oven and cook the chicken for roughly 18 minutes, until just about cooked through. Set the chicken aside.
- When the tomato mixture has simmered for a good while, place the chicken into the pot. Then, pour in the coconut milk over. Add in the fish sauce. Stir everything together and let the curry simmer for another 15 minutes or so. Give it a taste to see if you need more heat or seasoning.
- Serve the curry over rice with lime slices, chili peppers, cilantro and green onion.

113. Chicken And Dumplings

Serving: Makes 16 servings | Prep: | Cook: |Ready in:

Ingredients

- 1 Whole Chicken
- 6 cups flour
- 1 1/2 cups Self-Rising Flour
- 3/4 cup Shortening
- 3 cups Whole Milk

Direction

- Rinse chicken and place in a 10 quart pot.
- Fill pot with water and bring to a boil.
- Cook until chicken reaches internal temperature of 165 degrees F.
- Remove chicken from the broth and de-bone and then return chicken to the broth.
- In a mixing bowl, add flour, self-rising flour, shortening and milk. Mix and knead dough.
- Roll out dough, adding flour as needed. Cut into 2" X 2" squares.
- Bring chicken and broth to a rolling boil.
- Place squares individually into broth and chicken, then boil for 20 minutes, stirring occasionally.

114. Chicken And Pinto Bean Sauté

Serving: Serves 4 | Prep: | Cook: |Ready in:

Ingredients

- 1 medium onion, finely chopped
- 1 pound boneless, skinless chicken breasts, cut into 1-inch pieces
- 2 15-ounce cans pinto beans, well rinsed and drained
- 4 green onions, thinly sliced
- 1 teaspoon cumin
- 1/4 teaspoon cayenne pepper
- 1/2 teaspoon pepper
- 1/2 cup fat-free sour cream
- 4 flour tortillas

Direction

- Heat a large skillet sprayed with vegetable cooking spray over medium heat. Add onions and cook until golden brown, about 5 minutes. Add chicken and cook until browned.
- Add beans, green onions, and spices and cook until chicken is no longer pink and onions are tender.
- Serve with fat-free sour cream and warmed flour tortillas.

115. Chicken And Shrimp Meatloaf With Whole Grain Mustard Dipping Sauce

Serving: Serves 6 | Prep: | Cook: |Ready in:

Ingredients

- For the meatloaf:
- 1 tablespoon unsalted butter
- 2/3 cup onion, fine dice
- 1/3 cup red pepper, fine dice
- 1/3 cup celery, fine dice
- 1 tablespoon garlic, minced
- 1 1/2 pounds ground chicken, I used thigh meat
- 1/2 pound raw shrimp, peeled, deveined and cut into 1/2 inch chunks
- 1 1/2 teaspoons fresh thyme, minced
- 1 tablespoon Italian parsley, minced
- 1/3 cup bread crumbs
- 1/4 cup cream
- 1 egg
- Kosher salt and fresh ground pepper
- 1/2 cup saltines, ground, or smashed fine
- 2 tablespoons Italian parsley, minced
- For the dipping sauce
- 1/3 cup mayonnaise
- 1/2 teaspoon whole grain mustard
- 1/4 teaspoon lemon zest
- 1/2 teaspoon fresh lemon juice

Direction

- Place a sauté pan over medium heat and add the butter. When it melts add the onions, red pepper and celery. Season with a little salt and pepper. Sauté until translucent without browning them. Add the garlic and sauté until fragrant. Remove from the heat and let cool. In a large mixing bowl, if you have a stand mixer it works great, place the chicken, shrimp, bread crumbs, cream, egg, parsley and thyme. Add a 1 teaspoon of salt and a 1/2 teaspoon of pepper. Add the cooled veggies and mix until very well combined. Place a large pot, filled half way with water, on the stove and turn the heat to high. Place a 10 x 10 piece of plastic wrap on top of a 10 x 10 piece of foil. Place a quarter of the filling on the wrap and wrap it up being careful not to let the wrap roll into the interior of the loaf. Now roll the plastic wrapped loaf in the foil. Twist the ends of the foil until the loaf is tight. Repeat this process three more times with the remaining loaf mixture. When the water is boiling add loaves and reduce the heat to a simmer. Let simmer for 40 minutes. If they don't stay submerged you can turn them occasionally or put a wire rack on top of them. While they are cooking combine all the dipping sauce ingredients in a bowl and mix well. Check the loaves by inserting a cooking thermometer into the middle. It should read 165. If not cook longer. Combine the saltine crumbs and the parsley on a tray. Carefully unwrap the loaves, there will be lots of juice so you may want to do this on a plate. Then roll them in the crumbs. Slice and serve.

116. Chicken And Steak Skewers With A Tahini Yogurt Marinade

Serving: Serves 6 | Prep: 2hours45mins | Cook: 0hours20mins | Ready in:

Ingredients

- For the tahini-yogurt marinade:
- 2/3 cup plain, whole-milk yogurt
- 1/3 cup tahini, well-stirred
- 3 fat cloves of garlic, minced
- 1/2 teaspoon freshly ground cumin (or crushed cumin seed)
- 1 1/2 teaspoons paprika
- Grated zest and juice of 2 small lemons (about 3 tablespoons of juice)
- 3 tablespoons extra-virgin olive oil, plus more as needed
- 1 teaspoon kosher salt
- For the skewers:
- 1 1/2 pounds boneless skinless chicken thighs or breasts, cut into 1 1/2-inch cubes
- 1 1/2 pounds boneless top sirloin steak, cut into 1 1/2-inch cubes
- 1 pint cherry tomatoes
- 1-2 zucchini and/or summer squash
- 1 eggplant
- 1 red onion
- 1 pint peppadews (drained) or 1 red bell pepper
- Olive oil and kosher salt, for seasoning vegetables

Direction

- For the tahini-yogurt marinade:
- In a large bowl, whisk together all of the ingredients until smooth and emulsified. If you're using Greek or skyr yogurt, you may need to add a bit more extra-virgin olive oil to loosen the marinade.
- For the skewers:
- In a bowl or plastic zipper-lock bag, combine chicken with half of marinade. Repeat with steak. Cover and refrigerate for at least 2 hours, or up to 24 hours.
- Soak wooden skewers in cold water for 30 minutes before grilling.
- Remove the chicken and steak from the marinade, letting any excess drip off. Working one protein at a time, thread 5 or 6 cubes on each wooden skewer. (Tip: thread the cubes on 2 skewers so the pieces don't flip over on the

grill when you turn them). Let stand at room temperature while the grill heats up.
- Cut vegetables into bite-sized (abut 2-inch) pieces. (Leave cherry tomatoes and peppadews whole.) Toss vegetables in olive oil to generously coat, and season with kosher salt, to taste. Alternating with squash and cherry tomatoes, thread onto skewers. Repeat with red onion, eggplant, and peppadews or red peppers.
- Heat grill to medium-high and brush your grates clean.
- Grill each skewer until it reaches your desired degree of doneness (165F° for chicken, 125F° to 130F° for medium-rare steak). This should take about 3 to 5 minutes per side for the steak, zucchini, and eggplant skewers; and about 5 to 7 minutes per side for the chicken skewers. Remove from the grill and place on a platter; tent with foil to keep warm until all the skewers are complete.

117. Chicken And Veggie Curry

Serving: Serves 5 | Prep: | Cook: |Ready in:

Ingredients

- 1 pound of chicken breast, boneless and skinless
- 1 onion, chopped
- 3 carrots, chopped
- 1 can of chickpeas, drained and rinsed
- 1 can of coconut milk
- 1 tablespoon tumeric
- 1 teaspoon cumin
- 1 tablespoon fresh grated ginger
- 1 lime, juiced and zested
- 1/2 cup cashews, roasted
- 1/2 cup cilantro, chopped
- salt and pepper

Direction

- Cut the chicken and sauté in a Dutch oven with olive oil until brown. Add some salt and pepper.
- When chicken is cooked put on the side and reserve. Use same pot, add some olive oil, the onion and the ginger and cook for 4-5 minutes. When translucent, add the carrots and cauliflower. Add the coconut milk, turmeric, cumin, 1 1/2 tsp of salt and 1 tsp of pepper. Cook until veggies are tender 8-10 minutes.
- Add the chickpeas and chicken and cook for another 5 minutes and add lime juice and zest. Serve with roasted cashews on top and cilantro. I like mine spicy but my kids do not, so I added some chili flakes to my bowl.
- Et Voila, Bon Appetit!

118. Chicken And White Bean Stew With Rosemary

Serving: Serves 4 | Prep: | Cook: |Ready in:

Ingredients

- 1 tablespoon olive oil
- 1 strip of thick cut bacon or 3 strips of regular bacon
- 4 large boneless, skinless chicken breasts
- 2 cups AP flour
- 1 onion
- 1 sprig rosemary
- 1/4 cup tomato concasse, or crushed san marzano tomatoes
- 1 cup white wine
- 1 quart high quality chicken stock (homemade if possible)
- 1 16 oz can of navy or cannellini beans, drained
- salt and pepper to taste

Direction

- Heat olive oil over medium low heat in a large, covered saute pan. Chop the bacon finely (I truly feel a cleaver is the best tool for

this--it seems excessive, but it provides a consistency somewhere between a chop and a grind), add the bacon to the pan and begin to render the fat and crisp the meat. Remove the bacon with a slotted spoon and reserve.
- Cut your chicken breasts into large 1-2" chunks and toss with flour. Increase heat to medium high and add the chicken pieces to the hot bacon fat to brown a few at a time. Remove chicken from the pan once color starts to develop and reserve. Add more olive oil to the pan as needed.
- Reduce heat to medium. Slice the onion and add to the pan and sprinkle with salt. As the onion begins to sweat, scrape up the golden bits that have formed on the bottom of the pan. When the onions are soft, deglaze with the white wine and add the tomatoes and the rosemary. Let the mixture simmer for a few minutes.
- Return the bacon and the chicken to the pan, and add the chicken stock. Let the liquid come up to a simmer, and reduce the heat to low, partially covering the pan. The liquid should be simmering gently.
- Let this work for 45 minutes or so, stirring occasionally to make sure the chicken cooks evenly.
- When the liquid has reduced by half, and the chicken is cooked through and very tender, add the beans. If this makes the stew too thick, add some more chicken stock, or even a bit of water. Let this simmer until the beans are cooked through. Remove the rosemary stem, check for seasoning, and serve warm.

119. Chicken Drumsticks Wrapped In Pancetta

Serving: Serves 4 | Prep: | Cook: |Ready in:

Ingredients

- Fresh
- 8 chicken drumsticks
- 8 rashers of unsmoked pancetta
- 5 sage leaves
- 2 sprigs fresh rosemary
- From the storecupboard
- 2 cloves of garlic
- 2 teaspoons dijon mustard
- 2 tablespoons olive oil
- 100 milliliters white wine
- 1 pinch sea salt
- 1 pinch black pepper

Direction

- 1. Start Turn the oven to 180C/160C Fan/Gas 4
- 2. Skin Rinse the drumsticks under the tap and pat dry with kitchen paper. Remove the skin by pulling it towards the thin end of the drumstick.
- 3. Wrap With a sharp knife make 4 slits into each piece. Coat each drumstick with mustard, making sure some goes into the slits. Wrap a rasher of pancetta around each drumstick and place in an ovenproof dish.
- 4. Season Wash the rosemary and sage. Drizzle the drumsticks with olive oil. Sprinkle with the sage leaves and rosemary needles. Add the unpeeled garlic. Season with a pinch of salt and a generous grind of black pepper. Pour the wine over the drumsticks and put them in the oven for 45 minutes.
- 5. Baste Spoon the cooking juices over the chicken a couple of times while it's in the oven.
- 6. Check Make sure the meat is cooked by pricking it with a fork. If the juices that come out are clear, it's done. If they're still pink, put it back in the oven for a bit longer.

120. Chicken In White Wine With Mushrooms

Serving: Serves 2 people | Prep: | Cook: |Ready in:

Ingredients

- 2 tablespoons extra virgin olive oil
- 1 tablespoon butter
- 1/2 pound thickly sliced mushrooms, (I used a mix of white button and crimini, but let your imagination run wild!
- 2 garlic cloves, crushed
- 2 boneless skinless chicken breasts
- 1 cup white wine
- 1 teaspoon dried thyme
- 1/2 teaspoon sea salt
- 1/4 teaspoon freshly ground black pepper
- 1/2 cup chicken broth
- 1/2 cup heavy cream
- salt and pepper to taste

Direction

- In one skillet, heat 1 tbsp. of oil over medium heat. While it's heating, wash and pat dry the chicken breasts. Season with salt and pepper. When skillet is hot, brown chicken on all sides.
- Meanwhile, heat remaining tbsp. of oil and butter in another skillet, and when hot, add mushrooms, thyme, salt and pepper. Sauté until all the liquid has evaporated. Reduce heat and keep warm while chicken cooks.
- After chicken is thoroughly browned, add white wine, garlic cloves, and chicken stock. Bring to a boil, reduce heat and simmer until chicken is cooked, about 10 to 15 minutes.
- Remove chicken breasts, cover with foil and keep warm. Increase heat, and bring liquid in the skillet to a rapid boil until reduce to about a third. Add the heavy cream, reduce heat, and continue to simmer until thickened. Season to taste with salt and pepper.
- Slice chicken breasts, add mushrooms and spoon sauce over the chicken and mushrooms and serve.
- I like this served with creamy mashed potatoes and steamed asparagus, but serve with whatever starch and veg floats your boat.

121. Chicken Rillettes

Serving: Serves 8 | Prep: | Cook: | Ready in:

Ingredients

- 2 chicken legs, skin-on, each weighing about 1/2 lb.
- 1/2 tablespoon coarse sea salt
- 1/2 teaspoon dried thyme
- 8 green peppercorns, lightly crushed
- 1 bay leaf, torn in half
- 2 garlic cloves, sliced
- Plenty of inexpensive olive oil
- 1 tablespoon French wholegrain mustard
- 1 garlic clove, crushed
- 2 teaspoons finely chopped fresh marjoram
- Salt (if needed), and freshly ground pepper

Direction

- Sprinkle the chicken legs with salt and thyme, and rub into the meat. Distribute crushed peppercorns evenly over the chicken pieces. Press one half bay leaves and several garlic slivers onto the fleshy side of each of the two legs. Arrange the chicken legs in a non-reactive container, cover with plastic film, and refrigerate overnight, or up to 48 hours.
- Preheat the oven to 200 F. Rinse the chicken legs thoroughly, and pat dry with kitchen paper. Pack tightly in an ovenproof pan, and cover completely with olive oil. Bring to a simmer over a low heat. Place in the oven, uncovered, and cook for 3-4 hours, or until the fat has become clear, and the meat tender.
- Carefully lift the chicken legs out of the fat. Place in a deep, narrow dish. Pour in enough poaching fat to cover, and then a bit more. Make sure that the chicken juices that have accumulated at the bottom of the pan keep in place, and that they don't blend in with the fat as you pour. Refrigerate.
- Tip the remaining fat (with the juices, and now they may well be happily blended together) into a glass bowl. Refrigerate.

- The next day (or a couple of days later) remove the dish containing the chicken from the fridge. Let sit in room temperature until the oil is nearly liquid. Lift the chicken legs out of the oil, and place on a plate.
- Combine the oil from the chicken and the nearly solified oil from the fridge (without the juices that are sitting at the bottom of the glass bowl - put the bowl with juices straight back into the fridge) into a saucepan. Slowly bring to the boil. Strain, chill and refrigerate. (This chicken-flavored olive oil is an excellent cooking medium for meat, and even more so for potatoes. It will keep for a couple of weeks.)
- Pull the meat off the chicken legs. Discard skin and bones. Shred meat finely, either with hands, or using two forks. Place in a bowl, and mix with mustard, garlic, marjoram and most of the jellified chicken juices from the fridge. Season with salt (if needed), and freshly ground pepper.
- To serve: Either distribute between eight little individual ramekins, or spread on small toasts. Offer mayo, French-style gherkins, and crisp salad leaves on the side.

122. Chicken Stir Fry Wraps

Serving: Serves 2 | Prep: | Cook: | Ready in:

Ingredients

- ½ lb. (200g) boneless, skinless chicken breast
- 1 tsp. garlic, grated
- 1 tsp. ginger, grated
- 1 TBSP. sake
- 2 tsp. potato starch
- ½ red bell pepper
- 1 TBSP. Sesame oil
- 2 TBSP. soy sauce
- 1 TBSP. sugar
- 1 tsp. mint leaves, minced
- ½ tsp. sesame seeds
- 1 head Boston lettuce
- ½ zucchini, very thinly sliced using peeler (optional)

Direction

- Cut chicken in half horizontally, and slice thinly. Season with S & P. Put into a bowl; add grated garlic, ginger, sake, and potato starch. Marinade for 15 minutes.
- Meanwhile, Cut bell pepper in half lengthwise, remove the white pith inside, julienne.
- Heat sesame oil over medium heat. Add the chicken; cook, stirring constantly, until opaque. Add bell pepper and sugar; cook until glossy*, stirring constantly (for about 2 min). Add soy sauce, stir a little.
- Turn off the burner, add mint leaves. Garnish with sesame seeds.
- Serve in lettuce cups with zucchini.
- When it becomes glossy, it's a sign that the sweet taste has seeped into the ingredients. It's important to do before adding soy sauce. If soy sauce is added before sugar, it becomes very difficult for the sweet taste to absorb into the food.

123. Chicken Tikka Masala

Serving: Serves 8 | Prep: | Cook: | Ready in:

Ingredients

- 4 chicken breasts
- 1 bunch chopped coriander
- 4 garlic cloves
- 1 tablespoon garam masala
- 1 tablespoon red curry paste
- 1 tablespoon tandoori paste
- 1 cup greek yogurt
- 1 teaspoon salt
- 1 tablespoon grated ginger
- 2 tablespoons ghee
- 2 tablespoons sunflower oil

- 1 pint chopped canned tomatoes
- 1 pint coconut cream
- 1 pint chicken stock
- 1 red bell pepper
- 1 medium zucchini
- 2 red onions
- 4 tablespoons double cream
- 4 tablespoons toasted almond slivers

Direction

- Cut the chicken breasts into small pieces. Make a marinade by mixing the chopped coriander (save some sprigs for the garnish), red curry paste, tandoori paste, chopped garlic, gram masala, salt, grated ginger and yogurt. Mix the chicken with the marinade, cover with cling film and let it sit, for as long as you can, even overnight
- Heat the ghee with the oil in a non-stick deep pan. Fry the marinated chicken until it is nicely browned
- Meanwhile, chop all the vegetables into bitesize pieces, the onions in half-moons. Take the chicken out of the pan and add the onions. Cook until soft and add all the other vegetables
- Put the chicken back with the veggies, add the canned tomatoes, coconut and (homemade) chicken stock. Give it a nice stir and simmer for about 25 minutes.
- To serve: sprinkle with some fresh coriander, toasted almond slivers and some spoonfuls of double cream. Very nice with basmati rice or naan bread. Bon appétit!

124. Chicken With Black Truffles

Serving: Makes 2 chicken breasts | Prep: | Cook: |Ready in:

Ingredients

- 1 small fresh black truffle
- 2 boneless chicken breasts, skin on
- salt
- 1 gallon size plastic resealable storage bag
- 2 cups whole milk
- 4 sprigs fresh thyme
- 2 bay leaves
- 2 tablespoons butter, divided
- 1/4 cup dry white wine
- 1/2 cup chicken stock

Direction

- Place the chicken breasts skin side up on a cutting board. Use your fingers to gently pry the skin away from the breasts, making sure to keep the skin attached to the breasts. You simply want to create a small pocket of space between the skin and the breast meat.
- Using a mandolin or truffle shaver, shave half of your truffle into very thin disks. Place these disks underneath the skin of the chicken. The skin of the chicken should hold the truffles in place.
- Season the flesh side of the chicken breasts with salt, then place the chicken inside the gallon size bag. Add the milk, thyme, and bay leaves to the bag. Let the chicken marinate overnight, or for at least 4 hours.
- Set a large pot of water over medium heat. Use a thermometer to monitor the temperature of the water. When the temperature of the water is between 170 and 180 F, place the sealed bag of chicken inside the pot of water. Try to get rid of any large pockets of air inside the bag before adding to the pot.
- Continue to monitor the temperature of the water. Now that you have added the chicken, you want the temperature to stay between 145 and 155 F. Adjust the heat as necessary to achieve this temperature. Let the chicken cook for 1 hour.
- After 1 hour, remove the bag from the water. Remove the chicken from the bag, pat it dry with a towel, and let it rest momentarily on a large plate. Discard the bag along with everything inside of it. Set a skillet over medium heat, and add 1 tablespoon of butter.

When the butter is melted and beginning to sizzle, add the chicken skin side down. Let the chicken cook for 3-4 minutes. Use tongs to lift the chicken and check if the skin has browned nicely. When the skin looks brown and crispy, flip the chicken and cook the flesh side for 3-4 minutes. Remove the chicken from the skillet.
- Deglaze the skillet with white wine. When the wine has reduced by at least half, add the stock. When the contents of the skillet have again reduced by at least half, add the remaining 1 tablespoon of butter and whisk to incorporate. Season the sauce lightly with salt, taste, and adjust with more salt as necessary. Add the chicken back into the skillet. Shave the remaining half of the black truffle over the top of the chicken and into the sauce. Serve and enjoy.

125. Chicken With Fennel, Pernod And 40 Cloves Of Garlic

Serving: Serves 4-6 | Prep: | Cook: | Ready in:

Ingredients

- 1 3 1/2 pounds chicken at room temperature
- 1 1/2 teaspoons dried thyme or savory or a combination
- 1 bay leaf
- several sprigs of parsley
- pinch of dried rosemary (optional)
- lots of fresh tarragon
- salt freshly ground black pepper to taste
- fresh basil and fennel tops (optional)
- 1 small onion or large shallot, peeled and chopped (optional)
- 1/4 cup extra virgin olive oil
- 40 cloves of unpeeled garlic
- 2 tablespoons Pernod, Sambucca or other anise flavored liqueur

Direction

- Preheat the oven to 350 F. Rub the chicken inside and out with salt and pepper and the dried thyme.
- Place the bay leaf and half of the parsley, rosemary, tarragon, and other herbs if using and onion or shallot in the chicken cavity. Strew the rest of the herbs and onion or shallot in the bottom of an oven proof casserole just large enough to hold the chicken. Place the chicken on top of the herbs, breast side up.
- Combine the oil, garlic cloves and salt and pepper to taste in a small bowl, then pour over and around the chicken. Pour the Pernod over the chicken, cover and place the casserole in middle of the preheated oven. Roast for one hour. Raise the heat to 400F and uncover the casserole. Continue roasting until brown and the chicken is done, about 20 minutes. Test for doneness by piercing a drumstick with a fork. The juices should run clear rather than pink. Remove the chicken from the casserole and allow to rest 15 minutes before carving.
- Scoop the garlic into a bowl with a slotted spoon and set aside, covered with foil to stay warm.
- Strain the pan juices into a pitcher. The fat will rise to the top. When ready to serve spoon off as much fat as possible.
- Carve the chicken and arrange on a serving platter surrounded by the cooked garlic cloves. Pour the defatted juices over the top or pass the pitcher separately. To eat the garlic, squeeze interior out of the peel and spread on the chicken or on toasted French or peasant bread.

126. Chicken, Spinach And Pasta Al Forno

Serving: Serves 2 - 4 | Prep: | Cook: | Ready in:

Ingredients

- 1 pound spinach

- 1/2 pound dried short pasta, such as mezze rigatoni or penne
- 1 1/4 cups heavy cream
- 1 crushed garlic clove
- 1/2 teaspoon kosher salt
- Fresh ground black pepper, to taste
- 1 cup cooked chicken, in bite-size pieces
- 1/3 cup shredded Fontina cheese
- 1/3 cup grated Parmesan cheese
- 2 tablespoons butter

Direction

- Heat oven to 475 degrees.
- Bring a large pot of water (5 or 6 quarts) to a boil with 2 teaspoons salt.
- Drop spinach into the water and cook 1 minute; remove with a slotted spoon to a colander and drain. Put the spinach in a clean kitchen towel (careful, it's hot), roll it up and squeeze over the sink to remove as much water as you can. Chop spinach.
- Parboil the pasta until halfway cooked, 7 - 10 minutes depending on the size and thickness of the pasta. Drain.
- Stir together cream, garlic, salt, pepper, chicken, spinach and the cheeses in a large bowl; add drained pasta and mix together.
- Smear the butter over a 1-quart gratin or baking dish. Transfer pasta mixture to the gratin. Bake 12 minutes or so, until the cream is bubbling and edges of the pasta begin to brown. Cool 10 minutes before serving.

127. Chicken, Spinach, Tomato And Feta Pasta

Serving: Serves 4 | Prep: | Cook: | Ready in:

Ingredients

- Main Ingredients
- 8 ounces pasta - seashells, farfelle, penne, etc.
- 1 tablespoon olive oil
- 1 pound boneless skinless chicken breast
- 2 cloves of garlic smashed and chopped
- 1/2 cup chicken stock
- 10 ounces spinach
- 1 pint roasted cherry tomatoes - recipe belo
- 6 ounces feta cheese with Mediterranean herbs
- Roasted Cherry Tomatoes
- 1 pint cherry tomatoes
- 2 tablespoons olive oil
- 2-3 dashes sea salt

Direction

- Cook pasta according to directions - but make sure it is a bit al dente.
- Toss tomatoes, olive oil and salt together and roast in a 350 degree oven for about 30 minutes. Stir the tomatoes a couple times during roasting. When done take out and set aside.
- Heat a large sauté pan with olive oil over medium high heat. Once hot add chicken and garlic and lightly brown.
- Add chicken stock to sauté pan and scrape up any bits on the bottom of the pan.
- Add spinach to chicken and cover. Let cook until spinach has wilted.
- Toss tomatoes and almost all of the feta cheese in with the chicken and stir.
- Toss pasta in, stir and let cook a bit to finish cooking pasta and allow sauce to thicken - about 5 minutes or so.
- Serve with remaining feta sprinkled on top.

128. Chicken, Chile And Tomatillo Soup

Serving: Serves 10-12 | Prep: | Cook: | Ready in:

Ingredients

- 2 red bell peppers
- 10 tomatillos (about 1.5 pounds), husked and rinsed
- 3 poblano peppers

- 1-2 jalapeno peppers
- 3 tablespoons olive oil, divided
- 3 ears white corn, husked
- 6 garlic cloves, peeled
- 1 large onion, peeled and quartered
- 2 cups canned chopped tomatoes
- 1 tablespoon ground cumin
- 1 teaspoon ground corriander
- 1/2 teaspoon Spanish smoked paprika (Pimento de la Vera)
- 1 tablespoon chile powder
- 1 tablespoon ancho chile powder
- 6 cups chicken stock
- 2 1/2 pounds boneless, skinless chicken thighs
- 2 teaspoons dried oregano
- 3 cups cooked black beans
- 1 1/2 tablespoons adobo sauce from a jar of chipotle chilies
- 2 teaspoons kosher salt
- 3/4 cup cream
- 1 handful cilantro, chopped
- 1 cup grated Mexican cheese blend
- 1 avocado, diced
- 2 limes, cut in wedges
- 2 cups tortilla chips

Direction

- Heat oven to broil. Seed and slice the red peppers so that each slice lies flat. Put a splash of olive oil in the bottom of a roasting pan and wipe with a paper towel to oil the bottom of the pan. Spread cut peppers, whole tomatillos, whole poblano chilies and whole jalapeno chiles over the pan. Broil to blacken the skins of all the vegetables, turning to char all sides. Check frequently. It will take about 15 to 20 minutes total, but some vegetables will blacken more quickly. As the vegetables char, remove and put in a bowl and cover with plastic wrap. Let sit for 10 to 15 minutes to steam. Reserve any liquids that are left in the roasting pan or bowl to add to the soup later.
- Put the corn cobs in the roasting pan and broil, turning frequently so all sides of the cobs are lightly charred. Set aside to cool.
- While the vegetables are steaming and cooling put the garlic in a food processor and whirl until they are finely minced. Add onion to the food processor and pulse to coarsely chop. Heat 2 T olive oil in a large soup pot. Add onion and garlic mixture to the pot and sauté over medium heat for 15 minutes until they soften and begin to color.
- Stir in tomatoes, cumin, coriander, Spanish paprika, and chile powders to the onion and garlic mixture. Cook another 2 minutes.
- Add chicken stock, chicken thighs and oregano to the pot and bring to a boil. Reduce heat to medium-low and simmer for 15 minutes, until chicken is cooked. Remove chicken and set aside to cool, reserving all liquids.
- Return to the roasted vegetables. Using your fingers, slip the peels off the red peppers, the poblano peppers and the jalapeno peppers. Remove the seeds and discard. Chop the red peppers into 3/4" pieces. There is no need to remove the skins from the tomatillos, but you should remove and discard the hard core. Coarsely chop the poblano peppers, jalapeno peppers and tomatillos. Add the peppers, tomatillos, beans and any reserved liquid to the soup pot.
- When the chicken has cooled shred it and add it to the soup pot along with any reserved juices. Cut the corn from the husks and add it to the soup pot.
- Season with salt, pepper and adobo sauce to taste. Turn off the heat and stir in the cream. Serve in individual bowls and garnish with lime squeezes, cilantro, grated cheese and tortilla chips.

129. Chicken Pecan Quiche

Serving: Serves 8 | Prep: | Cook: | Ready in:

Ingredients

- 1 cup all-purpose flour

- 1 cup sharp cheddar cheese, grated
- 3/4 cup pecans, chopped
- 1/2 teaspoon salt
- 1/4 teaspoon paprika
- 1/3 cup olive oil
- 1 cup sour cream
- 1/2 cup chicken broth
- 1/4 cup mayonaise
- 3 large eggs, lightly beaten
- 2 cups cooked chicken, finely chopped
- 1/2 cup sharp cheddar cheese, grated
- 1/4 cup white onion, minced
- 1/4 cup scallion, finely chopped
- 2 tablespoons chives (or other fresh herbs), chopped
- 3-4 drops tabasco or other hot sauce
- 1-2 tablespoons freshly grated parmesan
- 1/4 cup pecan halves

Direction

- Combine first 5 ingredients in a medium bowl; stir well. Add oil; stir well. Firmly press mixture in bottom and up sides of a 9-inch deep-dish pie plate. Bake at 350° for 12 minutes. Cool completely.
- Combine sour cream and next three ingredients; stir with a wire whisk until smooth.
- Stir in chicken and next 5 ingredients.
- Pour chicken mixture over prepared crust. Sprinkle a layer of grated parmesan cheese on top of chicken filling.
- Arrange the pecan halves in radial lines on top of the parmesan-topped filling.
- Bake at 350° F for 55 minutes or until set. Let stand 10 minutes before serving.

130. Chicory Coffee Glazed Game Hen With Giardiniera Cabbage

Serving: Serves 2 | Prep: | Cook: | Ready in:

Ingredients

- Giardiniera cabbage
- 1.5 cups cauliflower, in small florets
- 1 large carrot, peeled then shaved into long ribbons with the peeler
- 1/2 cup white wine vinegar
- 1/2 cup olive oil
- 1/4 teaspoon crushed red pepper flake
- 1/4 teaspoon black pepper
- 1/2 teaspoon celery seed
- 1/2 teaspoon dried oregano
- 1/2 teaspoon dried thyme
- 1 bay leaf
- 1 teaspoon salt
- 2 tablespoons butter
- juice of 1/2 lemon (zest it before juicing, as you will use the zest for the hen)
- 1/2 medium head of green cabbage, thinly sliced
- pinch of salt and white pepper
- Chicory Coffee Glazed Game Hen
- 1 2lb Cornish game hen
- 3 tablespoons room temperature butter, divided
- 1/2 cup plus 1 tsp light brown sugar
- 1 tablespoon fresh thyme leaves
- zest of 1/2 lemon
- 1/2 cup strong brewed chicory coffee
- 1 tablespoon apple cider vinegar
- 1 teaspoon salt
- 1/2 tablespoon flour

Direction

- Giardiniera cabbage
- Place the cauliflower florets and carrot ribbons in a large mixing bowl. In a small saucepan, combine the vinegar through the teaspoon of salt and bring to a boil over medium high heat. Boil, stirring, just until the salt dissolves. Pour over the cauliflower and carrot and stir to coat. Let marinate for 1 hour at room temperature or 2 hours in the fridge. Can be made a day in advance.
- Melt butter with the lemon juice in a sauté pan over medium high heat. Add the cabbage and

toss to coat in the butter. Sprinkle with salt and white pepper and sauté, turning frequently with tongs, for about 5 minutes.
- Remove the marinated vegetables from the oil and vinegar with a slotted spoon and add to the warm cabbage, turning with tongs to combine.
- Chicory Coffee Glazed Game Hen
- Preheat the oven to 450F. Prepare a foil-lined, rimmed baking sheet.
- Using kitchen shears, remove the backbone from the game hen by cutting down either side of it. One the spine is removed, flatten the hen on a cutting board breast side up and press with the butt of your hand, then, with a sharp chef's knife, cut between the 2 breasts to create 2 equal halves. Alternatively, your butcher can do this for you. Pat the skin of the hen dry with paper towel.
- Combine 2 tablespoons of butter with 1 teaspoon of brown sugar, plus the fresh thyme and lemon zest and a pinch of salt. Gently separate the skin from the meat on the thigh and breast of each game hen half. Salt and pepper the skin and beneath the skin of the game hen, and spread the compound butter underneath the skin.
- In a small saucepan, combine the coffee, vinegar, 1/2 cup of brown sugar, and 1 tsp salt. Bring to a boil over high heat to dissolve the sugar and salt and set aside.
- Heat a dry cast iron skillet over medium-high. When hot, add a drizzle of olive oil and add the hen halves, skin side down. Cook for 4 minutes, then turn skin side up and sear for an additional minute. Remove from heat and transfer the hen halves to the prepared baking sheet. Reserve the pan juices (the mixture will be dark and that is OK.) Roast the hen halves in the oven about 20 minutes, until the juices run clear.
- While the hen cooks, complete the glaze. Combine the remaining 1 tablespoon of butter with the flour to make a beurre manié. Add the reserved coffee mixture to the cast iron skillet with the pan drippings from searing the hen, and bring to a boil over medium-high heat, whisking occasionally. Cook until reduced by half, about 7 minutes. Add the beurre manié, whisking constantly, and cook an additional 2 minutes, or until the glaze coats the back of a spoon. Taste for salt and pepper and adjust seasoning as needed.
- Remove the hen halves from the oven and allow to rest, tented with foil to hold in the heat, 5-10 minutes. Plate each half over a mound of warm cabbage and spoon over a generous amount of coffee glaze (serve the remaining glaze on the side for dipping.)

131. Chile Verde With Chicken

Serving: Serves 4 | Prep: | Cook: | Ready in:

Ingredients

- 12 chicken thighs, boneless
- flour for dredging chicken
- 10-12 tomatillos, cleaned and halved
- 1 medium onion, quartered
- 5 cloves of garlic, smashed
- 1 jalapeño, halved
- 1 1/2 cups pepitas, (roasted pumpkin seeds)
- 1 1/2 cups chicken stock
- handful of torn cilantro
- 2 teaspoons toasted cumin seeds
- zest of one lime
- 1/2 a red onion, sliced into half moons
- 1 cup extra virgin olive oil

Direction

- Flour chicken lightly and sear in hot olive oil until browned and crisp. Remove to a plate.
- Roast at 375 - tomatillos, onion, garlic, and jalapeño in olive oil until soft. (About 20 minutes)
- Blitz in a food processor or blender, the pepitas, cilantro, cumin seeds, and lime zest, adding chicken stock to form a rough saucy paste.

- When veg is soft - cool a bit before adding to the cilantro paste and blitz again until incorporated. Loosen with a bit of stock if too thick. You want the sauce-not too thick, loose enough to be a saucy sauce. So add more stock if needed.
- In a 375 preheated oven, to a casserole add; the chicken, the sauce, red onion slices, and a few torn cilantro stems and leaves. Braise for about an hour, uncovered- the chicken will be softly cooked, and melty, while the bits above the sauce and stock will be nicely roasted.
- Serve with beans, charred corn tortillas, lime wedges, and chopped cilantro.

132. Chinese Chicken Salad

Serving: Serves 4 | Prep: | Cook: | Ready in:

Ingredients

- 1/4 head of cabbage, shaved on the Mandolin or cut very thin
- 4-5 ounces Spring Mix
- 2 boneless, skinless chicken breasts seasoned and sauteed until done
- 1/8 cup hoisin sauce
- 2 tablespoons rice wine vinegar
- 2 tablespoons soy sauce
- 1/2 tablespoon fish sauce
- 2 teaspoons toasted sesame oil
- 1 inch piece of fresh ginger, grated
- 4 green onions, sliced thin
- 1/4 cup toasted peanuts
- 4-5 stems of fresh basil, chopped
- 1/3 bunch of cilantro
- 1 bunch of mint
- 1 large can of Mandarin oranges
- Chinese Noodles to go around the plate (about 1 package or can)

Direction

- In a small bowl or jar, mix the hoisin sauce, rice wine vinegar, soy sauce, fish sauce, sesame oil, ginger and green onions together.
- Shred the chicken into bite sized pieces
- Pour the sauce mixture over the salad mixture and toss.
- Serve this mixture in a bowl or on a plate and sprinkle the Chinese noodles around the salad just before serving so they are nice and crispy.

133. Chipollini Cognac Chicken

Serving: Serves 4 | Prep: | Cook: | Ready in:

Ingredients

- 8 chicken drumsticks
- 8-10 cipollini onions, whole
- 1 shallot, finely chopped
- 8 small carrots, cut in half
- 2 handfuls sugar snap peas
- 1 cup sweet peas
- 1+2 tablespoons olive oil
- 1 tablespoon butter, unsalted
- 1 tablespoon flour
- 1 cup white vine
- 2 tablespoons cognac
- 3 stems fresh thyme
- salt
- pepper

Direction

- Season chicken drumsticks with salt and pepper.
- Preheat the oven to 350 F/180 C.
- Heat 1 tbsp. oil in a frying pan. Brown the meat very quickly over a high heat. Place the meat in a nonstick, ovenproof pot.
- Sauté the vegetables in the same pan for 5 minutes or just until slightly brown, over a high heat. Be sure not to discard the meat fat and browned bits from the pan, scrape them up with a wooden spoon for richer flavor.

Season with salt and pepper and place the vegetables over the meat.
- Add remaining 2 tbsp. olive oil and butter in your pan, add the flour and cook it for a minute or two (stirring constantly) to get rid of the lumps. Then add vine, cognac and thyme and bring to a simmer. Pour it over the meat and vegetables.
- Place the pot with the lid on in the heated oven and cook for 30 minutes.
- Remove the lid and broil for a few minutes, just until golden brown.
- You can mash some potatoes, like I did, mashed potatoes tastes great with this sticky, flavor rich chicken. Or if you want to upgrade the dish a bit, cook some polenta with butter.
- It's actually kind of classic chicken stew with a vine and cognac kick to it. You should definitely try this one, it tastes great!

134. Chutney Chicken Meatballs

Serving: Serves 6-8 | Prep: | Cook: | Ready in:

Ingredients

- 1 pound ground chicken
- 1/4 cup white rice
- 1/4 cup all-purpose flour
- 1/4 teaspoon ground cumin
- 1/4 teaspoon ground coriander
- 1/4 teaspoon ground cinnamon
- 1/4 teaspoon ground cardamom
- 1 clove garlic, pressed
- 1 egg
- 2 tablespoons minced green onion
- 1/4 teaspoon orange zest
- 3/4 cup plain Greek yogurt
- 1/4 cup mango chutney
- 2 tablespoons snipped mint
- lettuce leaves

Direction

- In a medium bowl combine the chicken and the next 10 ingredients with 1/2 cup water; mix well.
- Bring 6 cups water to a boil in a 4 quart pot.
- Form 1 Tbsp. meatballs and drop into the pot.
- When the water boils again, reduce the heat and gently simmer the meatballs, covered for 20 minutes.
- Combine the yogurt, chutney and mint in a small bowl and place on a platter.
- With a slotted spoon transfer the meatballs to the lettuce lined platter. Provide party picks for serving.

135. Classic Chicken Coconut Curry

Serving: Serves 4 | Prep: 0hours7mins | Cook: 0hours20mins | Ready in:

Ingredients

- 1 jar Masala Mama Coconut Curry Sauce https://food52.com/shop...
- 2 tablespoons oil or ghee
- 1¼ pounds boneless, skinless, chicken thighs, cut into bite sized pieces
- ¼ teaspoons red pepper flakes, more for additional heat (optional)
- ¾ cups coconut milk, more for a creamier curry
- Cilantro for garnish
- Salt and pepper
- Mama's Perfect Basmati Rice, https://food52.com/recipes...

Direction

- Heat oil in large sauce pan over medium-high heat. Once hot, add the chicken and sear lightly on all sides, about 7 minutes.
- Stir in Masala Mama's Coconut Curry Sauce*, coconut milk and red pepper flakes. Cover the pan with a lid and simmer for 10-12 minutes, or until the chicken is cooked through.

- The sauce should have a nice pouring consistency similar to heavy cream. If the sauce is too thick, add stock or water 1-2 tablespoons at a time until desired consistency is reached.
- Adjust salt to taste, garnish with cilantro and serve with rice or naan.

136. Classic Chicken Parmigiana

Serving: Serves 4 | Prep: 0hours10mins | Cook: 0hours40mins | Ready in:

Ingredients

- For the chicken Parmigiana:
- 3/4 cup all-purpose flour
- 1/2 teaspoon dried onion
- 1/2 teaspoon dried oregano
- 2 eggs
- 1 dash water
- 1/2 tablespoon minced garlic
- 3/4 cup seasoned breadcrumbs
- 1 tablespoon freshly grated Parmesan cheese
- 4 boneless, skinless chicken breasts
- Canola oil, as needed for pan frying
- For the assembly:
- 1 cup homemade marinara sauce
- 8 thin slices of smoked mozzarella
- 1 bunch fresh parsley, coarsely chopped as needed for garnish

Direction

- First, set up the breading line for the chicken with three big, shallow bowls. In the first bowl mix together the flour, dried onion, and dried oregano. In the second bowl, whisk together the eggs, water, and minced garlic. In the third bowl, mix together the breadcrumbs and Parmesan cheese. Have a plate handy on the end to hold the breaded chicken.
- Once the breading line is set up fill a cast-iron skillet with about 1 1/2 inches of canola oil and heat it over medium-high heat. Pre-heat the oven to 350°F. While the oil gets hot, put all 4 chicken breasts through the breading line. Use one hand to coat the chicken in the flour, the other hand to dip it in the egg wash mixture, then back to the first hand to coat it in the breadcrumbs. This keeps it as clean and neat as possible. Then just transfer the chicken to the plate once it is breaded.
- Pan fry the breaded chicken in the hot oil, cooking the first side for about 3 minutes to let it get super crisp and golden. Flip it over to get just as crispy and golden on the other side, about another 3 minutes. Once crispy and cooked through, remove them to a paper towel-lined plate to help soak up some of the excess oil.
- Move the chicken into a baking dish and top each piece with a 1/4 cup of marinara sauce. Then lay 2 slices of smoked mozzarella on each piece to finish assembling the chicken Parmigiana. Bake for 15 minutes, or until the mozzarella is melted and bubbling.
- Remove the baking dish from the oven and let the chicken rest for 1 or 2 minutes. Sprinkle the finely chopped fresh parsley on top for some green freshness and serve warm.

137. Coconut Chix Stix

Serving: Serves 4-6 | Prep: | Cook: | Ready in:

Ingredients

- FOR THE STIX
- 8 to 12 chicken tenders, 2 or 3 per person
- 2 eggs, whisked with a pinch of salt to let the whites relax and better incorporate with the yolks
- 1 1/2 cups all-purpose flour
- 1 1/2 cups Panko bread crumbs
- 1 cup unsweetened dried coconut (available from any natural foods store with a decent bulk bins section)
- Generous pinch of red pepper flakes

- 1 teaspoon sea or kosher salt
- 12 grinds from a pepper mill
- FOR THE DIPPING SAUCE
- 1 can unsweetened coconut milk
- 2 tablespoons Mae Ploy (sweet chili sauce)
- 2 tablespoons sesame oil
- 2 teaspoons lemongrass paste (available in a tube in the produce aisle)
- Juice of 2 limes
- 1" of grated fresh ginger
- 1/2 teaspoon sea or kosher salt
- 1 teaspoon Sriracha
- 1/2 cup scallion greens sliced 1/4" thick for garnish

Direction

- Preheat the oven to 350 degrees. Line a baking sheet with parchment.
- Pour the whisked eggs onto a plate. Scatter the flour over a separate plate.
- In a bowl, stir together the Panko, coconut, red pepper flakes, salt and pepper. Pour them out onto a third plate.
- Working with two tenders at a time, dip them into the egg, then into the flour, turning them over so that each side is covered. Dip them back into the egg, then lay them in the crumb/coconut mixture. Cover the tenders with the crumbs, pressing down firmly to adhere a good crust. I know, there's a whole lot of dipping going on, but if you follow this sequence, you'll have an excellent crisp crust as opposed to a soggy one, or one where approximately half of it won't stick to anything but your fingers. And if you use tongs, adherence of all the layers will be even better and your hands won't be a mess. Transfer tenders to the baking sheet. Discard the egg, flour, and crumbs.
- Bake for about 20 minutes, until the tenders are gently browned and a thermometer inserted in the middle registers 165 degrees.
- While the tenders are baking, make the dipping sauce. Whisk together all of the sauce ingredients, except for the Sriracha. First taste the sauce, then add drops of Sriracha if you need it to be hotter. I do. The sauce may appear on the thin side. Not to worry; the crisp, crunchy coating will nap it perfectly without picking up so much that it is overpowering.
- Serve the tenders alongside a bowl of the dipping sauce that you've garnished with thinly sliced greens of scallions. The chicken will be perfectly tender, the crust crisp with notes of sweet, and the sauce bright and spicy. You might never go back to shrimp.

138. Coconut Pecan Crusted Chicken Served With Sweet And Spicy Apricot Sauce

Serving: Serves 4-6 | Prep: | Cook: | Ready in:

Ingredients

- Coconut Pecan Crusted Chicken Breast Cutlets
- 6 Chicken breast cutlets (thin chicken breasts)
- 1 1/2 cups Shredded coconut
- 1 cup Chopped pecans
- 1/2 cup All-purpose flour
- 2 Eggs whisked with a tablespoon water
- 1 tablespoon Chopped fresh Italian parsley for garnish
- Sweet and Spicy Apricot Sauce
- 1/2 cup Apricot preserves
- 1-2 teaspoons Grated fresh ginger
- 2 tablespoons Sweet chili sauce from Thai Kitchen
- 1/4 cup white wine, sherry, saki or water

Direction

- Pre-heat the oven to 400F.
- In a food processor add the coconut and pecans and pulse until nicely ground together, like bread crumbs. Set aside. Per a lovely readers comments, a few tablespoons of panko can be added to the breading for a little extra texture and crunch.

- Set out three bowls. One with flour, one with egg wash and the last one with the coconut pecan mixture.
- Season the chicken with salt and black pepper. Lightly dust the chicken in the flour, then the egg wash and then press them into the coconut pecan mixture. Place them on a platter. Cover with plastic wrap and refrigerate for about 15-30 minutes. This step can be done in the morning and then baked in the evening for dinner.
- Transfer the chicken to a parchment lined baking sheet. Place the baking sheet in the pre-heated oven for about 20-30 minutes, depending on thickness or until the chicken is done. I cook my chicken until the internal temperature reaches about 160F. I highly recommend having a meat thermometer handy for cooking poultry and meat.
- Once the chicken is done, take the chicken out of the oven and let it sit for about 5 minutes before serving.
- For the sauce: In a bowl mix together all the ingredients. You can lightly warm the sauce in a small pan stove top or in the microwave. Don't over warm or the sauce will be too runny. The sauce will thin once it's paired with the warm chicken.
- To serve: Ladle a bit of the sauce onto four plates. Place a piece of chicken on the sauce and garnish with chopped fresh Italian parsley. Serve with coconut rice and fresh greens with a sesame dressing.

139. Collard Greens With Smoked Turkey Leg

Serving: Serves 4-6 | Prep: | Cook: |Ready in:

Ingredients

- 2 bunches collards, or mix with mustard or other hearty, healthy greens.
- 1 smoked Turkey leg.
- 2 teaspoons red pepper flakes
- 4 cups chicken stock
- 1 tablespoon hot sauce, like Franks.
- 1 tablespoon apple cider vinegar
- salt and pepper to taste.
- 2 cloves garlic, minced.

Direction

- In a large pot add turkey leg and stock, bring to boil, reduce to low and simmer 30 minutes.
- Add collards (if using fresh make sure and clean well, remove stems, and chop),garlic, and pepper flakes turn heat to medium and cook another 20 minutes.
- Remove turkey leg and shred meat, remove bones and skin, and add meat back to pot. Serve with a drizzle of vinegar, hot sauce, and a bit of s&p!

140. Coq Au Vin

Serving: Serves 4 | Prep: | Cook: |Ready in:

Ingredients

- 1 whole chicken, broken down into 8 pieces
- flour as needed, for dredging
- salt and pepper, to taste
- 2 tablespoons unsalted butter
- 4 tablespoons brandy
- bouquet garni (4 inch carrot stick, 4 inch leek (split it half), 1 sprig of thyme, 1 bay leaf)
- 3 garlic cloves, peeled and crushed
- 1 cup red wine
- 2 cups chicken stock
- 2 pieces bacon, chopped into 1/4 inch pieces
- 18 pearl onions, peeled
- 10 button mushrooms, quartered

Direction

- Season the chicken pieces with salt and pepper.

- Place the flour in a shallow dish and dredge each piece of chicken, shaking off any excess. You want to get a good dredging because ideally, the flour that ends up on your chicken will ultimately be what thickens up your sauce throughout the cooking process.
- In a large Dutch oven heat the butter under medium high heat. Add the chicken, in batches, and cook until both sides are browned nicely. Set the chicken aside on a plate.
- Add bacon pieces to Dutch oven and cook until fat is rendered and bacon is crispy. Drain all but 2 tablespoons of fat from pot. Add the brandy and ignite. Cook until flame dies out.
- Return chicken to pot and add bouquet garni, garlic, wine, and chicken stock. Bring to a boil and then reduce to a simmer. Cover and let simmer for about 45 minutes to an hour. Or until chicken is tender and sauce is thickened.
- About 20 minutes before ready to serve, add in pearl onions and mushrooms.
- Season with salt and pepper.

141. Cornish Hens With Potatoes, Porcinis And Tarragon En Papillote

Serving: Serves 2-4 | Prep: | Cook: | Ready in:

Ingredients

- The Hens
- 2 cornish hens
- 2 tangerines
- 1 head of garlic
- 4 tablespoons butter
- 1/2 bunch French taragon
- 1/4 cup White Wine
- 1/4 cup chicken stock
- 2 ounces dried porcini mushrooms
- Potatoes, Tarragon and Garlic en Papillote
- 1/2 bunch tarragon
- 3-4 medium Yukon Gold (or similar, thin-skinned) potatoes
- 5-6 cloves of garlic
- 2-3 tablespoons butter

Direction

- The Hens
- Prep. Step: put porcinis in 2 cups of water to soak (they require at least an hour of soaking prior to beginning this recipe). Preheat the oven to 450 degrees. Put a little wire rack in a roasting pan for the birds to rest on. Peel the garlic cloves - all 20 or so of them!
- Readying the birds: wash them in cold water and pat dry with paper towel. Season them outside and in with a lot of salt and pepper. Rub them all over with a lot of butter. Put half a tangerine, a few sprigs of tarragon, and a peeled and smashed clove of garlic or two in the cavity of each bird. You don't want the cavities stuffed though, there should be some air in there - we're trying to get an aromatic tangerine/tarragon/garlic steam bath type thing happening in the bird's cavity - we're not trying to slow the cooking process by stuffing it full. Truss the birds tightly. Put them on the wire rack/roasting pan combo, breasts down. Arrange garlic cloves around the birds, ideally a few under the rack underneath them as well.
- Cooking the birds: Put the birds in the oven at 450 for 30 minutes. Remove from the oven, flip breasts up, lower oven to 350. Pour the white wine and the chicken stock over the birds and brush them with a little more butter. Put them back in the 350 oven (NOTE: this is when you put your packet of potatoes, tarragon, garlic and porcinis in the oven, described below, if you want it all done together), probably for only another 20-30 minutes but you simply have to keep checking with a meat thermometer, aiming for about 160-165 in the fattest part of the bird you can fine (it will come up another 5 degrees when you take them out of the oven and let them rest). Baste at least every 10 minutes.
- The gravy: Right after you first put the birds in the oven at 450, drain the porcinis and reserve the water in which they have been soaking.

You use the porcinis themselves in the second part of the recipe, below, but for the gravy you're going to reduce the soaking liquid. To do this, put it in a sauce pan, squeeze in the juice of the other tangerine, and just boil it all down for about 30 minutes - until has reduced by about half, but not until it is really as thick as you ultimately want it. When the birds are finished, splash a little cold white wine (or chicken stock, or water) into the pan they've been in and scrape like mad (deglaze it, in other words). Skim some of the grease off, then pour the remaining drippings and the cloves of garlic in with the reduced porcini liquid. Reduced the combined porcini liquid and pan drippings, whisking it all the while, for about 6 minutes at a furious boil. It should be thick enough to coat a spoon at that point. Strain and season it. Meanwhile your birds have been resting and your little packets of potatoes have been roasting, so once you're done with the gravy you can serve.

- Potatoes, Tarragon and Garlic en Papillote
- Potato and garlic pre-boil: Before you begin prep. of the birds, when you're just putting the oven on to preheat (in Step 1, above), put the potatoes in a pot with the garlic cloves and just barely cover in cold water. Put this on the stove and bring it to a boil, then boil for 10 minutes (no more - this is just a pre-cooking step). Drain the potatoes and slice them into rounds about as thick as your pinky. Slice the garlic cloves in half.
- Making the packets: (N.B. If you're fancy, you will know how to make little packets of vegetables and what have you out of lovely honest parchment paper tightly sealed around the edges already. You will probably even know that you have to brush the parchment with water before you put the little packets into the oven, so that they won't scorch, since they're going to be in there for 30 minutes or more. I'm not even going to talk to you since you already know everything. HOWEVER, if you don't already know what en papillote means and/or you're not OCD-level nostalgic, the recipe works just as well with aluminum foil, so that's how I'm going to explain it).Draw out a sheet of aluminum foil as long as your arm (so it's about twice as long as it is wide) and spread it shiny side up on the counter. Smear it with butter, but leaving an inch or two band un-smeared all around the edge. Make a pile 1 or 2 levels deep of potato rounds on one side (long-ways), then pile on tarragon leaves, then the garlic cloves, the porcini mushrooms, and a couple hunks of butter, then more tarragon leaves, then another layer or 2 of potato rounds. Fold over the aluminum on top of this packet and crimp it tightly around the edges, so you have a little, sealed, square packet of potato, tarragon, garlic, porcini and butter.
- Cooking and serving the packets: Throw the packets in the oven with the hens when they are put BACK into the oven at 350. They need a minimum of 30 minutes cooking time, but it's pretty hard to overcook them, so don't worry about it - just take them out when you're done with the birds and the gravy, they'll be fine. I like to put them on a platter and open them table side by slitting them down the middle with a sharp knife, as this allows the steam out, which is very fragrant.

142. Country Stuffing

Serving: Serves big family! | Prep: | Cook: | Ready in:

Ingredients

- 2 loaves toasted white bread or 1 crusty Italian bread, cut into cubes
- one bunch celery, cleaned and sliced
- 2 large onions, chopped
- 1 pound of breakfast sausage
- 1/2 cup parsley leaves and/or fresh herbs(whatever you have on hand thyme and oregano are my favorites)finely chopped
- juice of one lemon
- ground pepper to taste

Direction

- Directions: toast the bread in a hot oven.
- In a large skillet brown the breakfast sausage add herbs, then add onions, let cook for about five minutes, add celery then add bread cubes.
- Add the juice of one lemon
- Using a large casserole place ingredients in and cook for about an hour at around 350(or whatever temp you are cooking your turkey) until crispy and golden.

143. Creamy Gnocchi With Braised Chicken And Winter Vegetables

Serving: Serves 4 | Prep: | Cook: | Ready in:

Ingredients

- 8 ounces cremini/baby bella mushrooms
- 2 medium parsnips
- 2 medium carrots
- 1 cup (generous) 1/2"-3/4" cubes of butternut squash (about 6 oz.)
- 1 medium-large broccoli crown (about 6 oz.)
- 1/2 tablespoon butter
- 1/2 tablespoon olive oil
- 4 smallish skinless, boneless chicken thighs (about 3/4 lb.), trimmed of excess fat
- kosher salt and freshly ground pepper
- 2 garlic cloves, minced
- 1/2 tablespoon minced fresh sage
- 1/4 cup dry white wine
- 1 1/2 cups chicken broth, divided
- 1 17.5 oz. package gnocchi (I used De Cecco brand)
- 1/4 cup half-and-half
- 1/4 cup mascarpone cheese
- 1/4 cup all-purpose flour
- chopped fresh parsley, for serving

Direction

- Prep all of the vegetables. You are going to add them to the pan at different times, so—except for the carrots and parsnips—keep them in separate bowls. Wash and stem the mushrooms, and pat them dry; quarter them if they are small and cut them into 6 or 8 pieces if they are large. Peel the carrots and parsnips and cut them on the diagonal into 1/3" coins. Separate the broccoli crown into bite-site florets.
- Heat the butter and olive oil in a 12" skillet over medium-high heat. Pat the chicken dry and sprinkle it on both sides with salt and pepper. When the pan is hot, add the chicken and cook until browned on both sides, flipping once, about 3-4 minutes per side. Remove the chicken from the pan, place on a plate, and tent with foil.
- Add chopped mushrooms to the pan and cook until they release their juices and the juices have mostly evaporated, about 5 minutes total.
- Add the garlic and sage and stir for 30 seconds to 1 minute, just until fragrant, then pour in the wine and scrape up any brown bits. Boil for 1 minute.
- Return the chicken thighs and any accumulated juices to the pan, and also add the carrots, parsnips, and 1/4 cup of the chicken broth. Turn the heat down to medium-low, cover, and braise for 5 minutes. After the carrots and parsnips have cooked for 5 minutes, add the butternut squash to the pan, stir, put the lid back on, and cook for 15 more minutes. Then add the broccoli, stir, put the lid back on, and cook for 5 additional minutes.
- While the vegetables are braising, cook the gnocchi according to the package directions, drain, and set aside. Meanwhile, in a small measuring cup, combine the half-and-half with 3/4 cup of the chicken broth. In a different cup, whisk the flour into the remaining 1/2 cup of broth.
- After the broccoli has cooked for 5 minutes, remove the chicken, place it in your serving bowl, and shred it with 2 forks. Pour the half-and-half / broth mixture into the pan and also add the mascarpone cheese. Turn the heat up

to medium-high and stir until smooth. When the liquid starts simmering, add the flour/broth mixture and stir until thickened. Add the whole thing to the serving bowl, dump in the gnocchi, and toss gently to coat everything evenly. Season to taste with salt and pepper, and serve immediately. Top each serving with a small handful of parsley.

144. Creamy Sun Dried Tomato + Parmesan Chicken Zoodles

Serving: Serves 6 | Prep: | Cook: | Ready in:

Ingredients

- 1 tablespoon butter
- 1.5 pounds skinless chicken thigh fillets, cut into strips
- 4 ounces fresh semi-dried tomato strips in oil, chopped
- 4 cloves garlic, peeled and crushed
- 1 1/4 cups thickened cream, reduced fat or full fat (or half and half)
- 1 cup shaved Parmesan cheese
- Salt to taste
- Dried basil seasoning
- Red chilli flakes
- 2 large Zucchini (or summer squash), made into Zoodles (use a vegetable grater if you don't have a Zoodle grater)

Direction

- Heat the butter in a pan/skillet over medium high heat. Add the chicken strips and sprinkle with salt. Pan fry until the chicken is golden browned on all sides and cooked through.
- Add both semi-dried and sun dried tomatoes with 1 tablespoon of the oil from the jar (optional but adds extra flavor), and add the garlic; sauté until fragrant. (While the chicken is browning, prepare your Zoodles with a Zoodle maker OR with a normal vegetable peeler.)
- Lower heat, add the cream and the Parmesan cheese; simmer while stirring until the cheese has melted through. Sprinkle over salt, basil and red chili flakes to your taste.
- Stir through the Zoodles and continue to simmer until the zoodles have softened to your liking (about 5-8 minutes) and serve.

145. Creamy Chicken With Lemon And Rosemary

Serving: Serves 4 | Prep: | Cook: | Ready in:

Ingredients

- drizzle of olive oil
- 4 chicken thighs (about 600g)
- salt and pepper
- 1 tablespoon butter
- 1/2 onion, finely chopped
- 1 teaspoon crushed garlic
- 100 grams mushrooms, sliced
- 100 grams diced bacon
- 1 tablespoon flour
- 2 teaspoons very finely chopped rosemary
- 1/4 cup marsala wine
- 2 tablespoons lemon juice
- 300 milliliters chicken stock
- 1/2 cup cream

Direction

- Heat a drizzle of olive oil in a griddle pan. Season the chicken thighs with salt and pepper and cook over a high heat to brown on both sides. Leave them for a good few minutes so that they are well browned, then set aside.
- Melt the butter in a deep saucepan over a medium heat. Sauté the onion and garlic, then add the mushrooms and bacon. Cook for a few minutes before stirring in the flour and rosemary.

- Stir in the masala wine and lemon juice. Add the chicken stock and cream and stir to combine.
- Add the chicken thighs back to the pan. Bring to the boil, then reduce the heat and allow to simmer for about 30 minutes, stirring occasionally, until the sauce has thickened and the chicken is cooked through. The chicken can be turned over halfway through.
- Check the seasoning then serve with rice, potatoes or roasted veggies.

146. Crispy Chicken Thighs With Chicken Fat Fried Rice

Serving: Serves 4 | Prep: 0hours30mins | Cook: 1hours10mins | Ready in:

Ingredients

- 1 tablespoon canola oil
- 4 bone-in, skin-on chicken thighs
- 1 pinch kosher salt, plus more as needed
- 1 pinch freshly ground black pepper, plus more as needed
- 1 tablespoon Microplaned (or very finely grated) fresh ginger
- 2 large garlic cloves, Microplaned or minced
- 1/2 large yellow onion, finely diced
- 1 bunch scallions, finely chopped
- 2 medium carrots, peeled and finely diced
- 1/2 cup frozen peas
- 2 cups cooked white or brown rice, short- or medium-grain, cold
- 1 tablespoon soy sauce, plus more to taste
- 1 tablespoon unsalted butter (more canola oil works, too)
- 4 large eggs

Direction

- Add the oil to a large, heavy skillet, preferably cast-iron. Set over medium heat. Season the chicken thighs all over with salt and pepper. Add them to the skillet, skin side-down. Cook without moving until the fat has rendered and the skin is super golden brown and crispy, 15 to 30 minutes. Adjust the heat as needed, reducing to medium-low if the skin begins to burn before it gets evenly brown. Turn the thighs over and continue cooking until the other side is browned and the meat closest to the bone is cooked through, 15 to 20 minutes. When the chicken is done, transfer it to a plate, and pour the rendered fat into a heatproof glass or bowl. Leave the heat under the skillet on.
- Add 1 tablespoon chicken fat to the pan, then the ginger and garlic. Stir-fry for 1 minute until very fragrant. Add another 1 ½ tablespoons fat, along with the onion, scallion, carrot, and a big pinch of salt. Stir to combine, then cover the pan. Cook covered for 5 minutes, stirring halfway through. Uncover the pan and cook for another 3 minutes or so, until the vegetables are mostly tender. Add the peas and stir-fry to thaw and cook, about 2 minutes. Add the rice, soy sauce, and a little more chicken fat (or all of it!). Season to taste with salt, pepper, and more soy sauce. Turn the heat down to low while you cook the eggs in a separate pan.
- Add the butter or oil to a nonstick skillet and set on the stove over medium heat. Crack the eggs into a bowl, season with a pinch each of salt and pepper, and beat with a fork until smooth. When the butter has melted and is starting to foam, pour in the eggs. They should sizzle. Cook, stirring slowly but constantly, until the eggs are just set—this should only take a minute or so. Add the eggs to the rice and gently stir to incorporate so they're evenly distributed in big pieces.
- Nestle the chicken thighs on top of the fried rice and serve hot.

147. Crispy Grilled Chicken With Blueberry Barbecue Sauce

Serving: Serves 6 | Prep: 0hours20mins | Cook: 1hours30mins | Ready in:

Ingredients

- For the blueberry BBQ sauce
- 3 garlic cloves, minced
- 1/4 cup finely diced vidalia onion
- 2 tablespoons olive oil
- 2 cups ketchup
- 1/4 cup water
- 3 tablespoons apple cider vinegar
- 2 tablespoons tomato paste
- 1 tablespoon Worcestershire sauce
- 1 tablespoon soy sauce (gluten-free if necessary)
- 1/3 cup light brown sugar
- 2 tablespoons chili powder
- 1 tablespoon ground cumin
- 1 tablespoon coarsely ground black pepper
- 1 teaspoon dry mustard
- 1/2 teaspoon cayenne pepper
- 3 cups fresh blueberries
- For the chicken
- 2 2 1/2-pound fryer chickens, cut into pieces
- 2 teaspoons kosher salt
- 2 teaspoons ground black pepper
- 2 tablespoons butter, melted
- 1 1/2 cups blueberry barbecue sauce, above

Direction

- For the blueberry BBQ sauce
- In a heavy bottomed saucepan over medium heat, sweat the garlic and onion in the olive oil until soft, about 5 minutes.
- Add the ketchup, water, vinegar, tomato paste, Worcestershire sauce, and soy sauce. Stir until combined.
- Add the brown sugar, chili powder, cumin, pepper, mustard and cayenne and stir until combined.
- Let simmer on low heat, stirring frequently for 30 minutes.
- Fold in the blueberries, and continue cooking over low heat for an additional 30 minutes
- Serve warm, or cool. Refrigerate in an airtight container for up to one week.
- For the chicken
- Preheat a gas grill to medium, set up for indirect cooking. Or light a charcoal grill set up for indirect cooking.
- Season the chicken with salt and pepper. Place the chicken pieces, skin side up on the grill.
- Cook the chicken with the grill cover on. Rotate the chicken every ten minutes for even cooking. Baste with the butter. Do not flip the chicken, or the skin will stick to the grill. Cook to 160° F, checking the temperature with an instant-read thermometer. The chicken pieces will not all cook to the same temperature at the same time. As the pieces are complete, move to a platter.
- When all the chicken is cooked, return to the grill, again, keeping the chicken skin side up. Coat with barbecue sauce. Close the grill and cook 2 minutes. Arrange chicken on platter and serve with additional sauce for dipping.

148. Crispy Roast Chicken With Truffle Butter

Serving: Serves 3 | Prep: | Cook: | Ready in:

Ingredients

- one whole organic chicken
- 1/4 cup truffle butter, room temperature
- 1 lemon
- 1 bunch fresh thyme
- 2 tablespoons extra virgin olive oil
- salt
- pepper

Direction

- Wash and dry inside and outside of chicken.
- Preheat oven to 450 degrees.

- Gently slide index finger under skin of each side of breast and thighs, slowly detaching skin from meat.
- Carefully slide the truffle butter in between the skin and meat of the chicken in all 4 places.
- Cut the lemon in half and put both halves inside the cavity of the bird. Put the thyme inside the cavity with the lemon.
- Rub skin with olive oil and season generously with salt and pepper.
- Place chicken in roasting pan and roast until skin is golden and crispy and temperature of chicken is 170 degrees.

149. Crock Pot Chicken Stock

Serving: Serves 3 liters/12 cups | Prep: | Cook: | Ready in:

Ingredients

- 1 cooked chicken carcass
- 2 carrots, washed and trimmed
- 3 celery stalks (including leaves), washed
- 1 whole onion, washed
- 1 bay leaf
- 4-6 peppercorns
- 1 handful parsley (optional)
- water

Direction

- Chop the carrots into 2 inch pieces. Chop the celery stalks in half length-wise. Chop the onion into 4 pieces; you can include the outer brown skin, which helps to color the stock. Add all of the vegetables, chicken carcass, bay leaf, peppercorns, and parsley if using (I say optional because I don't always have parsley available so I've made the stock with and without it) into a large crock-pot. Fill with water to 1 inch from the top of the pot (keep in mind that not much liquid evaporates from a crock-pot). The amount of water you use will depend on the size of your crock-pot. Cover and cook on low setting for 4-8 hours, or overnight.
- After 4-8 hours, turn the crock-pot off and place lid off-center so the stock can cool. When the pot is warm enough to handle, discard vegetables and carcass. Strain the stock using a fine-sieved strainer. Use for a recipe like chicken soup or freeze for later use.

150. Crunchy Apple And Brussels Sprout Salad

Serving: Serves 8 | Prep: | Cook: | Ready in:

Ingredients

- Salad
- 16 ounces Brussels sprouts
- 8 ounces cooked, shredded chicken
- 2 crisp, tart apples, diced (such as Macoun, Honeycrisp, or Granny Smith)
- 3 ounces dried cranberries
- 1 shallot, thinly sliced and then diced
- 2 ounces pecans, toasted and broken into pieces
- 2 ounces extra sharp cheddar cheese, coarsely grated
- zest from half an orange (optional)
- Dressing
- Juice from 1 grapefruit
- 1 teaspoon Dijon mustard
- 2 ounces extra virgin olive oil

Direction

- Salad
- Rinse the Brussels sprouts. Cut off the ends and remove any damaged leaves. If you have a food processor, set it up with the slicer blade and enjoy the pure joy of dropping the sprouts down the shoot. If you don't have a food processor, thinly slice the sprouts (a sharp knife or mandolin works well). Once the Brussels sprouts are all sliced, give them a good bath in a salad spinner or large bowl to

get all the trapped grit out. Spin or drain and pat them dry.
- Combine all of the salad ingredients in a large bowl. Top with dressing and toss to coat salad with dressing.
- Dressing
- Combine all of the dressing ingredients in a jar and shake to combine. Taste and adjust as necessary.

151. Cumin And Mustard Roasted Chicken With Fruit

Serving: Serves 4 | Prep: | Cook: |Ready in:

Ingredients

- 1 Whole organic chicken, backbone removed, cut into 8 pieces, extra skin and fat trimmed
- 1 tablespoon Olive oil
- 1 tablespoon Unsalted butter
- Salt
- Pepper, fresh ground
- 1 1/2 teaspoons Ground cumin
- 1/2 cup Dry white wine
- 16-18 slices of mixed dried fruit – apricots, peaches, pears, apples and prunes
- 1-2 tablespoons Chopped Italian parsley for garnish
- 4 teaspoons Dijon mustard

Direction

- Preheat oven to 450°F.
- Prepare chicken if your butcher hasn't pre-cut it. Wash and dry the chicken pieces and trim off all fat and extra skin. Salt and pepper the side with the skin.
- In a skillet, warm olive oil and butter on medium high heat. Swirl to combine, and when butter stops sizzling, place the chicken in the skillet, seasoned side down, to brown and crisp skin for 3 – 4 minutes. While that side is browning, season the top side with salt, pepper and cumin.
- After the first side is nicely browned, turn chicken pieces over and brown the other side for 2 minutes. Add white wine and spread mustard on top of each piece.
- Place 2 pieces of dried fruit on top of each lightly mustard-coated piece. Put 2 – 3 pieces of fruit on each of the breasts, depending on the size of the fruit. You want to essentially cover the top of the chicken.
- Place the skillet in the oven and roast for 15 – 18 minutes. Check doneness with a thermometer; it should read 160 to 165 degrees.
- Remove chicken pieces to a platter, keeping the fruit on top. Pour any juices left in the skillet on top of the chicken.
- Let rest for 10 minutes, sprinkle chopped parsley on top, and serve with love.

152. Curried Chicken Mulligatawny Soup

Serving: Serves 6 - 8 | Prep: | Cook: |Ready in:

Ingredients

- Curried Soup
- 3-4 pounds bone-in chicken breasts
- 1-1/2 tablespoons ground coriander
- 1 tablespoon ground cumin
- 2-1/2 teaspoons ground turmeric
- 1-1/2 teaspoons kosher salt
- 5 whole cloves
- 1/4 teaspoon dried red pepper flakes
- 1 large yellow onion, cut in thin rings
- 4 garlic cloves, minced
- 1 teaspoon fresh ginger, grated
- 4+2 cups low sodium chicken broth
- 1 can chickpeas, drained
- 1/4 teaspoon whole cumin seed
- 1/2 teaspoon canola oil
- Garnishes
- 1/2 cup shredded unsweetened coconut, lightly toasted

- 1/2 cup roasted peanuts, chopped
- 1/2 cup raisins
- 1   lemon, cut into 8 wedges
- 1/2 cup Major Gray Apricot Chutney
- 1/2 cup plain yogurt
- 1/4 cup fresh cilantro leaves, coarsely chopped

Direction

- The original recipe is cooked in a clay pot but any large Dutch oven will work. If you're using a clay pot, soak the top and bottom of the clay cooker in water for at least 15 minutes, then drain.
- In a small bowl combine the coriander, turmeric, cumin, salt and cloves. Set aside. Cut the onion slices thinly, mince the garlic and grate the ginger.
- Remove the skin from the chicken breasts and arrange them slightly overlapping in the clay cooker (or Dutch oven if you're not using the clay pot). Sprinkle the spices over the chicken. Cover the chicken with the onion slices, garlic and ginger. Pour 4 cups of chicken stock over everything, cover tightly and place in a cold oven. Set the temperature to 400 degrees.
- Cook for 2-1/2 hours. Remove the chicken pieces from the soup and debone the meat. Return the meat to the soup. Add 2 more cups of chicken broth and half the can of the drained chickpeas. Mash the remaining chickpeas coarsely and add them to the soup also.
- Toast the 1/4 teaspoon of cumin seeds in a small skillet over medium high heat for 1 minute. Add 1/2 teaspoon of canola oil to the skillet and continue to toast the spice for another minute. Watch carefully! The cumin can burn quickly. You want to add a toasty taste so if you feel the seeds are done before the minute is up, remove them. Add the toasted cumin to the soup. Replace the top and put it back into the oven for another 30 minutes.
- Place all the garnishes in separate bowls arranged around the table so everyone can customize their soup with the garnishes of their choice.

153.   Curried Smoked Turkey Salad

Serving: Serves 4 | Prep: 0hours0mins | Cook: 0hours0mins | Ready in:

Ingredients

- 1 teaspoon Patak's Garlic Relish
- 1/2 cup mayonnaise
- 1 pound smoked turkey breast, cut into 1/4-inch dice
- 1/4   medium red onion, finely chopped
- 2   celery ribs, cut into 1/4-inch dice
- 1/4 cup flame or golden raisins (dried cranberries wouldn't be bad, either!)
- 1 teaspoon freshly ground black pepper, to taste
- 4 handfuls mixed greens (be generous)
- 1 splash Olive oil, for sprinkling
- 1 splash Balsamic vinegar, for sprinkling
- 1/3 cup coarsely chopped walnuts, toasted
- 4   slices cranberry (or raisin) pecan bread, toasted and buttered

Direction

- Make the mayonnaise: mix the garlic relish and mayonnaise, and adjust to taste, adding more garlic relish for more curry flavor.
- Combine the turkey, onion, celery, raisins and black pepper, and then, little by little, add in the mayo, folding it together with a spoon. The salad should just come together, but not be too wet. Only season with salt if necessary (smoked turkey is usually salted).
- To serve: sprinkle a bowl of greens with a little olive oil and balsamic vinegar (the curry mayo also acts as additional dressing so use oil and vinegar sparingly!). Serve a generous scoop of the turkey salad on top of greens, top with a handful of the chopped walnuts, and a little

more black pepper. At Iris Cafe, they serve this salad with a piece of toasted cranberry pecan bread from Pain d'Avignon, in the Essex Street Market.

154. Curried Turkey And Potato Hand Pies

Serving: Makes 6 hand pies | Prep: 0hours5mins | Cook: 0hours5mins |Ready in:

Ingredients

- 1 whole egg, lightly beaten with 1 Tb water

Direction

- Cook

155. Curried Peanut Chicken And Date Stew

Serving: Serves 3-4 | Prep: 0hours30mins | Cook: 0hours20mins |Ready in:

Ingredients

- 1.25-1.5 pounds boneless chicken thighs
- 2 tablespoons oil
- 1 tablespoon minced or crushed garlic
- 2 teaspoons grated ginger root
- 3/4 cup chopped onion
- 1/2 cup chopped green bell pepper
- 1 cup pitted medium dates, halved
- 14 1/2 ounces can of diced tomatoes
- 1 cup hot, prepared chicken broth (or hot water and 1 bouillon cube)
- 1/4 cup natural peanut butter (smooth or chunky)
- 2 teaspoons Sriracha sauce (or more for more spice)
- 1 teaspoon garam masala (or substitute--see below)
- 1 tablespoon soy sauce
- 2-3 tablespoons chopped cilantro
- Salt and pepper to taste

Direction

- Cut chicken thighs into four pieces each. Salt and pepper to taste. Sauté in 1 T. of oil at medium high heat until seared. Set aside.
- Sauté the onions and green pepper in the remaining tablespoon of oil until soft. Add garlic, ginger root and dates and sauté for 30 seconds.
- Mix peanut butter, soy sauce, can of tomatoes and sriracha into the hot broth and add to the sautéed onions, peppers, garlic and ginger. Add garam masala, or substitute 1/4 tsp. cinnamon, 1/4 tsp ground coriander and 1/2 tsp ground cumin if garam masala is not available.
- Add chicken pieces to the pan and cook covered on medium low for about twenty minutes, until the chicken has absorbed some of the flavor of the sauce. You may add more liquid (broth or water if needed). After it has cooked through, uncover the pan and raise the heat to medium for a few minutes to reduce the sauce. Check seasoning.
- Mix in the chopped cilantro, saving a tablespoon or so to garnish the dish.

156. Deep Dish Chicken Pot Pie

Serving: Makes 1 pie | Prep: | Cook: |Ready in:

Ingredients

- 1 rotisserie chicken, meat removed from bone
- 2 cups sliced fresh carrots
- 2 cups fresh green peas
- 1 clove garlic, chopped
- 1/3 cup butter
- 1/2 medium Spanish or yellow onion, chopped

- 1/3 cup flour
- 1/2 teaspoon salt
- 1/2 teaspoon black pepper
- 1 pinch celery salt
- 1 3/4 cups low sodium chicken broth
- 2/3 cup 1% milk
- 1 egg white
- 2 refrigerated pie crusts

Direction

- Preheat the oven to 425 degrees F. In a medium saucepan, boil the carrots and peas together for about 15 minutes, then strain and set aside.
- While the peas and carrots are boiling, melt the butter in a large non-stick skillet on medium heat. Add the garlic and onion and cook for 10 minutes.
- Add the salt, pepper, and flour to the skillet. Stir everything together, then slowly stir in the broth and milk. Let this simmer for about 8 minutes (the mixture should thicken).
- While the gravy is simmering away, unroll and press a pie crust into the bottom of your casserole or pie dish. Brush the crust with a little bit of egg white.
- Alternately add peas & carrots and chicken to the pie crust. Pour the gravy on top, making sure to evenly drizzle over the filling.
- Add the top crust and press the edges together to seal. Using the tip of a sharp knife, cut 4 slits in the top. Brush the top crust with egg white. Bake for 30-35 minutes and allow to cool 5-10 minutes before diving in.

157. Deliciously Cheesy Crumb Chicken Casserole

Serving: Serves 6 | Prep: | Cook: | Ready in:

Ingredients

- Casserole
- 3 cups diced leftover chicken or lemon herb rotisserie chicken
- 1 1/2 cups brooccoli cuts, steamed lightly
- 1/2 cup sliced canned mushrooms, drained
- 1 1/2 cups cream of mushroom soup, undiluted
- 1 1/2 cups cream of chicken soup, undiluted
- 1/4 cup milk
- 2 teaspoons butter, melted
- 2 tablespoons Italian seasoning
- 2 teaspoons sea salt
- 1 teaspoon freshly ground black pepper
- 8 ounces Rotini pasta, cooked al dente, drained
- 2 tablespoons butter for buttering casserole dish
- Cheesy Crumb Topping
- 12   stale multi-grain Italian loaf slices
- 6   Sharp American Cheese Slices

Direction

- Casserole
- Preheat oven to 350 degrees.
- Butter casserole dish with 2 tablespoons butter.
- In large mixing bowl combine diced chicken, broccoli cuts, mushroom, cream of mushroom soup, cream of chicken soup, ¼ cup milk melted butter, Italian seasoning, sea salt and black pepper. Stir lightly until combined. Add pasta and mix well. Pour into a 4 quart buttered casserole dish. Set aside.
- Cheesy Crumb Topping
- Place cheese slices while still in wrappers in freezer while you prepare the bread.
- Take the bread slices and tear into pieces and place in mixing bowl. Each slice should be torn into 4 to 6 pieces
- When all are torn remove cheese slices from freezer and unwrap.
- . Place ½ of torn bread pieces in food processor. Take 3 slices cheese, tear into 6 pieces and place on top of bread. Process for 1 to 2 minutes until bread is chopped into fine crumbs and cheese is integrated into crumbs.

- Remove from processor and repeat with remaining bread and cheese.
- After all bread and cheese is processed, spread crumb mixture over prepared casserole. Crumb topping should be about 1 to 2 inches thick on top of casserole.
- Bake at 350 degrees for 30 minutes until golden and bubbly.
- Variations include substituting any vegetables for broccoli such as carrots, green peas, etc. Celery can be substituted for mushrooms or added for an extra layer of flavor. Experiment and make it your family's own.

- Place the poultry pieces in a plastic or small paper bag with the instant flour and shake to coat the pieces.
- In a large sauté pan, melt the butter, add the poultry and sauté for a few minutes. Add the onion, garlic and mushrooms, cook another minute, then add the Sherry.
- Continue to cook another couple of minutes, then add the ham and tomato sauce.
- Stir in the parsley and broth and simmer until the mixture thickens a bit.
- Stir in the cheese and pour the mixture over the cooked pasta. Stir it around, adding more pasta cooking liquid if necessary. Garnish with more cheese and parsley.

158. Denny's Tetrazzini

Serving: Serves 4 to 6 (can easily be doubled) | Prep: 0hours0mins | Cook: 0hours0mins | Ready in:

Ingredients

- 8 tablespoons butter (one stick)
- 4 cups bite size pieces of cooked turkey or chicken
- 4 tablespoons instant flour (Wondra)
- 1 cup diced onion
- 2 cloves garlic, minced
- 1/2 cup finely diced ham
- 2 cups sliced mushrooms
- 8 ounces tomato sauce (your favorite)
- 1/2 cup dry Sherry
- 1 teaspoon black pepper
- 1/2 teaspoon salt
- 1/2 cup chopped parsley plus more for garnish
- 3 cups chicken or turkey broth
- 1/2 cup grated Romano cheese plus more for serving
- 1 pound pasta such as fettucini or linguini which has been preferably cooked in chicken broth but water is ok
- Save a little pasta water if needed

Direction

159. Dinner Salad With Roasted Chicken Thighs, Caperberries And Roasted Lemons

Serving: Serves 4 | Prep: | Cook: | Ready in:

Ingredients

- 4 chicken thighs with bone and skin
- 5.5 ounces baby spinach leaves
- 3-4 romaine lettuce leaves, washed, dried and torn into bite size pieces
- 1.75 pounds baby Yukon Gold potatoes – scrubbed, dried and cut into 2" chunks
- 2 tablespoons olive oil, plus more to drizzle on finished salads
- 1/3 cup caperberries, drained
- 2 whole lemons, washed, dried and cut in half
- 8 radishes, scrubbed clean and dried, trim if greens are not nice
- 1/2 cup sugar snap peas, washed, strings removed, and cut on a diagonal into slices
- 3 tomatoes, washed, dried and each cut into 8 wedges

- 4 small sweet peppers – yellow, orange or red, washed, dried, split in half lengthwise, seeds removed
- 3 scallions, cleaned and sliced, white, light green and some dark green parts
- garlic powder
- Maldon Salt
- sesame seeds
- freshly ground pepper

Direction

- Preheat oven to 425 degrees. Toss potatoes with 2 Tbs. olive oil and season with salt and pepper. Roast potatoes in the oven for 15 minutes. Then add the caperberries to the potatoes and toss and return to the oven for 20 – 30 minutes more.
- Meanwhile, wash and dry chicken thighs, removing all fat and extra skin on the edges. Season both sides with salt, pepper, garlic powder and sesame seeds, pressing them in to adhere. Place thighs on a rack on a rimmed baking sheet, add lemon halves in the corners of the baking sheet, cut side down and roast on the top shelf in the oven for 30 – 40 minutes.
- Prepare all the other vegetables.
- Distribute the spinach and romaine lettuce leaves evenly among four dinner plates. Place chicken thighs in the center and evenly distribute all the other vegetables around the chicken, putting one roasted lemon half on each plate and finishing with the scallions sprinkled all over. Drizzle olive oil on the vegetables in a circle around the chicken, and squeeze the lemon all around. Finish with some crushed Maldon salt and fresh ground pepper.
- Serve with LOVE and enjoy!! We paired this with an Alsace Riesling – perfect!

160. Don't Tell My Cardiologist Thanksgiving Leftover Sandwich

Serving: Serves 1 | Prep: | Cook: |Ready in:

Ingredients

- 2 slices challah, preferably homemade
- Good Jewish Chopped Chicken Liver
- Cornbread, Bacon, Onion & Apple Dressing (or your favorite stuffing recipe)
- Leftover Roast Turkey
- Cranberry Sauce
- Mayonnaise

Direction

- Spread each slice of bread with mayonnaise.
- Add a nice thick schmear of chopped liver on one of the slices.
- Press some dressing on one side of the sandwich.
- Spoon some cranberries over the dressing, let the juices sink in.
- Layer some turkey over the cranberries.
- Top with the other slice of mayonnaise's bread.
- Press down a little, just so you can fit it in your mouth. Cut it in half to look polite.
- Enjoy. Once a year. Maybe twice.

161. Duck Confit

Serving: Serves as desired | Prep: | Cook: |Ready in:

Ingredients

- 1 whole fresh duck
- kosher salt

Direction

- Butcher duck into its separate parts (2 legs, 2 breasts, 2 thighs, etc.).

- Remove all of the skin, except for skin on the breasts. On each breast, leave a layer of skin about the same size as the breast. Reserve all of the skin and fat. Salt duck parts liberally. (Alternatively, you could brine...See Brining recipe)
- Reserve all of the excess bones (i.e., backbone, etc.) for stock (either use now or freeze).
- Preheat oven to 200F
- Place all of the skin and fat into a 2 qt. Dutch oven (Le Creuset, Staub or other heavy pot that can go on the stove top or in the oven)
- Cook fat/skin over medium low heat until melted into oil with only crispy pieces of skin left in the melted fat/oil. When the crispy pieces won't cook down any more, remove the crispy pieces and discard or keep if you can find a use.
- Place all of butchered duck parts (other than pure bones for stock) into the Dutch oven with the duck fat. Make sure all of the duck parts are fully submerged in duck fat. With regular American ducks, the breasts are very skinny. You can keep them separate and pan sear, roast, etc. or just confit with the rest of the duck parts. It's up to you.
- Place Dutch oven in the oven uncovered and cook for 6 to 8 hours
- Remove from oven and let the Dutch oven sit on the counter until duck and duck fat has cooled (at least an hour).
- You can either pick all of the meat off of the bones (which I've done for the) or leave on the bones. I prefer to pick the meat off of the bones.
- Place duck meat submerged in duck fat in a Tupperware/Rubbermaid and put in the refrigerator. Duck meat will last for several weeks submerged in duck fat.
- Use duck meat in recipes that call for duck confit (like my Duck Confit, Caramelized Onion and Gruyere Sandwich recipe).

162. Duck Prosciutto

Serving: Serves 8 | Prep: | Cook: |Ready in:

Ingredients

- 2 Duck Breasts, boned. I bought mine from Whitehouse Meats on St. Lawrence Market.
- Salt. Pickling or kosher salt is best as it contains no additives and flow control chemicals. Enough to cover the duck breasts.
- Spices. I used a mixture of cracked black pepper and coriander.
- Cheesecloth
- String
- One non-reactive bowl, just large enough to hold the duck breasts without them touching the sides or each other.

Direction

- Fill the bowl about 1/2 inch high with salt. Place the breasts onto the salt, skin side up. Make sure they don't touch, then pour more salt between them until they are covered. Cover with plastic wrap and put into the fridge for a minimum of 24 hours, but no longer than 36.
- Take the breasts out of the salt. The color will be a deep red and the meat will feel dense. Wash the salt off the meat with cold water, then pat dry with a paper towel. Rub the meat side with the spice mixture and wrap them into a layer of cheese-cloth. Hang into a cool, dark room for 7-10 days. If they aren't completely dried and stiff feel squishy and raw, dry for a day or two longer.
- Slice thinly and enjoy

163. Duck A L'orange Tartlet

Serving: Makes 4 | Prep: | Cook: |Ready in:

Ingredients

- pie dough

- cold water
- 1 cup AP Flour
- 6 tablespoons Unsalted butter (or combo with leaf lard), in small pieces
- 1 pinch salt
- Pastry Cream, Candied Orange Zest, Duck Confit
- 1 Orange
- 1 cup milk
- 3 egg yolks
- 1 tablespoon Cornstarch
- 2 tablespoons Flour
- 1 pinch salt
- 1 tablespoon Butter, diced
- 4 teaspoons Sugar
- 1 cup sugar
- pomegranate seeds, dried
- 1 Duck Leg Confit

Direction

- Pie dough: Mix dry ingredients and cut in butter/lard pieces until the texture is sand-like with different sized butter clumps. Pour in 2 Tablespoons cold water and mix until dough forms larger clumps. I add up to 2 more Tablespoons to get the dough to the point where it can be compressed into a disk. Then cool for a couple hours in the fridge.
- Pastry Cream: Heat milk until steaming, and steep 3/4 of the zest off the orange (avoid pith) for 5-10 minutes covered (remove zest). Beat egg yolks with sugar until thickened and pale yellow, add cornstarch and flour and continue to beat until well mixed. Temper the egg mixture with hot milk 1/4 cup at a time while stirring until all the milk has been combined with eggs. Place over medium low heat and bring to a simmer stirring constantly until smooth and thick (careful of splatters). Remove from heat and butter and salt. Cover with cling wrap right on surface of cream in an airtight container in fridge.
- Candied zest: Finely julienne remaining orange zest (again, avoid pith). Then blanch in water (start with cold), and drain. Next, heat 1 cup sugar and .5 cup water to dissolve sugar and bring to a simmer. Add zest and simmer for 10 minutes. Then using a candy thermometer, I got the syrup up to 225 degrees and cook for another 3-5 minutes. Rest of a rack until dry/cool and spring with some sugar (optional).
- Duck: Got some at a nice market, although if this contest was a couple weeks later the ducks in the fridge might have been ready. Shred about 1 oz. per tartlet and crisp a minute at medium high heat on each side in a little of the duck fat.
- Cut rounds of pie dough, then using a smaller ring assemble tarts in preferred order. Again a little less pastry cream per tart, and I might reverse the cream and orange slices next time. If you like a little more sweetness you can save the syrup from the candied zest to drizzle.

164. Duck! It's Baby Eggs In Onion Nests!

Serving: Serves 3-4 | Prep: | Cook: | Ready in:

Ingredients

- Olive oil (extra virgin)
- 1 very large or 2 medium yellow onions
- Duck breast – cured and dried (I got mine from "Fabrique Delices" or in the alternative you could use proscuitto)
- 3/4 teaspoon sea salt
- a pinch of sea salt
- fresh ground pepper
- 2 handfuls baby spinach
- ½ red onion
- 3-4 quail eggs
- Utensils: muffin tin

Direction

- Preheat oven to 400 degrees.
- Sauté red onion in enough olive oil to cover bottom of pan until translucent and slightly golden. Add spinach and a pinch of sea salt

and toss lightly to coat spinach until spinach is softened and just begins to wilt. Turn off heat and set aside.
- Slice yellow onions as thin as possible (or use a mandolin if you have). Sauté w/ ¾ tsp. sea salt over medium high heat in enough olive oil to cover bottom of pan until crisp and deep caramel/mahogany in color (almost on the verge of getting burnt, but not quite).
- Take out a muffin tin and place a small portion of the browned yellow onions in each of three or four muffin tins. Press against sides to cover entire bottom and sides of tin. Add a layer of cooked spinach/red onion mixture; smooch out again and add the smoked duck breast (or prosciutto); pressing against the sides firmly. Crack a quail egg on top of each "nest."
- Bake in 400 degree oven for 7-8 minutes – until whites are cooked and yellows are still golden and silky.
- Remove from muffin tins (carefully) using a rounded tablespoon; top with fresh ground black pepper. Serve and enjoy!

165. Easy Indian Chicken Curry

Serving: Serves 3-4 | Prep: | Cook: | Ready in:

Ingredients

- 6 pieces Skinless Thighs with/without bones or Breasts
- 2 medium onions chopped
- 2 tomatoes chopped
- 1 tablespoon Ginger Garlic paste
- 1 tablespoon ground Cumin
- 1 tablespoon Ground coriander
- 1 teaspoon Turmeric
- 2 teaspoons Garam Masala
- 2 teaspoons Red Chilli powder/cayenne (or according to your heat preference)
- 1 tablespoon Salt (or to your taste)
- 5 tablespoons oil
- 1 cup Water

Direction

- Preheat the oven to 400 degrees F. In a skillet heat oil and add the onions. Cook until golden brown. Then add the Ginger garlic paste. Cook for a couple of minutes and then add the tomatoes. Follow with salt and all the dry spices and cook about 5 minutes until the spices release their aroma (about 5-10 minutes on medium heat). You have the basic curry masala ready.
- Now puree the mixture in a blender/grinder. Transfer into an oven proof dish and add the chicken pieces. Mix them properly. Add water and bake them covered in the oven for about 35-40 mins until all the chicken is fully cooked. Boneless pieces will take shorter time. Adjust the seasonings. Enjoy with Rice or Rotis/Naans!

166. Easy Oven Baked Chicken Shawarma Recipe

Serving: Serves 2 | Prep: 0hours20mins | Cook: 0hours20mins | Ready in:

Ingredients

- 1/4 tablespoon ground cumin
- 1/4 tablespoon turmeric powder
- 1/4 tablespoon ground coriander
- 1/4 tablespoon garlic powder
- 1/4 tablespoon paprika
- 1/6 teaspoon ground cloves
- 3 boneless, skinless chicken thighs, sliced into small pieces
- 1/9 cup extra virgin olive oil
- 1/6 teaspoon cayenne pepper
- 1 large onion, thinly sliced
- 1 large lemon juice
- Salt to taste

Direction

- Preparation- Mix all the ingredients for the spice mix in a small bowl and set aside.- Put the chicken breasts in a large bowl, season with the Shawarma spices, onions, lemon juice, olive oil and salt. Toss them all together to make sure the chicken pieces are evenly coated. Cover with a cling film and store overnight in the fridge (or at least 3 hours).
- Instructions
- Remove the marinated chicken from the fridge, let it reach to room temperature.
- Spread the marinated chicken and the onions on the baking tray. Make sure all the chicken thighs are lying flat and not on top of each other. Put to bake in 30 minutes.
- Meanwhile, prepare the sauce to your preferences. I myself used a simple Greek Tzatziki sauce to enhance the chicken's flavor.
- I enjoyed my chicken shawarma in pita pockets, a few stems of arugula, and finally some drizzles of tzatziki sauce and olive oil. Be creative all you want.
- Notes- It is sure much more tasty if the chicken is marinated and let sit for 1 day beforehand in the fridge. Simply defrost it on the next day before cooking. - The chicken can also be frozen in its marination – as long as the meat has not been previously frozen – for up to 3 months.

167. Easy And Customizable Hasselback Chicken

Serving: Serves 2 people | Prep: | Cook: | Ready in:

Ingredients

- 2 chicken breasts
- 1/4 cup zucchini chopped
- 1/4 cup red pepper chopped
- 1/4 cup yellow pepper chopped
- 1/4 cup onion chopped
- 1/4 cup tomato sliced
- 1/4 cup fresh lemon sliced
- 2-3 red potatoes diced with the skin on
- Garnish with feta or parmesan cheese

Direction

- Preheat your oven to 400 degrees.
- Cut 6-7 slits (crosswise) into each chicken breast.
- Carefully transfer the chicken to a cookie sheet.
- Stuff each slit with your lemon and veggies in any order you like. You may use as much or as little veggies as you desire. Season each stuffed chicken breast generously with olive oil, salt, and pepper.
- Surround the stuffed chicken with the diced potatoes and leftover lemon and vegetables (optional). Season the potatoes, lemon, and vegetables with olive oil, salt, and pepper.
- Top the chicken and potatoes with fresh dill.
- Transfer the cookie sheet to the oven and cook for 20-25 minutes or until the chicken is fully cooked. Once the chicken is cooked I sprinkle some parmesan cheese on top and let it rest for 5-10 minutes before serving.
- NOTES: You don't have to worry about how deep your cuts are in the chicken so long as you don't cut all the way through it! You only stuff a little bit of the vegetables into the chicken which means you won't use an entire zucchini, pepper, onion, etc. I mixed in the leftover vegetables and lemon in with the potatoes that surrounded the chicken. If you don't want to use the leftover vegetables in this dish, plan to use them up in another recipe so they don't go to waste! I like to sauté the leftover veggies with some andouille sausage and cabbage! The smaller you dice the potatoes the faster they will cook. Worse case, if your potatoes are not fully cooked by the time your chicken is finished, allow the chicken to rest and pop the potatoes back in the oven for another 10 minutes or so. If you don't care for the vegetables I chose for this recipe, you can simply swap them out for the ingredients you enjoy most!

168. Filipino Chicken Porridge (Arroz Caldo)

Serving: Serves 6 | Prep: | Cook: | Ready in:

Ingredients

- 1 tablespoon canola oil, plus more for frying
- one 1-inch piece of ginger root, peeled and finely chopped
- 1 small onion, chopped
- 6 cloves garlic, smashed, peeled, and minced, divided
- 1 to 1 1/2 pounds boneless, skinless chicken thighs, sliced
- 2 tablespoons fish sauce
- 1 cup short grain rice
- 4 cups chicken broth
- Green onions, thinly sliced, as garnish
- Fried garlic flakes, as garnish

Direction

- Heat canola oil in a large pot or Dutch oven over medium heat. Add the ginger, onion, and 3 cloves of garlic and cook until the onion is translucent, about 3 minutes.
- Add the chicken and cook until browned, about 5 minutes.
- Add the fish sauce and let simmer for a few minutes, then add rice and simmer a few minutes more, stirring often.
- Add the chicken broth and bring to a boil. Lower heat and let simmer, stirring frequently until the chicken and rice are cooked through, about 25 to 30 minutes.
- Meanwhile, make fried garlic flakes: Heat a few tablespoons of canola oil in a skillet over medium-high heat. Add the remaining 3 cloves of minced garlic and fry until a deep golden brown. Transfer the flakes to a paper towel and set aside.
- Serve arroz caldo with fried garlic flakes and green onions sprinkled on top.

169. Filipino Chicken Adobo

Serving: Serves 4 | Prep: | Cook: | Ready in:

Ingredients

- 2 pounds bone-in chicken pieces (I like dark meat)
- 1 cup palm vinegar or cider vinegar
- 1 cup water
- 2 tablespoons soy sauce (a light one like Kikkoman, not 'Soy Superior')
- 4 bay leaves
- 1 tablespoon whole black peppercorns
- 5-6 whole cloves of garlic (I like to smash them slightly with the side of a knife)
- 2 teaspoons salt
- 1/2 teaspoon ground black pepper

Direction

- Combine and stir all the ingredients in a non-reactive pot or Dutch oven. Bring the whole thing to a simmer over medium heat. Do not stir the mixture, cover and simmer over medium low until the meat is cooked through, about 30 minutes for dark meat.
- When the meat is cooked through, remove it from the pot. Turn the pot with the sauce in it to medium high, and boil until the sauce reduces by about half and is quite thick. Remove from heat.
- Meanwhile, heat a few tablespoons of vegetable oil over medium high heat in a large saucepan. Add the chicken. If you have a splatter screen, use it. You can also cover it and just lift the lid when you need to turn the chicken pieces. Fry until they are crispy golden brown all over.
- Remove the chicken to a serving platter. You can either pour the sauce over directly, or use a strainer to strain out the bay leaves, garlic and peppercorns. Serve with steamed white rice.

170. Filipino Style Chicken Rice Porridge

Serving: Serves 6 | Prep: | Cook: | Ready in:

Ingredients

- 1 piece shallot, minced
- 1 tablespoon garlic, minced
- 2 tablespoons ginger, sliced thin
- 6 pieces chicken drumstick
- 4 cups chicken stock
- 1 1/2 cups jasmine rice
- 1 tablespoon fish sauce
- 1 tablespoon soy sauce

Direction

- Pat dry the chicken drumsticks with a paper towel. Season the chicken with salt and pepper. Put a little olive oil on a large pot on medium to high heat and fry the chickens until brown. This will take about 10 minutes. Make sure the oil is hot before putting the chicken. Oil might splatter so be careful. Set aside on a plate.
- Using the same pot, fry the garlic, shallots and ginger for about 3 minutes on medium heat. Make sure to scrape those brown bits on the pot from the chicken. That's some great flavor! :)
- Add the rice and mix for about 2 minutes to absorb the flavors. Add the chicken stock and bring to a boil.
- Once boiling, place the chicken back to the pot with all the drippings from the plate. Let it simmer for about 30 minutes. What I usually do is to cover the pot for about 15 minutes. Then simmer it uncovered making sure to mix it every once in a while so that the rice won't stick at the bottom. On the 20 minute mark, add 2 cups of water and mix. Add another cup of water until the desired texture is thick but soupy like a rice porridge. I added a total of 4 cups on mine.
- Add fish sauce and soy sauce. Mix. Salt and pepper to taste. To serve it, put the rice porridge in a bowl, top it off with chopped chives and fried garlic. You can even add some chicharon. Squeeze some lemon before serving. Enjoy!

171. Frogsicle Pops With Basil And Meyer Lemon

Serving: Serves 2-4 | Prep: | Cook: | Ready in:

Ingredients

- 1 pound frog legs
- 1 tablespoon capers packed in salt
- 1/3 cup clarified butter or ghee
- 1/4 cup superfine flour (Wondra)
- 12   basil leaves
- 4   meyer lemons, cut into wedges
- sea salt

Direction

- Begin by soaking the capers in cold water to rinse the salt off. Set aside
- Using a sharp paring knife or utility knife cut through the tendons of each frog leg and scrape down the bone to completely clean them. I'd like to say "save the scraps for another use" but I can't think of one. This will leave you a knob of flesh at the top
- In a pie pan spread out your flour and add some sea salt. Give the legs a good dusting of flour
- Heat the butter in a saute pan (this would be a good time to drain the capers)
- Working in batches saute the legs in the butter until cooked through, set aside
- Roll up the basil leaves into cigarette shapes and quickly chiffonade them
- Add the capers and the basil to the butter in the pan and give it all a quick toss
- Spoon the butter onto individual serving plates and arrange the leg pieces

- Serve with lemon wedges

172. Fusion Sticky Rice With Star Anise Chicken, Shiitake, Edamame, And Sunchokes

Serving: Serves 6-10 | Prep: | Cook: | Ready in:

Ingredients

- 2 cups Japanese sticky/sweet rice (soaked in water to cover by 2 inches, 4 hours or overnight, then drained)
- 2 T. canola oil
- 3 T. minced peeled ginger
- 6 T. minced light green and white scallion parts
- 3/4- 1 cup sliced fresh shiitake mushroom caps
- 5 ou. Sweet Italian sausage(pierced with fork a few places to keep from exploding)
- 1 cup chopped unpeeled Jerusalem artichoke, alone or combined with julienned sweet fried tofu skin (aburaage) and julienned Japanese flat omelet
- 1 cup cooked shelled edamame
- 13 ou. coconut milk (I prefer Nuoc Cot Dua))
- 1 cup +heated chicken stock (that 1 tsp. Lapsang Souchong has steeped in 30-60 minutes, then strained)
- 3 T. oyster sauce (Hop Ling Sung is excellent)
- 1 T. soy sauce
- 3 T. dry cocktail sherry or sake or Chinese rice wine
- 2/3 tsp. Kosher salt
- Add chili paste to taste if you wish, but I don't use it here
- STAR ANISE CHICKEN (optional)
- 4 chicken thighs, bone-in, skin-on
- 1/3 cup soy sauce
- 1/8 cup dark brown sugar
- 1 Tablespoon dry sherry (not "cooking sherry")
- 4 thin quarter sized peeled slices fresh ginger, smashed with side of knife and chopped
- 3 whole star anise or equivalent pieces
- 1/2 Tablespoon chili flakes
- 1 teaspoon minced garlic
- 1/3 cup o.j. or 3 T. frozen OJ concentrate plus 2 T. water

Direction

- Heat oil till hot, add ginger, then scallion, and stir fry a few minutes. Add shiitakes and sauté 5 minutes till soft.
- Remove ginger- shiitakes. Over medium heat, sauté sausages till done. Cool and cut lengthwise into quarters and then slice across in 1/3 inch slices.
- Return shiitakes, scallions and ginger to sausage pan. Mix well. Add Jerusalem artichoke and edamame and mix well. Pour coconut milk and stock over rice, then soy sauce through salt, stirring to coat well. Bring to boil.
- Turn heat to simmer, cover, till liquid is absorbed. Taste (rice should be chewy) but if not ready, add more coconut milk, stock, or water; cover and let cook till rice is chewy/al dente.) Add shredded cooked chicken to taste, somewhere near the end of the rice cooking.
- Taste and add more seasonings as needed. Serve as is or stuffed into Inari (fried tofu skin pockets.)
- CHICKEN: In a saucepan just big enough to fit four bone-in skin-on chicken thighs, heat a little canola oil to hot. For ~ 4 minutes, sear chicken thighs, skin side down. Turn over and sear 3 minutes. Remove from pan. Add to pan soy through o.j. Bring to a boil, stirring to dissolve the sugar, turn to simmer. Return thighs to pan, turn to coat with sauce, cover on low simmer for 20-30 minutes, turning once more, till meat easily pulls away from bone. Turn off, remove thighs from pot and let cool ~ 5-10 minutes. Discard skin and bones and put into upright narrow container. Top with sauce and refrigerate overnight. The next day, remove and discard the layer of solid fat that

has settled on the top. Shred the chicken into small pieces. Reheat the chicken with sauce, remove the chicken from the sauce (reserve to cook with later) and fold the chicken into the completed sticky rice. Serve.
- **When reheating sticky rice, you need water or liquid to create steam; otherwise the rice will be hard.

173. Garlicky Parmesan Corn Flake Baked Chicken Tenders

Serving: Serves 4 to 6 | Prep: | Cook: |Ready in:

Ingredients

- 1 1/2 pounds boneless skinless chicken breasts
- 1 tablespoon minced garlic
- 1 egg
- 3/4 cup milk
- 1/2 teaspoon Mrs. Dash Southwest Chipotle seasoning (you can substitute with any Cajun-blend seasoning if that's not available)
- ground black pepper, to taste
- 3/4 cup crushed cornflakes
- 1/2 cup seasoned bread crumbs
- 1/4 cup fresh grated parmesan cheese
- Olive oil cooking spray

Direction

- Pound the chicken breasts with a mallet until they are about 1/4 inch thick. If they are very thick to start with, you can also butterfly the breasts instead. Cut the chicken into strips and set aside.
- Add the minced garlic to a bowl, and mash it into a paste with the back of a spoon. Crack the egg into the bowl then add the milk, Chipotle seasoning and black pepper to taste. Mix well, then add the chicken.
- Cover and marinate in the refrigerator for about one hour. Meanwhile, you can prepare the coating.
- Fill a quart Ziploc bag with cornflakes and close. Crush the cornflakes finely using a pestle (or the palm of your hand). After crushing them, measure how much you have, and crush more if needed.
- Pour the cornflakes onto a large plate, then add the seasoned bread crumbs and grated Parmesan cheese. Mix well.
- Preheat the oven to 375 degrees.
- Line a large baking sheet with crumpled aluminum foil and spray with olive oil.
- When the chicken is done marinating, dredge each piece through the coating and place them evenly apart on the baking sheet.
- Spray the chicken lightly with olive oil. Cook for 20 minutes, turning once halfway through.

174. Gin Brined Turkey

Serving: Serves 6-8 | Prep: 0hours0mins | Cook: 0hours0mins |Ready in:

Ingredients

- 1 12 to 14 pound turkey
- 1 liter high-quality gin
- 1 liter water
- 2 cups kosher salt
- 1/4 cup honey
- 3-4 sprigs fresh sage, rosemary, and thyme, crushed
- 1 lemon and 1 lime, sliced thin
- 1 apple, quartered
- 4 cloves garlic, crushed
- 1/2 teaspoon juniper berries
- 1/2 teaspoon peppercorns

Direction

- In a very large working bowl, combine gin, water, and salt. Stir with a wooden paddle to dissolve the salt. Add the honey and stir to dissolve as well.
- Add all the aromatics to the brine: the thyme, rosemary, sage, juniper berries, peppercorns,

lemon, lime, apple, and garlic. Make sure the fruit and the garlic are slightly crushed so they will release their flavors.

- Put the turkey in a brine bag and then put it in a food safe large bucket, ice chest, or big bowl. Pour the brine over the bird, seal the brine bag and put it in the fridge. If you have the bird in an ice chest, pack it with ice.
- Let the bird hang out in the brine for at least 24 to 48 hours. Four hours before you are going to roast the bird, remove it from the brine. Rinse, pat dry with paper towels and place in the roasting pan.
- For crispy skin, it is important to return the turkey to the fridge for a couple of hours uncovered so the skin has time to dry out. Bring the turkey out of the fridge at least an hour before you roast it — your turkey will turn out better for it.
- I always add compound butter under the skin of my turkeys. You can also rub the skin with oil and salt and pepper. Be sure you have turkey broth in the base of your roasting pan for basting. I added a few shots of gin as well to flavor the broth and the future gravy.
- It never hurts to stuff some aromatics inside the bird — I put an apple, a lemon and an onion inside my bird — all halved or quartered.
- Use your preferred roasting method, or use what we did: Preheat your oven to 450°F, then reduce the temperature to 350°F and roast the turkey for 80 minutes, basting intermittently. Check on the turkey and roast for another 35 to 40 minutes — or until breast is 150°F and the thighs are 165°F. Let rest 20 minutes before carving. Use the gin flavored drippings to make a ginny gravy. Happy Ginsgiving!

175. Ginger Chicken Meatballs With Bok Choy

Serving: Serves 4 | Prep: | Cook: | Ready in:

Ingredients

- 2 cloves garlic, minced
- 1 1/4 pounds ground chicken
- 1 tablespoon soy sauce
- 2 1/2 teaspoons fresh ginger, finely grated
- 4 scallions, thinly sliced (plus more for serving)
- 1 1/2 cups chicken broth
- 2 tablespoons coconut oil
- 1 bunch bok choy, chopped
- 1/2 teaspoon red pepper flakes (** more depending on your heat level)
- 1/2 teaspoon kosher salt
- 1/2 teaspoon freshly ground black pepper

Direction

- In a medium bowl, combine the garlic, chicken, soy sauce, ginger, scallions. (Note: Be careful not to over mix)
- Scooping out by the tablespoonful, form mixture into 1"-diameter meatballs
- Heat oil in a large skillet over medium-high heat. Add meatballs and cook, turning occasionally, until golden brown all over, 8–10 minutes. Transfer to a plate
- Combine bok choy and red pepper flakes, along with a pinch each salt & pepper in skillet, and cook over medium-high heat until the greens are crisp & tender (~ 5 minutes)
- Add the meatballs and broth.
- Bring the broth to a boil, reduce heat, and simmer until the meatballs are cooked through (~ 5–8 minutes)
- Serve sprinkled with more scallions

176. Ginger Chicken W/ Braised Baby Bok Choy

Serving: Serves 1 | Prep: | Cook: | Ready in:

Ingredients

- 2 teaspoons vegetable oil
- 1/2 teaspoon toasted sesame oil
- 1 small onion, chopped

- 1 garlic clove, sliced thinly
- 6 ounces cremini (baby bella) mushrooms, sliced
- 2 teaspoons soy sauce
- 2 teaspoons rice vinegar
- 1/4 teaspoon hot sauce
- 1/2 inch chunk of ginger, peeled and sliced into very thin strips
- 2 baby bok choy, cut in half lengthwise
- 1 boneless, skinless chicken breast

Direction

- Heat oil in large skillet and sauté onion until soft, 4-5 minutes. Add garlic and cook 5-6 minutes more. Add mushrooms and cook until they are soft and have released their juices, 8-10 minutes.
- Add soy sauce, hot sauce, vinegar, & ginger, stirring to combine.
- Add baby bok choy, cut side down. Cook 2 minutes, then flip over and cook 2 minutes on the other side. Remove from skillet and set aside.
- Add chicken to skillet, stirring to coat in sauce. Cover and cook 4-5 minutes on each side until cooked through.

177. Goat Cheese And Chicken Stuffed Peppers

Serving: Serves 4-6 | Prep: | Cook: | Ready in:

Ingredients

- 4 Bell Peppers, Deseeded and Halved
- 1 tablespoon Olive Oil
- 4 ounces goat cheese
- 4 ounces canned green chilies
- 1 cup Salsa
- 2 1/2 cups Cooked shredded chicken
- 2 cups Zucchini
- 1/2 cup Cilantro, chopped

Direction

- Preheat oven to 425 and line a large baking pan with parchment paper.
- Cut the peppers in half from top to bottom and scoop out the seeds and place them in the pan with the inside of the pepper facing up.
- Drizzle the peppers with olive oil and sprinkle with salt and roast for 15 minutes.
- While the peppers are roasting combine the goat cheese, green chilies, salsa, chicken, zucchini and cilantro and mix until combined.
- After you pull the peppers out of the oven fill each one with about a ½ cup of filling and bake for another 15-20 minutes.
- Top the peppers with guacamole and chopped cilantro and serve immediately.

178. Grandma Ray's Oyster Stuffing

Serving: Serves 8 | Prep: | Cook: | Ready in:

Ingredients

- 1 Loaf of High quality bread, crust on and cut into 1 inch cubes
- 1/2 cup Butter
- 2 cups Celery, diced
- 2 cups Onion, diced
- 6 Eggs, slightly beaten
- 1/2 cup Parmesan cheese, grated
- 1/2 cup Flat-Leaf Parsley, coarsely chopped
- Salt, to taste
- 1 teaspoon freshly ground pepper
- 1 cup pecans, toasted and chopped
- 3-4 cups Homemade Chicken Stock
- 1 pint, fresh oysters

Direction

- Cube bread and allow to sit for several days to get stale. (Alternately, toast in 200 degrees oven until slightly brown) In skillet, melt butter. Sauté onions and celery until translucent. Add to bread mixture. Add beaten eggs, parmesan cheese, chopped parsley, pecans, salt and pepper. Mix well. Add 3 cups of chicken stock and stir to moisten all. If needed, add more stock until mixture is very moist. Add oysters and stir gently. Turn into greased casserole dish and bake, uncovered for 40 minutes at 350 degrees

179. Grandpas Chicken Noodle Soup From Scratch

Serving: Serves 5 | Prep: | Cook: | Ready in:

Ingredients

- Chicken Stock
- 1 Whole free range chicken, with the skin, (about 3 1/2 pounds), rinsed, giblets discarded
- 2 Carrots, unpeeled cut into large chunks
- 3 Organic celery stalks and leaf cut into chunks
- 2 Large white onions, quartered
- 1 Head of garlic, take it and just cut in in half
- 1 Turnip, quartered
- 1/4 bunch FRESH thyme
- 2 Bay Leaves
- 8 Whole black peppercorns
- Soup
- 2 tablespoons Extra virgin Olive Oil
- 1 Medium Yellow onion chopped
- 3 garlic cloves, minced
- 2 2 medium carrots, cut diagonally into 1/2-inch-thick slices
- 1 Bay Leaf
- 4 fresh thyme sprigs
- 8 ounces Wide egg noodles (found in Kosher foods section)
- 1 1/2 cups shredded cooked chicken
- 1 handful fresh flat-leaf parsley, finely chopped
- 2 dashes Kosher Salt
- 3 dashes Freshly Ground Black Pepper
- 1 pinch Flat-leaf Parsley
- 2 quarts 2 quarts chicken stock, recipe follows

Direction

- For the Stock: Place the chicken and vegetables in a large stockpot over medium heat. Pour in only enough cold water to cover (about 3 quarts); too much will make the broth taste weak. Toss in the thyme, bay leaves, and peppercorns, and allow it to slowly come to a boil. Lower the heat to medium-low and gently simmer for 1 to 1 1/2 hours, partially covered, until the chicken is done. As it cooks, skim any impurities that rise to the surface; add a little more water if necessary to keep the chicken covered while simmering. Carefully remove the chicken to a cutting board. When it's cool enough to handle, discard the skin and bones; hand-shred the meat into a storage container and put in the fridge. Carefully strain the stock through a fine sieve into another pot to remove the vegetable solids. Store the stock, place the pot in a sink full of ice water and stir to cool down the stock. Cover and refrigerate overnight. In the morning take a spoon and remove all the fat from the top.
- For the Soup: Place a soup pot over medium heat and coat with the oil. Add the onion, garlic, carrots, celery, thyme and bay leaf. Cook and stir for about 6 minutes, until the vegetables are softened but not browned. Pour in the chicken stock and bring the liquid to a boil. Add the noodles and simmer for 5 minutes until tender. Fold in the chicken, and continue to simmer for another couple of minutes to heat through; season with salt and pepper. Sprinkle with chopped parsley before serving.

180. Granny Karate's 'Korean' Chicken Remedy Soup (For The Bachelor's Lady's Cold)

Serving: Serves 4-6 generous bowls | Prep: | Cook: | Ready in:

Ingredients

- 2 whole chicken breasts - about 1 lb.
- 3 celery stalks, cleaned and chopped
- 2 carrots, cleaned, peeled and chopped
- 1 1/2 yellow onions, chopped
- 1 teaspoon whole allspice
- 1 teaspoon whole peppercorns
- 6 tablespoons pearl barley, rinsed
- 1/2 bunch of fresh parsley, leaves removed. Keep the stems.
- 1 -3 dashes coconut aminos, soy sauce or tamari
- 10 cups chicken broth (I use Imagine brand, plus a combination of 1-2 cups of frozen leftover homemade chicken stock if I have it on hand)
- 2 small bay leaves
- 1/3 cup kimchee per serving, as garnish

Direction

- Prepare all the ingredients and have them in place.
- Pour the chicken broth into a large saucepot and bring to a boil.
- Place the chicken breasts, spices, chopped vegetables and parsley stems into the boiling broth. Reduce the heat to medium-low, cover, simmer for 30 minutes
- Remove chicken from the broth; slice or shred, and place chicken back in broth.
- Drain the rinsed barley and place in the soup.
- Boil gently for 1 hour and remove from heat.
- Ladle desired amount of soup into individual serving bowls. I put a ladle of soup into a strainer over the bowl and fish out the peppercorns and allspice. Then I throw the chicken and vegetables into the bowl. Top with 1/3 cup of chopped up kimchee, a dash or two of coconut aminos and some chopped parsley leaves.

181. Greek Chicken With Herbed Yogurt Sauce

Serving: Serves 4 | Prep: | Cook: | Ready in:

Ingredients

- 1 cup plain low-fat yogurt
- 2 tablespoons finely grated lemon peel
- 1 ½ tablespoons lemon juice
- 2 tablespoons oregano and parsley, finely chopped
- 1 clove garlic, minced
- ¼ teaspoons salt
- ¼ teaspoons ground pepper
- 1 pound chicken breasts, boneless, skinless

Direction

- Combine the yogurt, lemon peel and juice, oregano, parsley, garlic, salt and pepper.
- Put the chicken into a dish and spread about ¼ cup of the yogurt sauce over the chicken. Cover with plastic wrap and refrigerate several hours or overnight. Cover and refrigerate the remaining yogurt sauce.
- Place the chicken on a rack in a baking pan and bake in a preheated 375°F oven for 30 minutes.
- Turn the oven on to broil and continue cooking about 5 minutes, until the chicken is browned and cooked through. (Adjust the rack higher if necessary)
- Spoon the remaining yogurt sauce over the chicken and serve with veggie confetti salad.
- Per serving: 229 calories, 38 gm protein, 7 gm carbohydrate, 4 gm fat, 1 gm sat, 1 gm mono, 96 mg cholesterol, 1 gm fiber, 273 mg sodium

182. Green Diva Casserole

Serving: Serves 4 | Prep: | Cook: | Ready in:

Ingredients

- 1 large leftover chicken breast, small dice
- 1 head of broccoli, cut into florets
- 2 zucchini, small dice
- 8 ounces package of pasta (macaroni, egg noodle, or penne)
- 2 (15oz) cans of cream of chicken soup
- 15 ounces milk
- 1/3 cup Romano grated cheese, divided
- 1 cup frozen or fresh peas if in season in your garden
- 4 slices of bacon, crisped and crumbled
- 1 teaspoon garlic powder

Direction

- Prepare the pasta to al dente. Blanch the broccoli in the pasta water. Discard the water and drain the pasta and broccoli well.
- In a large bowl, stir together the cream of chicken soup and milk with half of the Romano cheese. Season with garlic powder, salt and pepper to taste.
- Place the zucchini, peas, chicken, bacon, cooked pasta and broccoli in the sauce and stir gently.
- Pour the contents of the bowl into a casserole dish. Sprinkle with the remaining Romano cheese. Cover the dish with foil.
- Bake your Green Diva in a 350ºF oven for 30 - 35 minutes. After baking, let the casserole stand on the stove to let the sauce cool slightly and thicken.

183. Grilled Apricot, Honey, And Habanero Pepper Chicken Wings

Serving: Serves 6 | Prep: | Cook: | Ready in:

Ingredients

- 4 lbs of chicken wings 1 tbsp fresh ginger and garlic 1 tbsp of lemon pepper salt to taste
- 4 pounds 4 lbs of chicken wings
- 1 tablespoon 1 tbsp fresh ginger paste
- 1 tablespoon 1 tbsp fresh ginger paste
- 1 tablespoon lemon pepper
- Pinch salt
- Sauce 1 cup apricot preserve or jam 1/2 cup fresh orange juiced 1 tbsp soy sauce 2 habaneros crushed 1/4 cup honey 1 tbsp olive oil
- 1 cup apricot preserve or jam
- 1/2 cup fresh squeezed orange juice
- 1 tablespoon soy sauce
- 2 habaneros crushed
- 1/4 cup honey
- 1 tablespoon olive oil

Direction

- Marinate the chicken wings for at least 3 hrs.
- After 3 hours put them on the grill
- While the chicken is grilling put the sauce on the heat and let it boil about 15 min,
- once the chicken wings are done dip the wings in the sauce and put them back on the grill for about 3 min just so the sauce gets candid on the wings, make sure you have some wet wipes cause this is going to get messy, very very delicious! Enjoy!

184. Grilled Chicken Bread Salad

Serving: Serves 8 | Prep: | Cook: | Ready in:

Ingredients

- 3/4 of a loaf of day-old crusty, rustic bread, cut into 1-inch thick slices
- 2 large tomatoes (about 1 pound), trimmed and cut in half
- 1 large red bell pepper, halved and seeds removed
- 1 large green bell pepper, halved and seeded
- 1 large red onion, sliced into large rings
- 1/4 cup extra-virgin olive oil
- 1/4 cup red-wine vinegar

- 3 tablespoons water or vegetable stock
- 1 tablespoon capers, rinsed
- 4 4 oz. boneless, skinless chicken breasts
- 1/2 bunch fresh basil leaves, shredded (about 1/4 cup)
- freshly cracked black pepper and kosher salt, to taste

Direction

- Prepare grill for medium-high direct heat. Place bread slices on grate and grill 1 to 2 minutes per side or until golden brown. Remove and set aside to cool slightly before cutting into large chunks.
- Place tomatoes, cut side down, peppers and onion on grate and grill 2 to 3 minutes or until lightly charred. Remove and set aside to cool slightly before cutting into large chunks.
- Place chicken breasts on grill and cook, 5 to 6 minutes per side or until fully cooked. Remove and let stand 30 minutes before chopping into bite-sized pieces.
- In a large salad bowl, whisk together oil, vinegar, water and any liquid released from the grilled tomatoes. Add bread, vegetables and all the remaining ingredients except the basil and toss to coat. Let salad stand at room temperature at least 1 hour, tossing every 20 minutes. Add the chopped chicken and basil and toss just before serving.

185. Grilled Chicken Tacos

Serving: Serves 4 | Prep: | Cook: | Ready in:

Ingredients

- 400 grams chicken breasts
- 1 large red bell pepper
- 2 red onions
- 2 cups shredded lettuce
- salt, pepper to taste
- paprika to taste
- thyme to taste
- olive oil
- balsamic vinegar
- 1 lime
- 2 spring onions
- 1/2 cup sour cream
- fresh chives, finely chopped
- tortillas

Direction

- Prepare chicken: wash and dry chicken meat (I used chicken breast meat). Season with salt, pepper, paprika and thyme. Massage the spices into the meat and cover evenly. Peel and finely slice an onion and add to the chicken meat. Lastly, add a tablespoon of olive oil and spread across the meat, covering it evenly. Set aside to rest in an airtight container for an hour or overnight.
- Prepare vegetables: Wash and dry bell pepper, then cut into slices and season with salt and pepper. Add a sprinkle of olive oil and coat evenly. Peel and finely slice an onion. Wash and shred lettuce and spring onion. Cut lime into quarters.
- Put sour cream into a jar, season with salt & pepper and add finely chopped chives. Combine well.
- Preheat the grill or a grill cast iron skillet (this is what I used). Remove onions from the chicken meat, but don't toss. When the grill is hot, place chicken meat on grill and cook on medium for about 8 minutes, then turn and cook on the other side for an additional couple of minutes, until the meat is cooked through. While the chicken is cooking, heat a pan on medium and add the marinated sliced onions. Cook on medium, stirring frequently, until the onions become crisp. Then, add a splash of balsamic vinegar, combine well and remove from heat. Remove chicken from grill and set aside to rest. Place bell peppers on the grill and cook until they soften and begin to blacken on the edges. Remove and set aside. Warm tortillas on the grill for a minute on each side.

- Cut chicken meat into smaller pieces or slices. Place a handful of shredded lettuce on a taco, add grilled chicken, grilled bell pepper, crispy onion slices and sliced red onion, a spoon of sour cream and a piece of lime. Repeat and serve.

186. Grilled Chicken And Mixed Greens Salad

Serving: Serves 1 | Prep: | Cook: | Ready in:

Ingredients

- 2 cups cups fresh mixed greens
- 1 cucumber
- 1 bell pepper
- 1 carrot
- 1 tablespoon canned corn
- 50 grams grilled chicken (breasts / file)
- parmesan
- 1 slice stale bread
- balsamic vinegar
- olive oil
- lemon
- salt, pepper to taste

Direction

- First things first. If you are not using a pre-grilled chicken file, then first season your chicken and put it in a hot pan to grill on both sides for a couple of minutes. Remove from heat and set aside to cool, then cut into smaller bites.
- Cut the stale bread slice into cubes and put into the pan to toast for a couple of minutes. When toasted, set aside to cool.
- Wash and drain the mixed greens. Use any kind of lettuce you like, or a mixture of it.
- Peel and slice the cucumber. Wash and slice your bell pepper (I had a light-green variety in my garden). Peel the carrot and cut into thin slices (or grate it). Cut cherry tomatoes in half.
- For the dressing, pour in a bowl or small jar olive oil and balsamic vinegar (1:3 ratio), add a squeeze of lemon juice or water, a small pinch of salt and some pepper. Mix well with a whisk or shake in a jar until well combined.
- Assemble your salad. In a bowl, place your washed salad greens, cucumber and bell pepper slices, halved cherry tomatoes, carrot sticks and a tablespoon of canned corn. Add chicken bites and bread croutons.
- Top the salad with some shaved parmesan cheese and the balsamic dressing.

187. Guinea Hen With Salsa Verde

Serving: Serves 6 | Prep: | Cook: | Ready in:

Ingredients

- Guinea Hen Breast
- 6 Guinea Hen breasts
- 1 tablespoon olive oil
- Salt
- Thyme
- Salsa Verde
- 4 cups loosely packed parsley leaves
- 2 cups loosely packed arugula leaves
- 1 cup loosely packed mint leaves
- 1 cup olive oil
- Salt
- 1/4 cup minced shallot
- 1/2 cup red wine vinegar
- Fresh cracked pepper

Direction

- Guinea Hen Breast
- Season the Guinea Hen Breasts evenly and generously with salt and let marinate for at least 6 hours before cooking them.
- Heat the olive oil in a medium-sized skillet over high heat for a minute until it just begins to smoke.

- Add the Guinea Hen, skin side down, to the skillet, then remove the skillet from the heat until the pan stops sizzling.
- Return to low heat, stirring the pan often and cooking for 15 to 20 more minutes while slowly rendering the skin of the Guinea Hen.
- Flip the breast over and finish cooking through, 1 to 2 minutes, adding a handful of thyme to the pan. Allow to rest for 2 minutes before carving and topping with salsa verde.
- Salsa Verde
- Finely chop the parsley, arugula, and mint, mixing them in a large bowl with the olive oil and a generous seasoning of salt to taste.
- Mix the shallot with the red wine vinegar and a hearty dose of fresh black pepper in a separate mixing bowl.
- Allow the shallots to macerate in the vinegar for 10 minutes while the greens break down in the oil.
- Add the shallot mixture to the greens and mix well with a fork, adjusting the seasoning as desired. Salsa Verde should be full flavored and well-seasoned, but highly acidic to bring out the dish it garnishes.

188. Hainanese Chicken Rice

Serving: Serves 4 to 6 | Prep: 0hours30mins | Cook: 0hours45mins | Ready in:

Ingredients

- Chicken and rice
- 1 whole chicken, 3 to 4 pounds
- 1 1/2 tablespoons kosher salt
- 1 three-inch piece of ginger, thinly sliced into 5-6 pieces
- 2 garlic cloves
- 1 bunch scallion
- 2 star anise
- 1/4 teaspoon ground white pepper
- 1 tablespoon sesame oil
- 2 tablespoons vegetable oil
- 2 shallots, minced
- 2 garlic cloves, minced
- 1 one-inch piece of ginger, minced
- 2 cups jasmine rice, rinsed 2 to 3 times to rid it of its excess starch
- 2 teaspoons soy sauce
- 1 tablespoon sesame oil
- 1/2 teaspoon kosher salt
- 2 pandan leaves, optional
- 1 cucumber, sliced, to garnish
- 1 bunch cilantro, to garnish
- Chili sauce
- 5 tablespoons sriracha sauce
- 3 tablespoons chicken broth, from above
- 1 teaspoon soy sauce
- 2 teaspoons lime juice, can be substituted by rice vinegar
- 1 garlic clove, minced
- 1 one-inch piece of ginger

Direction

- Trim any excess fat off the chicken, especially those around the nether-end. Reserve the fatty trimmings. Season the chicken with salt, making sure to season the cavity well. Stuff the chicken with the ginger, garlic, scallions, and star anise. Place the chicken in a large pot, and fill it with water until the chicken is completely submerged (around 4 quarts). When the water starts boiling, turn it down to a simmer, place the lid on the pot, and allow the chicken to cook for 20-25 minutes. (20 minutes is a good time for a 3-pound chicken in my experience.)
- When the chicken is done, remove it from the pot and transfer it to an ice bath. Leave it in the ice bath for 1 minute to halt the cooking process. Remove the chicken from the ice bath, and rub it all over with sesame oil. Let it rest while you prepare the rice and sauce.
- Meanwhile, add the ground white pepper into the chicken cooking broth, and boil until it has reduced by half.
- In a separate pot or saucepan, render the fat off any chicken trimmings you had from earlier by heating it over low heat for about 5

minutes. Then, discard the trimmings. Add in the vegetable oil, and sauté the minced shallots on medium heat for 2-3 minutes until aromatic, then add the minced garlic and ginger and continue sautéing for another minute or so, careful not to let the garlic burn. Then, add in the washed rice and give it a final sauté for a further 1-2 minutes.

- Add the soy sauce, sesame oil, salt, and whole pandan leaves to the rice. Then, pour in the reduced chicken broth until the rice is submerged by ½ an inch of broth. Cook this over high heat until it boils, then turn it down to a simmer and cook, covered, for 15 minutes, or a little more if needed. When cooked, the rice should be glistening and fluffy, with the individual grains of rice still distinguishable. When done, let the rice sit uncovered for 5 minutes to let it steam, then season to taste.
- While waiting for your rice to cook, you can make the sauce by mixing together the sriracha, chicken broth, lime juice, minced garlic, and ginger. Prep the cucumber and cilantro garnishes and carve up the chicken at this point too.
- To serve the rice, you can go traditional and shape it into little mounds using a small Chinese bowl. Serve it with a few slices of chicken, the chili dipping sauce, and garnish with cucumber slices and a few sprigs of cilantro. Oh, and don't forget to serve up some of that aromatic chicken broth as a soup too!

189. Hanoi Inspired Fried Chicken Wings

Serving: Serves 2 hungry people as a main or 4 as an appetizer | Prep: | Cook: |Ready in:

Ingredients

- For the wings
- 2 1/2 pounds whole chicken wings
- 2 tablespoons soy sauce
- 1 cup peanut or neutral oil, may need more depending on your frying vessel
- 1/2 cup rice flour
- For the glaze
- 1 tablespoon minced ginger
- 1 tablespoon minced garlic
- 2 tablespoons water
- 3 tablespoons granulated sugar
- 2 tablespoons fish sauce
- 1 tablespoon plus 1 teaspoon sambal oelek (ground red chile paste - I like Huy Fong brand)
- 1 handful chopped cilantro, for garnish
- 4 lime wedges, for garnish

Direction

- Rinse the chicken wings and cut into three sections: wing, drumettes and tips. Reserve tips for your stock bag. You should end up with a little more than 2 pounds of edible chicken pieces.
- Place chicken in a large bowl with the soy sauce. Toss well to coat and proceed, or you can cover and leave in the refrigerator for a few hours.
- Set aside 1 tablespoon each of minced ginger and garlic for the glaze. Also, set up a metal rack over a baking sheet near your frying station for your wings.
- When you are ready to fry, add peanut oil to a large, deep cast iron pot (such as a French oven) and turn to medium. The oil should come up about 1 1/2 to 2 inches high on the sides, so you may need more or less than 1 cup of oil depending on your frying vessel. Place a deep-fry thermometer in the pot and bring oil to between 350 and 375 degrees F.
- While you are waiting for the oil to heat, add 1/2 cup rice flour to a large bowl. Add wings one at a time and toss with your fingers to lightly coat each piece with flour. Set coated wings aside on a baking tray.
- When the oil is ready, add half the wings and immediately turn the heat up high to compensate for the temperature drop. Once the oil returns to around 350F, dial the heat

back down. The main goal is to try to keep the temperature as close to 350 as you can. If you have the temperature at around 350 (and you fry relatively small batches -- I fried 10 at a time), each batch of wings should take 6-8 minutes to cook through and get golden brown. Using tongs, remove each piece and set on the rack to drain and cool. Check your oil temperature and fry the second batch using the same method.
- Now make your sauce. In a wide skillet (nonstick is nice here) heated to medium, add 3 tablespoons of the frying oil. (Feel free to use fresh oil if you prefer.) Sauté the garlic and ginger until translucent, slightly golden and aromatic. Add 2 tablespoons of water and 3 tablespoons granulated sugar. Stir to combine and cook until the sugar melts and the sauce becomes foamy and glossy, about 2-3 minutes. Add 2 tablespoons fish sauce and cook an additional 2-3 minutes. The glaze should be slightly thickened by now. Finally, add 1 tablespoon plus 1 teaspoon of sambal oelek. Taste and add additional sambal oelek, if desired. Give the sauce a last stir to combine and add all the chicken pieces back to the skillet. Turn the pieces several times to coat with the glaze.
- Pile the chicken wings/drumettes in a serving bowl and garnish with cilantro. Serve with lime wedges for a nice hit of acidity and additional chile-garlic sauce for chile heads.

190. Harissa Turkey With Pomegranate Cous Cous

Serving: Serves 2 | Prep: | Cook: | Ready in:

Ingredients

- Turkey
- 2 turkey breast escalopes
- 2 tablespoons Harissa paste
- 1 splash olive oil
- 1 pinch salt and pepper
- Pomegranate Cous Cous
- 1 cup cous cous (uncooked)
- 1- 1.5 cups boiling water
- 1 Pomegranate (seeds from)
- large handfuls fresh coriander, chopped
- 2 tablespoons balsamic vinegar
- 1 pinch salt and pepper
- 4 tablespoons Natural Greek yoghurt (garnish: optional)

Direction

- Preheat the oven to 200C. In a roasting tray, lay the turkey escalopes out. Cover in the Harissa paste, some olive oil, salt and pepper, and bake in the oven for 15 minutes.
- Meanwhile, in a mixing bowl, put boiling water over the couscous and cover for at least 5 minutes (or until the couscous is cooked). Add the pomegranate, coriander, dressing to the cooked couscous, season to taste, then set aside.
- Remove the turkey from the oven, and serve with the couscous and a few generous tablespoons of Greek yoghurt (optional)

191. Harvest Stuffing

Serving: Serves at least 10 as a side dish | Prep: | Cook: | Ready in:

Ingredients

- For the Corn Bread
- 1 cup cornmeal
- 1 cup flour
- 1/3 cup granulated sugar
- 1 tablespoon baking powder
- 3/4 teaspoon kosher salt
- 1 egg
- 1 cup milk
- 1/3 cup (5 1/2 tablespoons) butter, melted, or vegetable oil
- For the Stuffing/Dressing

- 2 16-20 oz. loaves French or Italian bread
- 1 turkey, of any size
- 1 stick butter, divided
- 1 large yellow onion
- 1 stalk celery
- 2 whole carrots
- Kosher salt
- Coarse ground pepper
- 5-10 leaves of dried fresh sage, rubbed between palms into a pile of fluff, or 1 tablespoon dried sage

Direction

- As early as possible the day before Thanksgiving, turn the oven to 400 degrees. Grease a 9" baking pan, casserole or round cake pan.
- Place the cornmeal, flour, sugar, baking powder and salt in a medium mixing bowl and stir together. Add the egg, milk and melted butter; with a rubber scraper, stir and fold all ingredients together until moistened, being careful to not over mix.
- Pour into the prepared pan and bake for 15 to 20 minutes or until a toothpick poked into the middle comes out clean. Allow to cool.
- Cut the French bread into cubes, pile onto two cookie sheets and set aside.
- Heat oven to 400 degrees. Melt half a stick of butter in an oven-safe Dutch oven or a 4-quart casserole with a tight-fitting lid. Remove the giblets from the turkey, along with the "Pope's nose," and rinse with cold water; place in the Dutch oven. (Rinse the turkey with cold water, place in a roasting pan and put the whole thing inside a plastic trash can liner; keep refrigerated until ready to roast.)
- Cut off the root end of the onion and discard. Carefully cut through the peel and two layers of the onion; put this section into the Dutch oven, peel and all. Dice the center of the onion and reserve, refrigerated in a plastic bag until needed. Wash celery and chop off the entire leafy top of the stalk; place in Dutch oven. Remove three or four of the outer ribs of the celery stalk; wash and slice, then refrigerate the slices in a plastic bag until needed. Cut the top off the carrots and discard; place carrots in the Dutch oven. Sprinkle with 1 tsp. of kosher salt and 1/2 tsp. pepper. Place in oven and roast uncovered, stirring occasionally, until turkey and vegetables are browned, about 1 1/2 hours.
- Bring three quarts of water and two teaspoons of kosher salt to a boil. When turkey parts and vegetables have caramelized, carefully pour or ladle the hot water into the Dutch oven. Turn the oven down to 200 degrees and allow stock to simmer for an hour. Put the cookie sheets of French bread into the oven to dry, stirring once or twice. Let stock cool to room temperature, taste it and correct the seasoning by adding additional salt, pepper or water, and refrigerate. Put bread cubes into a very large mixing bowl, coarsely crumble the cornbread over the bread and set aside, uncovered.
- On Thanksgiving morning, strain the turkey stock through a colander and discard everything except the turkey neck; bring the stock to a simmer over medium-low heat. Melt 1/2 stick of butter over low heat in a small saucepan; stir in the reserved onions and allow to cook slowly until soft, about five minutes. Pour over dried bread cubes and stir in the reserved sliced celery. Sprinkle with three tablespoons of the freshly-rubbed sage, then ladle over enough of the stock make the bread moist without being soppy wet. Mix well. Taste, and add more sage, salt and pepper if needed. Strain, reserve and refrigerate the remainder of the stock for making gravy.
- Remove turkey from refrigerator and fill both ends of the bird loosely with the stuffing. Roast according to directions on wrapper. Place remainder of the stuffing into a buttered casserole, top with the turkey neck, cover and refrigerate until one hour before serving; reheat at 350 for about an hour. Remove stuffing from turkey before carving it; mix with reheated dressing if desired.

192. Hearty Chicken Harvest Dinner

Serving: Serves 4 | Prep: | Cook: |Ready in:

Ingredients

- ¾ pounds chicken breasts, boneless, skinless
- 1 tablespoon olive oil
- Olive oil spray
- 1 medium onion, thinly sliced
- 2 bell peppers, yellow or red, sliced
- 1 garlic clove, minced
- 1 14-16 ounce can diced tomatoes, low-sodium
- ? cups chicken stock, low-sodium or white wine
- 1 tablespoon each oregano and basil
- 1 cup canned cannellini beans, rinsed and drained

Direction

- Over medium heat, sauté the chicken in olive oil in a nonstick pan until golden brown. Remove from pan.
- Spray pan with olive oil, add onion, peppers, garlic and sauté until onions are translucent, 3-5 minutes.
- Add tomatoes with juice and stir. Place the chicken over mixture, add stock and sprinkle with herbs.
- Cover the pan and simmer for 30 minutes, stirring occasionally. To test when chicken is done, poke a knife in meat and juices should run clear.
- Mash half of the beans, then add to pot and stir into liquid until sauce thickens. Add the rest of beans and simmer for 5 minutes more. Serve in bowls with green salad and crusty bread.
- Per serving: 324 calories, 28g protein, 29g carbohydrate, 8g fat, 2g sat, 4g mono, 78mg cholesterol, 6g fiber, 293mg sodium

193. Hill Country Honey Bacon Quail

Serving: Serves 4 | Prep: | Cook: |Ready in:

Ingredients

- 4 semi boneless quail
- 2-3 slices of bacon (mine were very long so I used 2)
- 1/4 cup finely diced shallot (one very large shallot)
- 2 teaspoons fresh thyme
- 1 tablespoon olive oil
- 2-3 pinches aleppo pepper (or sub pepper flakes if you can't get your hands on aleppo - they will be spicier, a hint of heat is a good thing)
- 2-3 pinches salt
- 1 tablespoon honey
- 1/2 cup dry white wine
- 1-2 sliced green onions (I used 1 but ours are huge)

Direction

- Lightly season the quail on both sides with salt and set aside. Crisp the bacon up in a large non-stick skillet big enough to later accommodate the 4 quail. Remove it and set aside. Leave the fat in there.
- Add the olive oil to the pan and set the heat medium-high. Add the shallots and cook them until they are just clear, 3 or 4 minutes. Now push the shallots to the edges and add in the quail breast side down. Let them brown to just golden on one side. This won't take long, just a few minutes. You don't want to overcook the quail, they can get a bit of a livery flavor if you do, and they don't need anywhere near the cook time of other birds. Flip the quail and add the Aleppo pepper, thyme, honey and wine. Now turn the heat down a bit and let this all reduce to a nice glaze. Flip the quail back and forth a few times so that they get glazed all over, and taste for salt. They will

look like an odd shiny little dance troupe in the pan, which makes it more fun to cook them. Your total cook time will be around 10 minutes or so. In the last minute, add the green onions to just barely cook them, and finish them with the bacon that you have crumbled up.
- If the look of the whole quail weirds you out, half them to serve (over lentils is nice) or if you are a sick twist like me just arrange them doing the jitterbug on your plate and dig in.

194. Homemade Chicken Noodle Soup

Serving: Serves 6 | Prep: | Cook: | Ready in:

Ingredients

- 1 half chicken cut up and skin removed (or two chicken breast halves, bone-in, no skin)
- 12 cups water
- 3 cloves garlic, whole
- 1 onion, quartered
- 2 stalks of celery (chopped in 3 pieces each)
- 2 carrots (chopped in 3 pieces each)
- 3 bay leaves
- 1 bouquet of parsley or cilantro
- 6 shiitake mushrooms
- 4 green onions
- a handful of cilantro leaves
- Sambal Oelek chili paste

Direction

- Put the first 8 ingredients to a large stockpot, bring to a boil (high heat) and then reduce to simmer (medium-high heat).
- Simmer for 25-30 minutes, skimming from time to time and seasoning as needed.
- Chop chicken into large pieces and reserve.
- Strain the broth through a fine mesh sieve and discard the cooked veggies and herbs.
- After straining the broth, return it to a boil on the stove.

- Add two packages of unflavored Raman noodles—you can get the flavored kind and just throw away the little seasoning packet.
- Hakubaku makes the best organic dried noodles, including ramen, I found them at Cost Plus World Market.
- Stir periodically while that cooks, it'll take about three minutes.
- For your garnish, thinly slice six shitake mushrooms and four green onions, sliced thin on the bias and a few fresh cilantro leaves.
- When the Ramen is cooked, stir in the chicken, and then pour into bowls.
- Sprinkle the raw mushroom, onion and cilantro and stir in about 1/2 tsp. of Sambal Oelek chili paste to each bowl (the chili paste is spicy so use it at your own discretion).

195. Honey Vanilla Glazed Chicken Over Sweet Vanilla Rice

Serving: Serves 4 | Prep: | Cook: | Ready in:

Ingredients

- The chicken
- 4 bone in, skin on chicken thighs
- 1 cup AP flour
- 1 teaspoon salt
- 1/2 teaspoon black pepper
- Vegetable oil for pan frying
- 1/2 cup light brown sugar
- 1/2 cup honey
- 1 teaspoon vanilla extract
- 1/8 teaspoon cayenne pepper (optional)
- Sweet vanilla Rice
- 1 1/2 cups long grain rice
- 3 cups water
- 2 tablespoons honey
- 1 1/2 teaspoons vanilla extract, divided
- 1 tablespoon butter
- A pinch of salt
- 2 green onions, thinly sliced for garnish

- 1/2 cup chopped cashews for garnish

Direction

- The chicken
- Whisk the flour, salt and pepper together in a shallow bowl. Heat the oil in a large skillet. Dredge the chicken pieces in the flour mixture and Brown them in the oil on both sides until lightly golden. Remove and place in an appropriate sized baking dish.
- In a small sauce pan, combine the honey and brown sugar and gently heat until just boiling. Remove from the heat and stir in the vanilla and cayenne if using.
- Brush the tops of the chicken thighs with half of the glaze and bake in a pre-heated 325F oven for 20 minutes. After 20 minutes raise the oven temp to 350F and brush the thighs with the remaining glaze.(you'll probably have to re warm the glaze a bit in order to spread) Bake another 20 to 25 minutes.
- Sweet vanilla Rice
- In a medium sauce pan, combine the rice, water, honey, butter, salt and one teaspoon of the vanilla extract. Bring up to a boil and then simmer, covered for 15 to 18 minutes until the liquid is absorbed into the rice, stirring once or twice. Once done, remove from the heat and stir in that 1/2 teaspoon of vanilla extract.
- To serve, place 1/4 of the rice on each of 4 plates, top with a piece of the chicken and garnish with the green onions and cashews.

196. Honey And Garlic Chicken Stew

Serving: Serves 8 | Prep: | Cook: | Ready in:

Ingredients

- 1 Free range chicken, chopped in main parts
- 1/4 cup Olive oil
- 3 tablespoons Honey
- 2 teaspoons Ground cumin
- 2 teaspoons Ground turmeric
- 2 tablespoons Ground cinnamon
- 12 garlic cloves, chopped or grated
- 2 tablespoons sea salt
- 1 chilli, chopped
- 2 red onions, quartered
- 10 red small potatoes, halved
- 1 cup raisins
- 1 cup dried prunes
- water

Direction

- Mix all the spices into the olive oil. Place chopped chicken and cut vegetables into a big bowl and massage with a marinade. Keep in a fridge covered for 24-48 hours.
- Once ready to cook, remove from the fridge, stir once again, transfer to the slow cooker, cover with water and cook on a low heat for 6 hours.
- Serve with Basmati rice or bulgur.

197. Hot Smoked Paprika, Oregano Flower & Pepper BBQ'd Chicken

Serving: Serves 4-6 | Prep: | Cook: | Ready in:

Ingredients

- Chicken
- 1 Large Organic Chicken (I always try and go with the best quality you can afford and try and avoid buying from supermarkets)
- 1 Glug of Olive Oil
- Hot Chicken Rub
- 2 teaspoons Hot smoked paprika
- 1 teaspoon White Pepper
- 2 pinches Freshly Ground Black Pepper
- generous pinches Smoked Sea Salt
- 1 handful Dried/Fresh Oregano Flowers/Leaves
- 1 teaspoon Fennel Seeds

Direction

- Remove any string from the bird and rinse, place in a pan and drizzle with olive oil then combine all the hot rub ingredients together and sprinkle over and rub into the skin and legs of the bird.
- Allow to marinate if you have time for an hour or so or transfer straight to a hot BBQ. Place the lid on the BBQ and cook it breast side up- this saves the breast from burning .Cook for 20-25minutes and then slice into the thigh and side of the breast to see how thoroughly it's cooked through. Only serve when the juice from the chicken runs clear.
- Cook for a further ten minutes and check again. Allow to rest for at least 5 minutes before serving. You can also keep it warm on a higher shelf over the BBQ while you cook any sausages or vegetables.

198. Huckleberry Glazed Chicken Wings

Serving: Serves 4 | Prep: | Cook: | Ready in:

Ingredients

- 2 pounds chicken wings, split at the joints and tips removed
- 1/2 teaspoon Kosher Salt
- 1/4 teaspoon Fresh Ground Black Pepper
- 1/4 cup Fresh Huckleberries (or Blueberries)
- 1/4 cup Low-Sodium Soy Sauce
- 2 tablespoons Rice Wine Vinegar
- 3 tablespoons Light Brown Sugar
- 1 tablespoon Extra Virgin Olive Oil
- 1/2 teaspoon fresh minced Garlic
- 1/4 teaspoon Crushed Red Pepper Flakes
- 1/2 teaspoon Roasted Sesame Seeds
- 1/2 teaspoon Ground Ginger
- 1/8 cup sliced Green Onion

Direction

- Position the lower oven rack on the bottom third of the oven and preheat the oven to 450 degrees (F).
- Pat the wings dry and sprinkle them with kosher salt and ground pepper, to taste. Spread the wings out evenly in a 9x13 baking dish and bake the wings, flipping them over halfway through, for 40 minutes.
- While the wings are baking, combine in a food processor or blender the huckleberries, low-sodium soy sauce, rice wine vinegar, light brown sugar, olive oil, garlic, roasted sesame seeds, red pepper flakes and ground ginger. Blend until sauce is smooth. Transfer the huckleberry sauce to a small saucepan and simmer on low until slightly reduced.
- Once the wings are done baking, remove the wings from the baking dish and place them in the large bowl with the huckleberry sauce. Toss the wings until fully coated with the sauce and then return the wings to the baking dish to continue baking for 3-5 minutes until glazed.
- Plate the wings and garnish them with sesame seeds and green onion.

199. Huli Huli Wings

Serving: Makes about 15-18 wings | Prep: | Cook: | Ready in:

Ingredients

- Wings
- 1.5 cups Finely Chopped Pineapple
- 2 cups Huli Huli Sauce
- 3 pounds Chicken Wings, split and tips removed if preferred
- Huli Huli Sauce
- 1 cup Low Sodium Soy Sauce
- 2 tablespoons minced garlic
- 2 tablespoons minced ginger
- 1 juice of lime
- 2 tablespoons brown sugar
- 2 tablespoons ketchup

- 1 teaspoon Sriracha

Direction

- Wings
- Add pineapple and 1/2 of Huli-Huli sauce into gallon plastic bag.
- Add chicken wings, toss to coat. Seal bag removing all air.
- Marinate 25 minutes in refrigerator.
- Preheat grill to medium heat. Place on grill pouring excess marinade over wings. Grill 15-25 minutes or until chicken is no longer pink inside flipping once.
- Once cooked, remove from grill placing in large bowl with remaining Huli-Huli sauce. Toss to coat. Serve.
- Huli Huli Sauce
- Combine ingredients in sauce pan and bring to a boil. Simmer over medium heat until reduced to approx. 2 cups and sugar is completely dissolved. Remove from heat and split into two portions.

200. In The Midwest, We BAKE Chicken (with Lime, Spices And Garlic)

Serving: Serves 4-6 | Prep: | Cook: | Ready in:

Ingredients

- 8 bone in, skin on, chicken thighs and drumsticks
- 1 tablespoon kosher salt
- 2 tablespoons olive oil
- 2 tablespoons water
- pepper
- juice of 2 limes
- 2 teaspoons ground ginger
- 2 teaspoons curry powder
- 1/2 teaspoon cayenne pepper
- 2 cloves minced garlic

Direction

- Stir the kosher salt into 4 cups of water until dissolved. Pour over the chicken pieces in a plastic container with a lid and refrigerate for several hours or overnight.
- Pat chicken dry. Discard brine. Preheat oven to 400.
- Mix together oil, water, spices and minced garlic. Paint chicken with flavoring paste. Place on rimmed baking sheet covered with foil or on a rack (really, the rack is better but I don't have one). Bake with skin side up for about 40 minutes, until juices in the thigh run clear. If you have extra spice mixture you can baste the chicken, but leave at least 30 minutes for the skin to crisp. If necessary, turn up the heat to 450 for 5 or 10 minutes to be sure that the skin crisps.
- Enjoy with a cold beer!

201. Iranian/Persian Fesenjoon (walnut And Pomegranate Dish) With Rice

Serving: Serves 6-8 | Prep: | Cook: | Ready in:

Ingredients

- 2 cups Walnuts
- 1 Packed cup of grated (raw) or pureed (cooked) butternut squash or pumpkin
- 2.5 cups water
- 10-12 Dried golden plums (optional)
- 6 pieces Boneless, skinless chicken thighs (all visible fat trimmed)
- 1 Medium onion, minced
- 1 tablespoon Olive oil
- 1/2 cup Pomegranate molasses
- 2-3 tablespoons Brown sugar
- Salt and pepper to taste.

Direction

- Place the walnuts on a baking sheet and roast in a 350-degree oven for 5-10 minutes or until they start to change color. Let cool. This can be done ahead of time.
- Finely chop the walnuts to a coarse meal in a food processor.
- Put the walnuts, grated squash or pumpkin, dried plums (optional), and water in a medium pot. Add salt and pepper to taste. Cover and cook over medium heat for 30 minutes. Stir once or twice.
- Put the minced onions and olive oil in a small pot. Roll the chicken thighs and place them seam-side down on the bed of minced onions. Salt and pepper to taste. Cover and cook over medium heat for 10-12 minutes or until the onions start to caramelize.
- Add the pomegranate molasses to the walnut sauce. Add brown sugar, one tablespoon at a time, to the desired sweetness. Remove the chicken thighs to a side plate and scrape off the caramelized onions into the walnut sauce. Stir and adjust for the desired saltiness and sweetness. Place the pieces of chicken in the sauce. Cover the pot and simmer over medium low heat for another sixty minutes. If needed, add a tablespoon or two of water. Note: The sauce should not be too thin. If it is thinner than desired, leave the cover off during the last 15-20 minutes of cooking.
- Serve over parboiled and steamed Basmati rice. Left over khoresht (stew) freezes well.

202. Italian Chicken And Vegetable Casserole

Serving: Serves 12-18 | Prep: | Cook: | Ready in:

Ingredients

- Sauce
- 28 ounces DOP San Marzano tomatoes
- 6 ounces tomato paste
- 2 tablespoons rosemary
- 2 tablespoons thyme
- 2 tablespoons oregano
- 1 tablespoon white pepper
- 1 tablespoon black pepper
- 1 tablespoon ground cayenne pepper
- 1 tablespoon red pepper flakes
- 2 sweet onions, finely diced
- 2 red bell peppers, finely diced
- 2 tablespoons roasted garlic, minced
- Casserole and Assembly
- 4-5 cups head cauliflower, chopped large
- 4-5 cups broccoli, chopped large
- 8 ounces ricotta
- 8 ounces cream cheese
- 1 tablespoon white pepper
- 1 tablespoon oregano
- 1 egg
- 2 roasted chickens, rough pull meat
- 8 ounces shredded mozzarella
- 8 ounces shredded Italian 4-cheese mix

Direction

- Sauce
- Dice and start to caramelize the onion in some EVOO. About halfway through, add in the peppers. Half is used for the sauce; the other half for the dish.
- Put all of the ingredients for the sauce, including half of the onion and peppers, in a food processor and blend well.
- Casserole and Assembly
- The deli counters at most store do a nice job with roasting chickens, so I just buy two whole roasted chickens and pull the meat, which saves hours of roasting time.
- Layer 1: Pour a cup of sauce into the pepper and onions and place in the bottom of a large/tall casserole.
- Layer 2: Combine ricotta and softened cream cheese with an egg, white pepper, and oregano. Mix the broccoli and cauliflower into the ricotta mixture and layer onto the onions and peppers.
- Layer 3: 8 oz. shredded mozzarella.
- Layer 4: Mix 2 cups of sauce with the chicken, and layer onto the cheese.

- Layer 5: Add the remaining sauce; top with 8 oz. Italian cheese mixture.
- Cover and bake for 45 minutes at 350 F. Serve with a dusting of grated parmesan cheese.
- About 1/18 of this is a pretty reasonable serving, clocking in at only about 260 calories (12 g fat and 17 total carbs)

203. Italian Lemon Chicken Bowtie Pasta Salad

Serving: Serves 4 | Prep: | Cook: |Ready in:

Ingredients

- 1 box of bowtie pasta
- 1 large can of white meat chicken (12.5 oz)
- 1 large bundle of fresh asparagus, washed and cut into thirds
- 1/2 onion, minced
- 1 stalk celery, minced
- 1 tomato, cut into small pieces
- 1/3 cup lemon juice
- 1/4 cup olive oil
- 1 TBSP dried oregano
- 1 tsp lemon pepper
- 1 tsp minced garlic
- salt to taste

Direction

- Put your pasta on to boil in salt water. Mix the dressing of lemon juice, olive oil, oregano, lemon pepper and garlic in a bowl with a whisk. Place the chopped onion and celery in a bowl and sprinkle well with salt--this should sit about 10 minutes to draw out some of the water, which will give it a slight softer texture. After 10 minutes, rinse and toss into a large mixing bowl.
- . The asparagus should be fresh and green, not wilted--cut the bundle into thirds, place the pieces in a medium-sized pot and open the can of chicken--pour the chicken stock over the asparagus and add enough water to barely cover it, then a pinch of salt. Bring up to a simmer on medium heat and cook for no longer than 7 minutes--you want the asparagus done, but still firm. After the asparagus has finished lightly cooking, pour it into a strainer and rinse with cool water, set aside. Drain the pasta when done--again, you want it firm, not mushy--rinse with cold water.
- Add pasta, asparagus, and chopped tomatoes to the bowl with the celery and onions, pour the dressing over it and toss until it's distributed throughout. You can eat this pasta salad now, or chill for an hour for even better flavor serve it with stir-fried squash & zucchini and vegetable crackers.

204. Italian Style Breaded Chicken

Serving: Serves 2-4 (depending on the size of chicken) | Prep: | Cook: |Ready in:

Ingredients

- 2 Chicken Breasts, pounded to the same thickness & cut into 4 large pieces
- 2 Eggs
- 1 tablespoon Whole Milk
- 1/3 - 1/2 cups Dry Breadcrumbs (Make sure its gluten free if you are)
- 2 teaspoons Poultry Seasoning
- 1 teaspoon 21 Seasoning Salute
- 1/2 teaspoon Red Pepper Flakes
- 1/3 cup Parmesan Cheese
- 1 tablespoon Olive Oil
- Salt & Pepper

Direction

- Heat a skillet on medium/high heat and add oil to the skillet.
- Whisk Eggs and Milk together and place on a dish.

- Mix Breadcrumbs, Seasonings and Parmesan Cheese together and place on another dish.
- Take 1 Chicken Breast at a time and coat with wet mixture then dry mixture, dipping in every coating twice.
- Place all chicken pieces in the skillet and cover with a lid for 2 - 4 minutes.
- The chicken should start to become brown (if they are burning, turn down the heat) on the one side. Flip sides and let cook (can add more oil if needed) uncovered, for another 2 - 4 minutes until the chicken is golden brown and tender (making sure they are cooked all the way through). Enjoy!

205. Japanese Cream Stew (クリームシチュ)

Serving: Serves 8 | Prep: | Cook: | Ready in:

Ingredients

- 1 box of House Kokumaro stew cream sauce mix
- 2/3 pound chicken or pork
- 2 medium onions
- 2 medium potatoes
- 1 medium carrot
- 1/2 medium kabocha
- 1/2 cup sweet corn
- 3 1/3 cups water
- 1 1/4 cups milk
- 1 cup cheese

Direction

- Cut chicken or pork, onions, potatoes, carrot, and kabocha into bite sizes. Add onions, chicken or pork, potatoes, carrot, kabocha, and sweet corn to pan. Sauté in pan until lightly browned.
- Add 3 1/3 cups of water and bring to boil. Cook over low to medium heat for about 15 minutes, or until tender.
- Remove from heat. Break stew cream sauce mix into pieces and add to pan. Cook over low heat for about 5 minutes, or until sauce thickens. Add 1 1/4 cups of milk and cook over low heat for about 5 minutes.
- The stew is ready to serve. I love to serve mine over rice and sprinkle with cheese. Enjoy!

206. Jerk Chicken & Mango Kabobs

Serving: Serves 2-4 | Prep: | Cook: | Ready in:

Ingredients

- juice from 2 limes
- 1 tablespoon chili powder
- 1 teaspoon cayenne
- 1 teaspoon dried thyme
- 1/2 teaspoon allspice
- salt and pepper to taste
- 2 garlic cloves, minced
- 1 tablespoon brown sugar
- 1/4 teaspoon cinnamon
- 1 jalapeno, seeded and chopped
- 1 tablespoon olive oil
- 3-4 skinless and boneless chicken thighs, cut into strips/cubes
- 2 mangoes, cubed
- 1 red bell pepper, cut into chunks

Direction

- In a large plastic resealable bag, combine lime juice, cayenne pepper, thyme, allspice, salt, pepper, garlic, brown sugar, jalapeno, olive oil, and cinnamon. Seal bag and squish together to mix everything up. Add chicken thighs and marinate for at least 30 minutes.
- Light a grill under medium high heat. Put skewers together by alternating, chicken, mangoes, and red bell pepper.
- Grill for about 5 to 10 minutes, depending on the thickness of your chicken chunks, and

allowing chicken to become cooked throughout. Serve with fresh pineapple!

207. Judie's Beggar's Chicken

Serving: Serves 4-6 | Prep: | Cook: |Ready in:

Ingredients

- 1 Whole Chicken, 1.5 kg
- 10 grams tong sum (Codonopsis Pilosula)
- 10 grams dong quai (Angelica sinensis)
- 5 grams kei chee (Wolfberries)
- 10 grams ried longan flesh
- 3 teaspoons salt
- 1000 grams plain flour
- water for dough mixture
- aluminium foil

Direction

- Clean the Chicken and rub the whole chicken, inside & outside with half of the salt
- Heat up oven to 220°C. Put all the herbs + 1 Tbsp. Chinese Wine in a pot together with the 1 cup water and the rest of the salt and bring to a boil, reduce heat and simmer for further 5 minutes
- Place the chicken parcel in the center and bring the dough up to enclose the chicken securely and overlap the edges and knead to seal the dough crust close ...place it on a baking sheet and bake in the pre-heated oven for 2 hours
- When done, use a pestle or kitchen chopper and break open the flour dough crust, open the foil & bag/cling film carefully and tip the chicken and gravy into a serving dish, drizzle the balance of the Chinese Wine over the chicken and serve up as it is with a salad or served up with plain steamed rice and a stir-fried vegetable dish.

208. Kerala Chicken Stew

Serving: Serves 8 | Prep: 0hours10mins | Cook: 0hours45mins |Ready in:

Ingredients

- 2.5" Cinnamon stick
- 4 Cardamom pods
- 8 Cloves
- 20 Whole black peppercorns
- 1 teaspoon Garam masala
- 1/2 teaspoon Turmeric
- 1/4 teaspoon Fennel powder
- 1 teaspoon Finely ground black pepper
- 7 Thai green chilies, slit
- 35 Curry leaves
- 5 Cloves of garlic, minced
- 1 13.5 oz can of coconut milk
- 1/2 cup Coconut cream
- 150 grams Petite-cut carrots
- 400 grams Yukon gold potatoes, cut into bite-size cubes
- 1 tablespoon Lemon juice
- 300 grams Finely sliced yellow onions
- 1000 grams Boneless skinless chicken thighs, cut into bite-size pieces
- 3 tablespoons Coconut oil
- 1 teaspoon Ginger paste
- Salt, to taste

Direction

- Get all your ingredients ready for mise en place: Keep cinnamon, cardamom, cloves, and whole pepper together. Keep garam masala, turmeric, pepper powder, and fennel powder together. Keep minced garlic and ginger paste together. Keep coconut milk and coconut cream together. Keep carrots and potatoes together. Keep green chilies and curry leaves together. Keep chopped chicken in a bowl
- In a Dutch oven, heat the oil on medium, and fry the whole spices for a minute.
- Add onions and continue to fry for 10 minutes

- Add powdered spices and fry for a couple of minutes. Add oil as needed to prevent the spices from burning.
- Add minced garlic and ginger and fry until the raw smell goes.
- Add curry leaves and cook for 3 minutes. Watch out, as they may sputter. Turn down the temperature if it starts to sputter.
- Add carrots and potatoes and cook for 3 minutes.
- Add chicken and cook for 5 minutes.
- Add coconut milk, coconut cream, and salt
- Bring everything to a boil, then cover and let it simmer for 30 minutes.
- Finish with the lemon juice.

209. Kitchen Sink Chicken And Vegetable Curry

Serving: Serves 4 to 6 | Prep: 0hours30mins | Cook: 0hours30mins | Ready in:

Ingredients

- 2 tablespoons olive oil
- 1 small head cauliflower, broken into medium sized florets
- 1 medium eggplant, skin on, sliced lengthwise into 8 wedges
- salt and pepper for roasting eggplant and cauliflower
- 2 tablespoons oil - canola, vegetable, or olive oil
- 1 medium onion, chopped
- 2 cloves garlic, minced
- 2 stalks celery, sliced lengthwise and then chopped
- 2 tablespoons curry powder (Penzey's or The Spice Hunter)
- 1/4 teaspoon garam masala, for the sauce, plus extra to sprinkle on the eggplant and cauliflower
- 1 firm, tart apple or Asian pear, chopped
- 1 banana, chopped roughly
- 1 bay leaf
- 2 teaspoons tomato paste
- 2 to 3 cups chicken stock
- 2 cups cooked chicken, roughly chopped in bitesize pieces
- 1/3 cup dried black currants
- 1/2 cup dry roasted unsalted cashews, or other nutmeats

Direction

- Preheat the oven to 400 degrees. Prepare the eggplant wedges and cauliflower florets in a metal half sheet pan. Sprinkle with 2 TBS olive oil, salt, pepper and a little sprinkling of garam masala. Thoroughly mix with your clean hands. Place the vegetables in the lower third of the oven. After 15 minutes, turn the vegetables. After another 15 minutes, remove the eggplant, which should be tender yet firm and not falling apart. Keep the cauliflower in the oven for another 15 to 20 minutes, until browned. Remove from oven.
- In the meantime, heat the other 2 TBS. of oil in a large sauté pan or skillet over medium heat. Add the onion, celery, and garlic and sauté for about 8 minutes, but do not brown. Add the curry powder and the 1/4 TSP. of garam masala. Mix the spices into the onion mixture, and cook on medium low heat for a few minutes. Add the bay leaf, the apple, and the banana. Continue to stir until the spices cover all the contents of the pan. Add the tomato paste and chicken stock and mix well. Bring to a boil, then turn the flame down to simmer. Cover and cook for about 20 to 30 minutes, until the vegetables are tender. Remove from heat.
- Ladle a little less than half of the curry mixture into a blender or food processor and blend until pureed. Return the puree to the sauce pan with the unblended mixture, and mix the sauce so it is well incorporated. (Note: if you want a thinner finished sauce, use about one-third of the mixture for the blender.)
- Chop the cooled eggplant into 2" chunks. Add the eggplant, the roasted cauliflower, the

cooked chicken, and the currants to the curry sauce. Cover and cook over medium heat until the mixture is simmering lightly. Add the cashews and give a final stir, making sure all ingredients are well incorporated into the sauce.
- Serve over brown, basmati, or jasmine rice. This is delicious with a nice raita and some chutney.
- NB: The chicken may be omitted and you can use vegetable stock if you would like to make this curry vegetarian. Other vegetables such as potatoes and sweet potatoes can be given the roasting treatment and added to the curry mixture as noted above.

210. Korean Kimchi Quesadilla

Serving: Serves 1 | Prep: | Cook: | Ready in:

Ingredients

- 1 tablespoon butter
- 1/4 cup cabbage kimchi, chopped
- 1/4 cup chicken breast, shredded
- 1 flour tortilla
- 1/2 cup grated sharp cheddar
- 1/2 teaspoon sesame oil
- salt and black pepper to taste
- 2 tablespoons sour cream

Direction

- Mix kimchi and shredded chicken together. This way, any slight kimchi juice will be absorbed by the chicken.
- Add butter to a large skillet over medium-high heat. Place tortilla open face on the pan. On one side of the tortilla; add kimchi, chicken, cheese, sesame oil, and salt & pepper (to taste). Fold tortilla in half and cook until one side starts to turn golden brown (about 2 minutes per side). Once browned on one side, flip to the other side to brown.
- Slice into wedges and serve with a dollop of sour cream!

211. L'Orengue De Pouchins (Chicken In Orange Sauce)

Serving: Serves 4-6 | Prep: | Cook: | Ready in:

Ingredients

- 1 frying chicken, cut into pieces
- 2 large oranges, sliced but with the rind left on
- 2 tablespoons verjus
- 375 milliliters white whine
- salt and pepper
- butter or oil

Direction

- Heat a little butter or oil in a deep casserole or covered pot.
- Season the chicken with salt and pepper, dredge in flour, and brown in the butter. Remove the chicken to a plate and set aside.
- In the same pot, add the ginger and sauté it just until it begins to turn golden.
- Turn down the heat and add the orange slices and verjus and let cook a few minutes longer. (You can substitute lemon juice if you don't have verjus).
- Add the chicken pieces, and a little more wine if necessary to cover the chicken.
- Remove the cooked orange slices and serve hot.

212. Lamb Sausage, Feta And Mint Stuffing

Serving: Serves 12 | Prep: | Cook: | Ready in:

Ingredients

- 1 pound artisinal sourdough bread, cut into 3/4 inch cubes
- 1 pound lamb sausage (mild, not hot like a merguez)
- 1/2 stick of butter
- 2 cloves of garlic, finely minced
- 2 leeks, white and pale green parts only, thoroughly washed and cut into large dice
- 3 celery stalks, cut into medium dice
- 2 granny smith apples, peeld, cored, and cut into medium dice
- 1 cup dried cranberries
- 1 cup raw pistachio meats
- 1/3 cup finely sliced fresh mint
- 1 tablespoon finely minced fresh rosemary
- 1 tablespoon finely minced fresh thyme
- 1 tablespoon zatar (can be found in middle eastern markets, or through Penzeys)
- 2 eggs, beaten
- 1 1/2 cups low sodium chicken stock
- 1/2 cup finely minced fresh parsley
- 6 ounces feta cheese, crumbled
- olive oil
- kosher salt and black pepper to taste

Direction

- Preheat oven to 375F. Place bread cubes on sheet trays and bake until dry and just starting to turn golden, about 20 minutes. Remove from oven and place in a large mixing bowl.
- Remove sausage meat from casings, and sauté with a little olive oil in a skillet over medium high heat, breaking up large pieces with the back of a spoon, until cooked through. Remove from the pan with a slotted spoon and add to the bread cubes.
- Remove any lamb fat from the pan, return it to the heat, add the butter, then the garlic and sauté on low-medium heat until it just turns golden. Add the leeks, apples, celery, cranberries, pistachios, rosemary, thyme, za'atar, and mint, and turn heat up to medium. Season with salt and pepper and cook until the leeks and apples soften, about 10 minutes. When done, add to the mixing bowl with the meat and bread.
- Whisk the two eggs and add to the mixing bowl along with 1 to 1 1/2 cups low sodium chicken stock to moisten (how much will depend on the bread you use), add the fresh parsley, the feta cheese, and check again for seasoning.
- Preheat the oven to 350F. Butter a large glass or ceramic baking dish and fill with the stuffing. Top with a piece of buttered foil and bake for about 35-40 minutes, remove the foil and bake for another 10-15 minutes, until top is nicely browned.

213. Lemon Pepper Chicken Salad Sandwich

Serving: Makes 2 | Prep: | Cook: | Ready in:

Ingredients

- 3 chicken breasts
- 2 tablespoons Greek yogurt
- 1 half of a lemon (to taste)
- 2 tablespoons black pepper
- Cilantro (chopped)
- 2 tablespoons pecan chips
- 1 teaspoon minced garlic
- Garlic salt (to taste)
- Olive oil
- 4 slices Rye bread
- Kale (optional)

Direction

- Cook chicken breasts according to how you typically cook your chicken. I made my chicken breasts at 400 degrees and seasoned with garlic salt, black pepper for 35 minutes.
- Set warm chicken in bowl and drizzle olive oil over them.
- Add in chopped cilantro, minced garlic, Greek yogurt and pecan chips.
- Stir together while shredding the chicken pieces until well mixed together.

- Squeeze lemon half into mixture along with desired amounts of black pepper if you'd like more.
- Spoon mixture onto bread slices along with other desired items (I used kale).

214. Lemoniest Roast Chicken

Serving: Serves 4 | Prep: 48hours0mins | Cook: 1hours15mins | Ready in:

Ingredients

- Lemony brine for chicken
- 4 to 5 teaspoons kosher salt (corresponding to chicken weight, below)
- 1 tablespoon Microplaned (or finely grated) lemon zest
- 1 (4- to 5-pound) chicken, giblets and neck removed (or frozen for later)
- Lemony pan fixings and gravy
- 3 tablespoons unsalted butter, at a cool room temperature
- 2 teaspoons Microplaned (or finely grated) lemon zest
- Kosher salt and freshly ground black pepper
- 2 lemons, halved
- 3 tablespoons freshly squeezed lemon juice, adjusted to taste

Direction

- Brine the chicken: Combine the salt and lemon in a small bowl and rub them together with your fingers until the salt is lemony yellow and super fragrant. Massage this lemon salt all over the chicken (sprinkle a bit inside the empty cavity, too). Stick on a wire rack set over a sheet pan (or in a large bowl or baking dish) and stick in the fridge, uncovered, for at least 1 day or up to 2. (You can truss the chicken if you want, or not.)
- When you're ready to roast the chicken, remove it from the fridge, and heat the oven to 425°F. Pat the chicken all over with towels until it's totally dry.
- Add the butter and lemon zest to a small bowl and mix together until combined. Use a pastry brush or your hands to rub the lemon butter all over the chicken, then evenly season with salt and black pepper (you can go pretty light on the salt since it's already dry-brined).
- Transfer the chicken to a baking dish of your choice (I like a large cast-iron skillet). Stick one lemon half in the chicken's cavity, then place the remaining halves, cut side-down, in the pan around the chicken. Roast for 65 to 75 minutes, or until the juices run clear when you cut between the thigh and leg.
- Remove the pan from the oven and transfer the chicken and charred lemons to a cutting board with a deep juice groove (you can discard the lemon half inside the chicken). While that rests, pour the pan juices into a measuring cup or gravy boat, making sure to get all those crispy, golden bits stuck to the bottom of the pan (they're ultra-concentrated in flavor). Squeeze in a few drops of juice from one of the charred lemon halves on the cutting board, then add the 3 tablespoons lemon juice, and stir with a fork or tiny whisk. By now, some chicken broth has probably accumulated on the cutting board — pour all of that in (for me, this was about ¼ cup). Stir again and give it a taste. More fresh lemon juice, more charred lemon juice, both? Adjust the fat, acid, salt, and pepper until it's good enough to drink by the spoonful.
- Carve the chicken and serve with the charred lemons alongside and lemony gravy for pouring and dunking.

215. Lemony Chicken Noodle Soup

Serving: Serves 6 | Prep: | Cook: | Ready in:

Ingredients

- 1 chicken carcass
- 2 cups cooked chicken, shredded
- 2 tablespoons fresh rosemary
- 2 tablespoons fresh thyme
- 2 lemons, juiced
- 1 onion
- 4 stalks of celery
- 4 carrots
- 16 ounces crimini mushrooms
- 1/2 cup red quinoa
- 3/4 pound farfalle pasta
- salt and pepper to taste

Direction

- Bring water to a boil in a large soup pot. Place the chicken frame, along with some salt and a sprig of rosemary into the pot of water. Let simmer on medium or medium-low for at least an hour and a half.
- Strain the broth.
- Pour the strained broth back into the pot, and bring back up to a simmer. Toss in the carrots, celery, onion, mushrooms, chopped herbs, pepper, salt, lemon juice and lemon peel, and cover. Let simmer for another 15 minutes.
- Add in the uncooked red quinoa and cover, stirring occasionally.
- In the last 7-8 minutes of cooking, add cooked chicken and pasta. Once the noodles are cooked through, it's ready to serve!

216. Librarian's Turkey

Serving: Serves 12 to 18 | Prep: | Cook: | Ready in:

Ingredients

- 1 whole turkey, between 13 and 15 pounds
- 2 lemons
- 2 tablespoons garlic powder
- 1 cup tamari
- 1 cup water
- 5 onions, peeled and quartered

Direction

- Preheat oven to 350° F.
- Squeeze lemon over the top of the turkey and place rinds into cavity, season the outside of the bird with garlic powder and add tamari and water to the bottom of the pan.
- Place onions around turkey and season everything evenly with salt to taste then place in oven on lower rack.
- Baste the turkey every 30 minutes and cook for about 6 hours adding water as necessary to the bottom of the pan upon basting.
- Remove from the oven when the thighs are falling from the bird or can be pulled away with little to no resistance. Allow to rest for 30 minutes before serving, and do so alongside stuffing enhanced with onions from pan.

217. Lime Chicken Enchiladas With Roasted Red Pepper Herb Sauce

Serving: Makes 6 enchiladas | Prep: | Cook: | Ready in:

Ingredients

- Enchiladas
- 6 large whole wheat tortillas
- 3 boneless, skinless chicken breasts
- 1 pinch salt, to taste
- 1 pinch pepper, to taste
- 1/2 lime, juiced
- 3 1/2 ounces black olives, sliced thin
- 1 cup Monterey jack cheese, shredded
- 1 cup spicy cheddar, shredded
- 1/2 cup sour cream, to garnish
- Roasted Red Pepper Herb Sauce
- 6 ounces roasted red peppers
- 1 large tomato, chopped
- 4 cloves garlic, quartered
- 1/2 cup cilantro, roughly chopped
- 1 teaspoon ground Mexican oregano
- 1/4 teaspoon onion powder

- 1/4 teaspoon paprika
- 1/8 teaspoon cayenne pepper
- 1/4 teaspoon salt, to taste

Direction

- Preheat oven to 350 degrees F.
- Season both sides of chicken with salt and pepper and sprinkle with lime juice coating them.
- Place on a microwavable plate and cook just until no longer pink about 3 to 4 minutes per side.
- Let cool then using fingers shred apart.
- In a small bowl combine both cheese and mix well.
- Evenly place about half of each breast in the center of each tortilla, divide olives evenly between the six enchiladas then sprinkle 2 tablespoons of cheese mixture onto each.
- Tightly roll and fold each into an enchilada and place in an 8 x 11 baking dish seam side down.
- In a blender combine ingredients for sauce and pulse until smooth.
- Evenly pour over each enchilada then sprinkle remaining cheese evenly across the top.
- Cover with foil and bake about 25 minutes.
- Remove foil and bake another 5 minutes or so until golden and bubbly.
- Evenly garnish each enchilada with a dollop of sour cream.

218. Lime Cilantro Chicken Milanese

Serving: Serves 2 | Prep: | Cook: | Ready in:

Ingredients

- 4 boneless skinless chicken breasts, preferably organic
- 2 limes
- 1 handful cilantro chopped
- 1 tablespoon chives minced
- 1 1/2 tablespoons ground cumin
- 1/2 cup all purpose flour
- 1 cup breadcrumbs
- 2 eggs beaten
- 2 tablespoons red pepper flakes
- salt and ground black pepper
- olive oil

Direction

- Place your chicken breasts in a mixing bowl
- Add zest of one lime and juice of two limes
- Add the cumin, cilantro, chives and season it with salt and pepper to taste
- Mix well to ensure all the breasts are evenly seasoned
- Place your flour, eggs and breadcrumbs in three separate bowls
- Season the breadcrumbs with red pepper flakes and a pinch of salt
- Dredge the chicken breasts, one by one, first in flour, second in eggs, then in breadcrumbs. Set aside
- Drizzle olive oil on a skillet, medium heat, and cook for about 7 minutes on each side or until they're crispy and golden. You don't want to deep fry them, so take it easy on the amount of oil

219. Malawian Chicken Curry With Nsima

Serving: Serves 4-6 | Prep: 0hours20mins | Cook: 1hours0mins | Ready in:

Ingredients

- Chicken curry
- 3 tablespoons vegetable oil, divided
- 2 medium white onions, sliced into 1/4-inch half-moons
- 3 celery stalks, sliced 1/4-inch thick
- 4 garlic cloves, minced
- Kosher salt, to taste
- Freshly ground black pepper, to taste

- 4 large carrots, sliced in 1/4-inch rounds
- 1 (12-ounce) can tomato paste
- 1 (28-ounce) can whole peeled tomatoes
- 1/2 cup white distilled vinegar
- 1 lemon, juiced
- 1/4 cup yellow curry powder
- 5 pounds bone-in, skin-on chicken pieces
- 1 pinch granulated sugar (optional)
- Nsima
- 2 cups ufa (fine-ground white cornmeal)
- 5 1/2 cups water
- 2 tablespoons unsalted butter or margarine (optional)

Direction

- Chicken curry
- In a very large soup pot or Dutch oven, heat 2 tablespoons of the oil over medium heat. Add onions, celery, and garlic and season with a pinch each of salt and pepper. Cook for 4 minutes, or until vegetables are translucent, stirring occasionally with a wooden spoon.
- Add the 1 remaining tablespoon of oil and the carrots and tomato paste. Fry about 1 to 2 minutes, then add the whole peeled tomatoes, using a wooden spoon to break them up in the pot to 1/2-inch pieces. Add vinegar, lemon juice, and curry powder and mix together.
- Add the chicken pieces and season generously with salt and pepper; stir together with the tomatoey vegetables. Pour enough water in the pot to cover the chicken (you may need to add more as the stew reduces). Bring to a simmer, reduce heat to a low, and cover. It takes at least 1 to 1 1/2 hours for the chicken to become fully tender, but it can also stay on the stove all day. The longer it simmers, the stronger the flavors and the more tender the chicken will be.
- Taste and season with more salt and pepper as needed, and a pinch of sugar. Serve over nsima or cooked rice.
- Nsima
- In a saucepan, heat the water until lukewarm. Slowly mix in the cornmeal while stirring, avoiding lumps. Bring to a boil while stirring continuously. Lower heat and let the porridge gently ripple for 2 minutes; the mixture should look like thin transparent porridge. Continue stirring until the mixture is smooth and cooked through.
- If desired, the butter or margarine can be added at this point. Nsima can be served in a dish or scooped onto a plate as patties. Accompany with meat, fish, or vegetables.

220. Malaysian Chicken Curry

Serving: Serves 4 to 6 | Prep: 0hours15mins | Cook: 0hours45mins | Ready in:

Ingredients

- 6 shallots
- 8 garlic cloves
- 1 stalk lemongrass
- 1 (2-inch) piece ginger
- 5 dried red chiles
- 2 Thai red chiles, for extra spice (optional)
- 5 tablespoons oil
- 5 tablespoons Malaysian curry powder (usually labelled "meat curry powder"), I use Baba's or Alagappa's
- 1/2 teaspoon chile powder, plus more to taste
- 1 teaspoon kosher salt
- 1 cinnamon stick
- 2 star anise
- 10 to 15 curry leaves
- 2 1/2 pounds bone-in chicken thighs and drumsticks
- 4 cups water, or enough to cover chicken
- 3 medium potatoes, peeled and quartered
- 1 1/2 cups coconut milk

Direction

- In a food processor, blend the shallots, garlic, lemongrass, ginger, and both chiles until they form a smooth paste. (Alternatively, you can take the more traditional, and more laborious,

route—pounding it with a mortar and pestle until smooth.)
- Heat up the oil in a deep pot or wok set over medium heat. Add the blended paste and stir-fry until it turns fragrant and intensifies in color. This should take 6 to 8 minutes.
- Then, add the curry powder, chile powder, and salt, frying for another 3 to 5 minutes, or until the spice paste starts to glisten and split and you can see an oily film separate from the paste itself. This is the "pecah minyak" stage. (If your paste is cooking too quickly and starts to burn, add a teaspoon or two of water.)
- When the spice paste has reached the "pecah minyak" stage, add the cinnamon stick, star anise, curry leaves, and chicken. Mix and continue frying for 3 to 5 minutes, until the chicken is evenly coated in the curry paste. Then, pour water into the pot until the pieces of chicken are just covered. Cover the pot with a lid and let it simmer for 10 minutes. Add the potatoes, and simmer for another 25 to 30 minutes, until both the chicken and potatoes are cooked through.
- Finally, pour in the coconut milk. Give it a quick stir, and let the curry simmer for another 2 to 3 minutes. Taste the curry, adding more salt at this stage if necessary.
- The curry is best served hot. It's especially great with steamed white rice along with other Asian sides, or with Malaysian breads like roti canai or roti jala.

221. Mamie's Brunswick Stew

Serving: Serves group | Prep: | Cook: |Ready in:

Ingredients

- Chicken in pieces
- water just to cover
- Handful half shredded green cabbage
- one thin sliced russet potato
- large can tomatoes
- can baby lima beans
- can corn kernels
- can creamed corn
- Teaspoon bacon fat (optional)
- salt & pepper to taste

Direction

- In a large stockpot just cover chicken and cook through then remove cool and shred
- Add potato and simmer until cooked
- Add cabbage and simmer
- Put chicken back in
- Add can of tomato with liquied crushing the tomato
- Add beans and corn kernels along with seasoning
- Just before serving stir in creamed corn and serve with coleslaw and biscuits or hush puppies.

222. Maple Mustard Chicken Thighs

Serving: Serves 6 | Prep: | Cook: |Ready in:

Ingredients

- 8 bone in skin on chicken thighs (excess fat trimmed off)
- 1/2 cup whole grain mustard
- 1/2 cup dijon mustard
- 1/2 cup maple syrup
- 1/4 cup apple cider vinegar
- 4 cloves of garlic, minced
- freshly ground black pepper

Direction

- Preheat the oven to 375°.
- In a small bowl whisk together mustards, maple syrup, apple cider vinegar and garlic. After you get a smooth consistency add pepper to taste (I used probably 1/2 a teaspoon, you don't need a lot here).

- Arrange the chicken skin side up in a casserole pan (I needed to use two to fit them all) and pour 2/3 of the marinade over the chicken. Toss to fully coat the thighs.
- Roast chicken for about 50 minutes, after 35 minutes brush on the remaining marinade.

223. Maple And Mustard Glazed Turkey With Killer Gravy

Serving: Makes 1 large turkey and 5 cups gravy | Prep: | Cook: | Ready in:

Ingredients

- For the Flavored Basting Butter:
- 1/2 cup softened salted butter
- 2 tablespoons maple syrup
- 2 tablespoons Dijon mustard
- 1 teaspoon poultry seasoning
- For the Turkey and Gravy
- 1 16 pound or larger turkey
- 6 cups water
- 2 Carrots
- 2 Celery stalks
- 1 Onion
- 3 Bay leaves
- 1 Star anise pod
- 1/2 teaspoon whole black peppercorns
- Neck and giblets from the turkey
- 1 teaspoon salt, plus more to taste
- Pepper
- 1/4 to 1/2 cups sweet rice flour* or regular flour

Direction

- With an electric mixer, or with a wooden spoon and a bowl, mix the softened butter with the maple syrup, mustard, and poultry seasoning. Divide the flavored butter into two equal-sized portions and put one into a small covered container to keep at room temperature until roasting the turkey. Place the other half onto a square of plastic food wrap or wax paper and shape into a 3-inch log with a spatula or spoon.
- Wrap the butter and tidy up the shape, flattening the ends. Place it on a flat surface in the freezer, to freeze until solid.
- Several hours before roasting, take the turkey out of the refrigerator to bring to room temperature. Remove the neck and any giblets (often packed in a paper packet) from the cavity of the bird and reserve. Rinse the turkey and pat it dry with paper towels. Preheat the oven to 325°F.
- Remove the log of basting butter from the freezer and slice it into thin slices. Slide your fingers underneath the skin on the turkey breast and gently work your fingers back and forth to separate the skin from the meat. Then place the butter slices, one at a time, under the skin, spacing them out over the turkey breast. It will look lumpy, but when the butter melts and bastes the turkey meat, the skin will smooth right out again.
- Peel and chop the carrots, onions and celery into large dices. Place two of the bay leaves into the cavity of the turkey, then add the diced vegetables. Truss the turkey by tying the legs with kitchen twine, or by tucking the ends of the legs under the flap of skin at the tail end, if it has one. Tuck the wing tips under the back. If the legs come out from the flap during roasting, tie them together with kitchen twine. Place the turkey, breast side up, on a roasting rack inside a large roasting pan. Using your fingers, rub a thin layer (about a tablespoon) of the reserved soft glazing butter all over the turkey. Pour 2 cups of the water into the roasting pan around the turkey. If the roaster has a lid, put it on. Otherwise, cover the turkey with heavy duty foil, wrapping it firmly around the lip of the roasting pan to make a good tent for the turkey to steam in.
- Once the turkey is roasting, put the reserved neck and giblets into a saucepan. Cover with the remaining 4 cups of water, and add the bay leaf, star anise pod and peppercorns. Bring to a boil, then reduce the heat to low. Cover the saucepan and leave it to simmer

slowly the whole time the turkey is roasting. This will be the base for your gravy. The heart and gizzard add good flavor, but if your giblet packet contains the liver I would advise removing it as soon as it has come to a boil, and using it for another purpose (my cats love it), or leaving it out altogether. Leaving the liver in the broth to simmer for a long time will add a bitter taste to your gravy.

- Allow the turkey to roast for about 15 minutes per pound, or a little less, using the times for 'unstuffed' turkeys (the cut-up vegetables are much less dense than bread stuffing and still allow warm air to circulate inside the turkey). During the last hour of baking, periodically baste the bird with the remainder of the soft maple-mustard butter by brushing it all over the skin using a pastry brush. Insert a meat thermometer into the turkey breast, not touching the bone, and start checking the temperature after 3 hours. I find that by cooking the turkey this way, in a covered roaster with water in the bottom, it usually cooks faster than the recommended time because of the moist heat. It browns nicely if the roaster is large enough and has a lid, but if you find the turkey isn't browning enough, remove the lid (or the foil) during the last hour to half hour of the roasting time.
- While the turkey is resting, make the gravy: Pour the juices from the roasting pan through a strainer into a large saucepan. Also strain in the liquid from the simmering neck and giblets. With a large spoon, remove as much fat as you easily can from the top of the broth, leaving a few tablespoons in to add flavor to the gravy. (Reserve this combination of melted basting butter and turkey fat to use some of it instead of butter in the mashed potatoes, then refrigerate the rest to use for frying.) Add the reserved diced vegetables from the turkey to the broth. Bring to a boil, and allow to boil for 5 minutes (to get any extra flavor from the vegetables). Using a slotted spoon, remove the vegetables to a small serving bowl and keep warm. (Toss with a bit of butter and salt and pepper and serve alongside the turkey.)
- Add the salt to the broth. In a small jar with a lid, make a slurry of the 1/4 cup sweet rice flour by mixing it with about 1/2 cup water and shaking vigorously until there are no lumps.
- Bring the broth back to a boil, and pour the flour slurry in a slow stream while constantly whisking with your other hand. If it is not as thick as you like, make up some more flour and water slurry, and whisk in small amounts at a time until the gravy is thickened to your liking. Taste and season with pepper, plus more salt if needed. It may need up to a teaspoon more salt. (A gravy should be well salted, as its saltiness is diminished when combined with the mashed potatoes.) That is one killer gravy. Makes about 5 cups.
- Keep the gravy warm and return your attention to carving the turkey (or pass the job on to a willing volunteer, that is -- delegate someone).
- Kitchen Frau Tip: An easy way to carve the breast is to remove each breast-half in one piece, gently prying it loose from the breastbone with your fingers, then cut crosswise into slices.
- *Kitchen Frau Note: I find that sweet rice flour makes a foolproof and beautiful silky gravy. Any lumps easily whisk out of it and the texture never gets gummy. You can find sweet rice flour (different than regular rice flour) at health food stores, Asian import stores and sometimes in the gluten-free section of supermarkets. It is often labelled 'mochiko' sweet rice flour or glutinous rice flour in Asian markets. Even though it is ground from glutinous, or sticky, rice, it has no gluten in it and is not sweet -- it just binds gravy much better than regular rice flour and is lighter than wheat flour.

224. Matzo Ball Soup

Serving: Serves 6 to 8 | Prep: | Cook: | Ready in:

Ingredients

- For the fortified chicken stock
- 1 whole chicken
- 12 cloves garlic, divided
- 1/2 lemon
- 6 sprigs fresh thyme
- 2 sprigs fresh sage
- Olive oil
- Salt
- 32 ounces unsalted chicken stock
- 32 ounces water (replace water with chicken stock if your stock is homemade)
- 1 tablespoon whole black peppercorns
- 1 tablespoon whole coriander
- 1 yellow onion, large diced
- 1 bay leaf
- 1 cup loosely packed fresh dill
- For the matzo balls
- 2 medium carrots, washed and cut into 1/2-inch pieces
- 2 ribs of celery, cut into 1/2-inch pieces
- 2 cups cooked shredded chicken
- 4 eggs, lightly beaten
- 5 tablespoons chicken fat
- 1/2 teaspoon salt
- 2 tablespoons chicken stock
- 1 cup matzo meal
- 2 tablespoons seltzer
- A handful of chopped fresh dill sprigs to garnish

Direction

- Make the fortified chicken stock: Preheat the oven to 425° F. Stuff the cavity of the chicken with 4 smashed cloves of garlic, 1/2 lemon, 6 sprigs of fresh thyme, and 2 sprigs of fresh sage. Rub the outside of the chicken with olive oil, and season aggressively with salt. Place the chicken in a large Dutch oven or roasting pan, and cook for approximately 45 minutes, until the skin is golden and the dark meat is fully cooked. Set the chicken aside until it is cool enough to handle.
- Fill a large pot with the stock, water, peppercorns, coriander, onion, bay leaf, and 8 crushed cloves of garlic. Break the chicken down into pieces, making sure to capture and reserve all the fat and juices that are released. Discard the skin, reserve all of the meat, and place all bones and inedible bits into the large pot with the stock. Store the chicken meat in the refrigerator. You will need approximately 2 cups of shredded chicken for the soup, and any remaining chicken can be eaten as a snack or put to another use. Collect all fat and drippings from the roasted chicken and store it in the refrigerator (you will use some of this fat/drippings to make the matzo balls later). Set the stock pot over high heat. When the stock is boiling, reduce the heat to a very gentle simmer. Cook for 50 minutes. Add the dill and cook for 10 additional minutes. Strain the stock. Please note, the stock can be made ahead of time and stored in the refrigerator.
- Make the matzo balls: Add the reinforced stock to a large pot and set it over high heat. Set aside 2 tablespoons of chicken stock for the matzo balls. When the stock begins to simmer, turn the heat down to low. Add the carrots, celery, and shredded chicken. While the carrots and celery are cooking in the stock, make the matzo balls.
- Combine the lightly beaten eggs with the chicken fat. If you stored the chicken fat in the refrigerator and it has congealed, make sure to warm it until it becomes a liquid again before mixing it with the eggs. Add the salt and chicken stock. Add the matzo meal and mix with a rubber spatula until just combined. Add the seltzer and mix to combine. Store this mixture in the refrigerator for at least 30 minutes.
- Set a large pot of water over high heat until it boils. Reduce the heat to a gentle simmer. When the matzo mixture has been in the refrigerator for 30 minutes, you can lightly salt the boiling water, shape the matzo mixture into balls that are slightly bigger than a ping pong ball, and add them to the simmering water. Cook the matzo balls for 45 to 50 minutes. Transfer the matzo balls to the

chicken soup pot, garnish with fresh dill, and serve.

225. Mediterranean Potstickers

Serving: Makes 2 dozen potstickers | Prep: | Cook: | Ready in:

Ingredients

- Mediterranean potstickers
- 1 medium shallot, finely diced
- 2 cloves garlic, minced
- olive oil
- kosher salt and pepper
- 1 large chicken breast, marinated in Oregano, basil, parsley, salt and pepper, crushed red pepper, balsamic vinegar and olive oil, grilled, and chopped very fine
- 1 small jar artichoke hearts, drained and minced
- 3 cups fresh baby spinach, diced
- 1 cup feta cheese
- 2 dozen potsticker wrappers (these generally can be found frozen at the grocery store)
- neutral cooking oil for frying
- Greek yogurt-roasted red pepper sauce
- 1 cup Greek yogurt
- juice of 1/2 lemon
- salt and pepper, to taste
- 1 1/2 tablespoons honey, or to taste
- 1/2 jar roasted red peppers, minced

Direction

- Mediterranean pot stickers
- Cook shallot and garlic with olive oil, salt and pepper over low heat. Let it go until the shallot starts to caramelize.
- Add the marinated, then grilled, then finely chopped chicken. Let it warm for a minute or so.
- Add artichoke, dried oregano and a little crushed red pepper, and a squeeze of lemon juice. After a few minutes, add the spinach and remove from heat.
- In a large bowl, combine the chicken and artichoke mix with the feta cheese.
- Moisten the edge of a pot sticker wrapper with fingers dipped in water. Place a rounded tablespoon of the chicken mixture in the center, and fold the edges around the mix to create little half-moons.
- Make as many pot stickers as you plan to fry, and lay them out on a sheet pan.
- Bring the cooking oil to heat over just above medium. Frying about four pot stickers at a time, let each one go for about three minutes per side (I fried in oil that was just 1/2 inch deep), or until a slightly deeper version of golden brown. Drain on paper towels, season with kosher salt, and serve with Greek yogurt-roasted red pepper sauce.
- Greek yogurt-roasted red pepper sauce
- Combine the above ingredients, adjusting for saltiness, bitterness, and red pepper flavor. The roasted peppers will come through more as the sauce sits.
- Serve the fried dumplings with the creamy sauce. We also had some carrots — you know, for health.

226. Melissa Hartwig's Instant Pot Chicken Cacciatore With Zucchini Noodles

Serving: Serves 4 | Prep: 0hours25mins | Cook: 0hours25mins | Ready in:

Ingredients

- 8 boneless, skinless chicken thighs (about 2¼ pounds)
- 1 teaspoon dried oregano
- 1 teaspoon salt
- 1/4 teaspoon black pepper
- 1 tablespoon coconut oil
- 1 medium onion, chopped

- 1 red bell pepper, cut into 1-inch pieces
- 1 (8-ounce) package sliced mushrooms
- 1 (14.5-ounce) can Whole30-compliant diced tomatoes, undrained
- 1/2 cup Whole30-compliant chicken broth
- 2 tablespoons Whole30-compliant tomato paste
- 2 cloves garlic, minced
- 1 (10.7-ounce) package zucchini noodles or 2 small zucchini, spiralized
- Fresh chopped parsley (optional)

Direction

- SEASON the chicken with the oregano, ½ teaspoon of the salt, and the pepper. Add the coconut oil to a 6-quart Instant Pot. Select Sauté and adjust to Normal/Medium. When the oil is hot, add half of the chicken and cook, turning once, until browned on both sides, 4 to 8 minutes. Repeat with the remaining chicken. Select Cancel. Transfer the chicken to a plate.
- ADD the onion, bell pepper, mushrooms, tomatoes, broth, tomato paste, garlic, and remaining ½ teaspoon salt to the pot. Add the chicken. Lock the lid in place.
- SELECT Manual and cook on high pressure for 12 minutes. Use quick release.
- TRANSFER the chicken to a plate; cover to keep warm. Select Sauté and adjust to Normal/Medium. When the sauce is simmering, add the zucchini noodles. Cook, stirring frequently, until the sauce is thickened and the zucchini is crisp-tender, about 2 minutes. Select Cancel. Serve, topped with parsley if desired.

227. Melissa Hartwig's Instant Pot Sesame Chicken

Serving: Serves 4 | Prep: 0hours30mins | Cook: 0hours15mins | Ready in:

Ingredients

- 2 pounds boneless, skinless chicken breasts, sliced into thin strips
- 1/2 teaspoon black pepper
- 1 tablespoon plus 1 teaspoon arrowroot powder
- 3 tablespoons avocado oil
- 1/2 cup Whole30-compliant chicken broth
- 1/4 cup coconut aminos
- 1 tablespoon rice vinegar
- 2 teaspoons toasted sesame oil
- 1/2 teaspoon Whole30-compliant fish sauce
- 1/4 teaspoon red pepper flakes (optional)
- 1 (10.8-ounce) package frozen broccoli florets, or 4 cups broccoli florets, steamed (see Tips)
- 2 tablespoons sesame seeds, toasted (see Tips)
- 2 green onions, sliced

Direction

- PLACE the chicken in a medium bowl and sprinkle with the pepper. Add 1 tablespoon of the arrowroot and toss to coat.
- ON a 6-quart Instant Pot, select Sauté and adjust to Normal/Medium. Add the avocado oil. When it's hot, add half the chicken and cook, stirring once, until golden brown, about 6 minutes. Transfer to a plate. Repeat with the remaining chicken. Select Cancel.
- MEANWHILE, in a small bowl, whisk together the broth, coconut aminos, vinegar, sesame oil, fish sauce, and remaining 1 teaspoon arrowroot until the arrowroot is dissolved. Add red pepper flakes (if using).
- RETURN all of the chicken to the pot. Pour the sauce over the chicken. Lock the lid in place. Select Manual and cook for 6 minutes. Use quick release. Stir the chicken. Let stand until slightly thickened, 5 to 10 minutes. Meanwhile, cook the broccoli according to package directions.
- SERVE the chicken over the broccoli. Sprinkle with the sesame seeds and green onions.
- Tips: To steam fresh broccoli florets, combine in a microwave-safe bowl with 3 tablespoons water. Cover and microwave on high for 3 minutes or until crisp-tender. To toast sesame seeds, heat in a skillet over medium heat,

stirring, until fragrant and lightly browned, about 2 minutes.

228. Melly's Braised Holiday Chicken With Olives, Lemon And Apricots

Serving: Serves 6-8 | Prep: | Cook: |Ready in:

Ingredients

- Chicken Marinade
- 8 bone-in, skinless chicken thighs
- 2 tablespoons garlic, crushed
- 2 tablespoons ras-el-hanout
- 2 tablespoons dried cilantro
- 1 zest of 1 lemon (save for juice)
- 1 teaspoon cumin
- 1 teaspoon turmeric
- 2 teaspoons salt
- 3 tablespoons olive oil
- Chicken Braise
- 1/4 cup black olives, halved
- 1/4 cup green olives, pitted and halved
- 1 cup dried apricots, cut in half
- 2 preserved lemons, peels only, sliced thinly
- 1/2 cup white wine
- 1/2 cup chicken broth
- 1 juice of 1 lemon
- 1/3 cup brown sugar

Direction

- Chicken Marinade
- Combine all ingredients except chicken in a bowl. Combine thoroughly.
- Put chicken to a zip top freezer bag. Pour marinade over chicken, close bag and turn until chicken is coated. Marinate for 3-4 hours or overnight.
- Chicken Braise
- Preheat oven to 350 degrees. Add marinated chicken to a deep, heavy coated cast iron pot or casserole.
- Add olives, apricots and preserved lemon peel, scattering around the chicken.
- Pour white wine, chicken broth, and lemon juice around the sides of the chicken. The liquid should come up about 1/3 of the way up the side of the chicken.
- Sprinkle the brown sugar on top of the chicken.
- Cover and bake for 1 to 1 1/2 hours or until internal chicken temperature reaches 165 degrees.
- Serve with the sauce over polenta or rice.

229. Mini Duck Quesadillas W/Avocado Crema

Serving: Makes 24 mini quesadillas | Prep: | Cook: |Ready in:

Ingredients

- 1 large ripe avocado
- 1 teaspoon garlic powder
- 1 teaspoon onion powder
- juice and zest of 1 lime
- 1/2 cup Mexican Crema (or sour cream)
- salt & pepper to taste
- 1 pound duck confit, skin & bones removed
- 1 small jalapeño pepper
- 1 chipotle pepper in adobo
- 1 small red onion
- 1 teaspoon ground cumin
- 1 teaspoon ground turmeric
- 6 large flour tortillas
- 1/2 cup Queso Fresco
- 1 tablespoon canola oil
- edible flower petals or garnish (optional)

Direction

- Scoop flesh from the avocado and mash it with garlic powder, onion powder, lime juice and lime zest until smooth. Fold in the sour cream Salt and pepper to taste. Transfer to a piping bag and set aside.

- Shred duck meat with your hands (or 2 forks, if you prefer). Place duck meat in a skillet set over medium heat and cook 5 minutes, until warmed through.
- Mince the jalapeño, removing the seeds and ribs. Mince the chipotle pepper and red onion. Add the jalapeño, chipotle pepper, red onion, lentils, cumin, and turmeric to the skillet with the duck confit and fold thoroughly to combine. Salt and pepper to taste.
- Using a 2-inch round cookie cutter cut each large tortilla into 4 smaller ones. Fill each small tortilla with about 1 tablespoon of duck mixture, top with about 1 teaspoon of queso fresco and fold in half.
- Brush a small amount of oil onto a skillet set over medium heat and cook mini quesadillas until the insides are warm and the tortillas are lightly browned.
- Top each quesadilla with a dollop of avocado cream, Garnish with an edible flower petal and serve.

230. Mini Persian Rice Cakes (Tachin)

Serving: Serves 8 to 10 | Prep: | Cook: | Ready in:

Ingredients

- 1¾ cups long-grain basmati rice, rinsed
- 3 tablespoons kosher salt, divided
- 1 stick unsalted butter, melted and divided, plus more for greasing
- 1 medium yellow onion, diced
- 1 pound (3 medium) chicken breasts, cut into ½-inch pieces
- 1 cup whole Greek yogurt, divided
- 2 tablespoons dried barberries, plus more for garnish
- ½ teaspoons ground turmeric
- 2 tablespoons boiling water
- ¼ teaspoons saffron threads, ground
- 1 egg

Direction

- In a medium bowl, cover the rice with cold water and stir in 1 tablespoon of the salt. Let soak for 1 hour, then drain.
- Meanwhile, in a medium Dutch oven, heat 2 tablespoons of the butter over medium heat. Add the onion and cook, stirring often, until softened, 4 to 5 minutes. Add the chicken and continue to stir until cooked through, 5 to 6 minutes. Transfer to a medium bowl.
- To the chicken, add 2 teaspoons of the salt, 1/2 cup of the yogurt, the barberries and turmeric. Stir to combine, then set aside.
- In another medium bowl, combine the boiling water and the saffron. Let sit for 5 minutes, then whisk in 1 teaspoon of the salt, 2 tablespoons of the melted butter, the remaining 1/2 cup of the yogurt and the egg.
- Preheat the oven to 375° F and grease a non-stick muffin tin with butter. Bring a large pot of water to a boil; season with the remaining 1 tablespoon kosher salt. Add the soaked rice to the pot of boiling water and cook until just tender, 5 minutes, and then drain.
- To the bowl with the saffron mixture, stir in 3 cups of the cooked rice. You will be making wells for the chicken to go into. Divide the saffron rice between the 12 wells of the muffin tin (2 heaping tablespoons per well) and using a spoon spread up the sides.
- Divide the chicken mixture between each well of rice. Top each with the remaining plain rice (you may have a little leftover). Drizzle the remaining melted butter over the rice. Cover the tray with foil and bake, rotating halfway through, until golden, 2 hours.
- Let cool slightly, then run a mini offset spatula around the edge of each. Place a tray over the pan, then invert to release the tahini. Garnish with more barberries and serve.

231. Moroccan Chicken Tagine

Serving: Serves 4 | Prep: | Cook: | Ready in:

Ingredients

- 240 grams onions - chopped
- 1500 grams chicken thighs – cut into large chunks
- 2 cinnamon sticks
- 1/2 teaspoon turmeric
- 1 teaspoon black pepper
- 500 milliliters chicken stock
- 100 grams dried apricots
- 100 grams dried prunes
- 85 grams honey
- 1 teaspoon ground cinnamon
- 1 1/2 tablespoons almond flour
- 50 grams slivered almonds

Direction

- In a saucepan, heat a small amount of oil and sauté the onions until soft and then add into a large pot.
- Add the chicken with the cinnamon sticks, turmeric, and black pepper and pour in chicken stock.
- Cover with the lid and cook for 2½ hours on low-medium.
- Add the dried apricots, prunes, honey, cinnamon, and almond flour and stir until well combined. Cover with the lid and cook for another hour.
- In a dry pan, toast the slivered almonds. Serve the Tagine decorated with the toasted almonds.
- This dish can be served with our lima bean mash, cauliflower rice or pumpkin and cauliflower mash. A little bit of scd yogurt on the side is also delicious.

232. Mung Bean Rice Mosh Polo

Serving: Serves 4-5 | Prep: | Cook: | Ready in:

Ingredients

- 4 cups long grain basmati rice
- 2 1/2 cups Mung Beans
- 6 pieces Chicken with bones
- 1 Large Onion Chopped
- 1/2 cup Oil
- 1 tablespoon Garm Masala
- 2 1/2 tablespoons Coriender Powder
- 1/2 tablespoon Black Pepper
- 6 cups Water
- Salt to taste

Direction

- Fry onion in oil until golden brown, not burnt or else it will give burnt taste.
- Add chicken pieces in and fry with onion mixture for 5 minutes or until chicken changes color.
- Add the 6 cups of water at this point
- Add all the spices and salt
- When the chicken is cooked you have to remove it from the stock and put it aside. When there is about 5 cups of water in the pot add mung beans and let it cook for 10 minutes
- After 10 minutes or until mung beans are soft to your touch add in the rice that had been soaking in water for an hour. (Drain water from rice before you add it to the stock)
- Stir and then when the rice is almost fully cooked put back in the chicken on top of the rice- cover the pot and put in 500 degrees oven for 5 minutes.
- After 5 minutes lower oven heat to 425 degrees and let it bake in the oven for 30 minutes.
- Enjoy!

233. My Favorite Roasted Chicken, With Jerusalem Artichokes

Serving: Serves 4 | Prep: | Cook: |Ready in:

Ingredients

- 4 chicken legs or a 3-pound chicken, cut into serving pieces
- Salt and fresh ground pepper
- 3 tablespoons extra virgin olive oil
- 1 lemon
- 6 large garlic cloves
- 1 pound small jerusalem artichokes, peeled
- 1 pound small red potatoes, cut in half or quarters
- 6 large shallots, peeled and halved
- 2 tablespoons fresh thyme leaves
- 1 cup dry white wine
- 1 cup green olives, pitted

Direction

- Preheat oven to 400 degrees. Season chicken with salt and pepper, and rub with 1 tablespoon olive oil. Place chicken in a shallow roasting pan; set aside. Zest the lemon into long strips, and squeeze juice from lemon into a small bowl. Set aside juice.
- In a medium bowl, combine lemon zest, garlic, Jerusalem artichokes, potatoes, shallots, and thyme. Add remaining 2 tablespoons oil; season with salt and pepper. Toss to coat, and arrange in pan around chicken. Roast until chicken is golden brown, about 40 minutes.
- Remove from oven. Add reserved lemon juice, wine, and olives; stir up any browned bits on the bottom of roasting pan with a wooden spoon. Return to oven, and continue cooking until liquid has thickened slightly, 10 to 15 minutes. Remove from oven, and transfer to serving plates.

234. My Version Of My Mom's Chicken Paprikash

Serving: Serves 6-8 | Prep: | Cook: |Ready in:

Ingredients

- 3-4 pounds chicken cut up or any chicken parts (I used chicken drumsticks)
- 2 medium onions, diced
- 2 teaspoons paprika
- 1 teaspoon salt
- 1/2 teaspoon hot paprika
- 1/3 cup oil
- 1 fresh hot pepper
- 1 tablespoon hot peppers paste
- 2 tablespoons pepper/ tomato paste
- 4 cups chicken stock
- 4 tablespoons flour
- 4 tablespoons sour cream
- 1 (500g) or two packaging of gnocchi (homemade dumplings or noodles)

Direction

- Put chicken pieces into the large bowl with diced onion add paprika, hot paprika, salt, fresh hot pepper and oil. Mix all together and put on parchment paper covered baking sheet and bake on 375F for 25 minutes.
- When ready transfer everything into a large sauce pot, add chicken stock and water to just beryl cover the chicken.
- Add hot peppers paste, pepper/ tomato paste and bring to boil, reduce heat and simmer for 10-15 minutes.
- Make a slurry with flour and water and add to the pot with chicken, keep cooking for 10 minutes. Adjust seasoning.
- In this recipe, I used gnocchi and put them straight with chicken to cook them. (If I use noodles I will cook them separately)
- For the and put sour cream in the mixing bowl and add a ladle of hot sauce from chicken to temper sour cream, pour back to chicken paprikash and mix in. Take paprikash off the stove and serve

235. Nana's Chicken Salad

Serving: Serves 4-6 | Prep: 0hours20mins | Cook: 0hours20mins | Ready in:

Ingredients

- 16 ounces Chicken tenderloins
- 1.5 cups Chicken Broth
- garlic powder, salt, pepper

Direction

- For poaching the chicken, fill a medium-size pot with the raw chicken and add the broth, salt, pepper, and garlic powder making sure the chicken is covered. Turn the heat to medium-low.
- Bring the liquid to a low simmer, cover the pot and poach the chicken for about 20 minutes or until completely cooked through (center should be 165 ° and the juice clear). Make sure it stays at a low simmer and not a boil. While the chicken is cooking, cut up and measure out the salad ingredients and put in a large bowl.
- Using tongs or a slotted spoon remove the chicken onto a cutting board. Discard or save the broth for another use. Let the chicken cool slightly.
- Once cool enough to handle, chop or shred the chicken and place it in the large bowl with the other ingredients. Taste and add any ingredients as preferred.
- Put in the fridge for at least an hour or more so that the flavors can come together. Serve on croissants, bread, toast, lettuce, or with crackers on the side

236. Not My Grandmother's Chopped Chicken Liver

Serving: Serves enough | Prep: | Cook: |Ready in:

Ingredients

- 6 eggs, hard boiled & peeled
- 1 pound yellow skinned onions, minced fine
- 3 ounces unsalted butter
- 1 tablespoon grapeseed oil (substitute canola or safflower)
- 1/2 pound livers from pastured, free range chickens
- 2 tablespoons Cognac, dry sherry, white vermouth, or Calvados

Direction

- Chop the eggs very fine using a mezzaluna or the food processor. They should be fluffy. Put in a large bowl and set aside.
- In a large, heavy sauté pan, heat half the butter with the oil. Add the onions and sauté slowly until richly browned, but not burned. Salt and pepper generously while they cook.
- In the meantime, rinse and clean the livers well, removing connective sinew and anything yucky looking.
- When the onions have finished cooking, put them in the bowl with the eggs.
- Heat 1 oz. butter in the onion pan and sauté the livers until no pink remains. Do not brown or crisp. It's alright if they break up a bit. Salt and pepper generously.
- Remove the livers from the pan and deglaze with the booze. Pour the deglazing liquid into the bowl with the eggs and onions.
- Chop the livers with a mezzaluna (or use the food processor) and then gently fold the eggs, onions and livers together.
- Test and correct for seasoning. The flavor really blooms after chilling, so make this well in advance.
- Pack in ramekins or other serving dishes. Keep the dishes small – 4 oz. – and make sure to

freeze whatever will not be used within two days.

237. One Pan Roasted Chicken & Veggies

Serving: Serves 4-6 people | Prep: | Cook: | Ready in:

Ingredients

- 6-8 carrots
- 4 sweet potatoes
- 1 small onion
- 2 tablespoons olive oil
- 1/2 teaspoon sea salt (for veggies)
- 1 whole chicken
- 1 teaspoon butter
- 1/4 teaspoon sea salt (for chicken)
- 1/4 teaspoon Italian seasoning

Direction

- Preheat oven to 350°F and grease a large baking pan/dish with non-stick spray (olive/avocado/coconut varieties).
- Wash and peel vegetables then cut the sweet potatoes and onions into slices and cut the carrots into quarters, lengthwise, trying to cut the veggies at the same thickness to ensure even cooking.
- Add veggies to a large bowl and add the olive oil and sea salt. Toss all together.
- Spread veggies out in the pan. You can either place the chicken right on top or have the veggies surround the chicken.
- Rub the butter onto the chicken skin. Sprinkle on the sea salt and Italian seasoning evenly.
- Cook for two hours for a lightly bronzed, juicy chicken.

238. One Pot Sticky Coconut Chicken Curry

Serving: Serves 2-4 | Prep: | Cook: | Ready in:

Ingredients

- INGREDIENTS
- 1 pound chicken, bone-in and skin-on
- 2 large sized idaho potatoes, diced into chunks
- 8.5 ounces coconut milk
- 8 ounces vanilla yogurt
- 4 garlic cloves, minced or grated
- 5 dried chilies, +/- to taste
- 1 bouillon cube, low-sodium, crushed
- 2 teaspoons olive oil
- 3 bay leaves
- 1 teaspoon cumin
- 1 teaspoon paprika
- toasted sesame seeds, for garnish
- chopped cilantro, for garnish
- FOR THE CURRY PASTE
- 1 teaspoon tandoori
- 1 tablespoon curry powder or curry mix
- 1/4 teaspoon ground clove
- 1/4 teaspoon ground ginger
- 2 cardamom seeds
- splash of olive oil, to mix
- OR, you can buy a packet of pre-made, low-sodium curry paste

Direction

- Preheat the oven to 350 degrees. In a large pot that can go in an oven, heat the olive oil in the pot over a medium flame. Add the garlic, chilies, and powdered spices (listed in the first ingredient set) and cook for a minute or two, stirring continuously until the garlic is softened. Add the potatoes, stir again, and then add the curry paste and/or your homemade curry mixture (second ingredient list), stirring again.
- Add the coconut milk, yogurt, bay leaves, and bouillon cube and stir again, cooking for a

couple of minutes until everything is well-blended and sauce starts to thicken.
- In the pot, rest the chicken on top of the sauce and potato mixtures, so that the skin side is elevated out of the sauce. Season the top of the chicken (the skin) with black pepper and a little drizzle of olive oil.
- Place in the oven and cook, uncovered, until the chicken skin is crispy and browned on top and the meat is cooked thoroughly. You can use a meat thermometer, but figure about 40 minutes. This will vary depending on the type of chicken pieces you use; less time for wings, longer for thighs and legs attached.
- Garnish with sesame seeds and chopped cilantro. Serve with rice if you'd like.

239. Onion Marinated Grilled Chicken Breasts

Serving: Serves 4 | Prep: 0hours20mins | Cook: 0hours10mins | Ready in:

Ingredients

- 4 approximately 8-oz chicken breasts
- 1/2 large yellow onion
- 1 medium to large shallot
- 3 tablespoons olive oil
- 3 tablespoons water
- 2 tablespoons loosely packed fresh thyme leaves
- 1 1/2 teaspoons kosher salt (Diamond brand)
- extra virgin olive oil, smoked sea salt, and lemon wedges for serving

Direction

- Remove fat from chicken breasts if needed. Sandwich each breast in plastic wrap, and pound into an even 1/2-inch thickness. Transfer the breasts to a gallon zippered plastic bag.
- Roughly chop the onion (you should have about 3/4 cup) and the shallot (you should have about 2 tablespoons). Combine the onion, shallot, olive oil, water, thyme, and salt in a blender and blend until smooth. Pour the marinade into the bag with the chicken. Express the air from the bag, then gently massage and manipulate until all of the chicken breasts are coated. Refrigerate for at least 4 hours, and up to 24 hours.
- Prepare your grill for high heat, direct cooking. While the grill is heating remove the chicken from the fridge. Grill the chicken breasts (the marinade will cling, do not scrape it off), uncovered, for 2 to 4 minutes on each side (charcoal 2-3 minutes, gas 3-4 minutes). Take care not to overcook the chicken.
- Serve with a drizzle of olive oil, pinch of smoked sea salt, and spritz of lemon juice. If you're feeling fancy, top with your favorite fruit salsa or strawberry salsa fresca.

240. Ostrich Stuffed Peppers

Serving: Serves 2 | Prep: | Cook: |Ready in:

Ingredients

- 2 peppers (red, yellow, orange)
- 1 pound ostrich
- 1/2 red onion
- 1 teaspoon cumin
- 1 serrano chili
- 2 dashes feta
- 1 splash coconut oil
- 1 splash olive oil
- 1 dash salt & pepper

Direction

- Preheat the oven to 400F.
- Start by cutting the peppers in half and removing the insides. Be careful not to puncture the pepper while doing this otherwise it will leak in the oven. For extra effect, leave the stalk in place, cutting it in half as you halve the pepper.

- In a skillet and with a little coconut oil, sauté the garlic, chili, cumin and onions until soft. Turn the heat up a little to medium-high, add the ostrich and fry until brown. Season with the salt and pepper.
- Remove the ostrich from the heat, lay the peppers on a roasting tray and spoon the ostrich into the peppers. Drizzle with a little olive oil before placing in the oven and roasting until the peppers are soft and juicy with the edges beginning to brown, about 25 - 30 mins.
- Optionally, crumble a little feta on top and garnish with fresh cilantro.

241. Our Family Fried Turkey

Serving: Makes one 12 to 15 pound turkey | Prep: 0hours0mins | Cook: 0hours0mins | Ready in:

Ingredients

- For the rub
- 6 tablespoons salt
- 2 tablespoons Hungarian paprika
- 2 tablespoons granulated garlic
- 2 tablespoons black pepper
- 1 teaspoon cayenne pepper
- 1 teaspoon dried basil, crushed between your fingers
- 1 teaspoon dried oregano, crushed between your fingers
- 1 teaspoon onion powder
- 1/2 teaspoon ground thyme
- 1/2 teaspoon celery seed
- For the turkey
- 1 12 to 15 pound turkey (NO bigger than 15 pounds)
- 35 pounds peanut oil or a peanut/vegetable blend (about 5 gallons)
- 1 Turkey fryer with about a 30 quart capacity (preferably one with a handled basket as opposed to a hook)
- 1 frying thermometer
- Safety glasses
- Heavy duty gloves (welding gloves are great!)
- Water to figure out how much of that oil you'll need
- A propane tank to hook to your fryer
- The turkey rub

Direction

- For the rub
- Combine all ingredients and store covered until ready to use.
- For the turkey
- All right...let's get started. First you need to figure out how much of that 35 pounds of oil you'll need. To do this place the raw turkey in the basket of the fryer legs up and then place the basket in the fryer. Fill the fryer with enough water to cover the whole turkey. (You want to wash the turkey anyway, don't you?) Pull the turkey and basket out and take a mental image of how far up the fryer the water level is. This will be the amount of oil you'll need. Dry the fryer and fill with the oil. Oh and don't forget...this is an outdoor project away from decks and anything else that might catch fire!
- Bring the turkey indoors, dry it with paper toweling inside and out and rub it thoroughly, inside and out with the rub. Let that turkey rest for about an hour. You probably won't need all of the rub, but better to be safe than sorry.
- Now hook up your fryer to the propane tank, turn on the tank and wait until the oil reaches a temperature of 360F. Depending on the weather, this could take anywhere from 30 minutes to an hour. Once that's done place your rubbed turkey back into the basket, legs up, and wearing gloves and glasses SLOWLY lower the basket into the hot oil.
- Now set a timer. Standard frying time is 3.5 minutes per pound, so a 15 pound turkey will take between 52 and 53 minutes to cook.
- After cooking time is done, slowly lift the turkey filled basket out of the oil and let drain

for a few minutes. Let rest for about 15 minutes before carving.

242. Overstuffed Chicken & Broccoli Quesadillas

Serving: Serves 4 | Prep: 0hours5mins | Cook: 0hours20mins | Ready in:

Ingredients

- 1 tablespoon vegetable or olive oil
- 1 cup chopped onion
- 2 cups chopped broccoli
- Kosher salt and freshly ground black pepper
- 1 cup roughly chopped spinach or kale
- 1/2 teaspoon minced garlic
- 1 teaspoon chili powder
- 2 tablespoons minced fresh cilantro (optional)
- 2 cups shredded cooked chicken (see Author Notes)
- 4 teaspoons unsalted butter, divided
- 8 (8-inch) flour tortillas
- 3 cups (12 ounces) shredded white cheddar, or another type of combo or shredded cheese
- Guacamole, sour cream, and salsa, for serving

Direction

- Heat a large skillet over medium-high heat and add the vegetable or olive oil. Add the onion and broccoli, season with salt and pepper, and sauté for 3 minutes until the vegetables start to soften. Add the spinach, garlic, and chili powder and stir for another minute until you can smell the garlic, the spinach is wilted, and everything is well combined. Stir in the cilantro if using, turn the mixture into a bowl, and stir in the chicken until everything is blended.
- Wash and dry the skillet (or grab a new skillet). Place the skillet over medium heat and add a half teaspoon of butter. Place a tortilla in the pan. Sprinkle 2 tablespoons of the cheese mixture over half of the quesadilla, and distribute 1/8 of the chicken and vegetable mixture over the cheese. Top that with another 2 tablespoons of the shredded cheese. Flip the bare half of the tortilla over the filling, cover the pan, and sauté for about 2 minutes until the bottom is golden and the cheese has started to melt, then use a spatula to flip the half-moon quesadilla. Continue to cook, uncovered, until all of the cheese is melted and the underside is browned, 2 to 3 minutes. You can cook two at a time, if you nestle them in the pan with the flat sides of the half-moons abutting each other.
- Remove the quesadilla to a cutting board and let it sit for a minute before you slice into 2 or 3 wedges. Repeat until all of the quesadillas are cooked. Serve with guacamole, salsa, and sour cream.

243. Pad Thai From Kris Yenbamroong

Serving: Serves 1 to 2 | Prep: 0hours30mins | Cook: 0hours3mins | Ready in:

Ingredients

- 4 ounces dried rice stick noodles (1/8 to 1/3 inch wide)
- 2 tablespoons sugar
- 2 tablespoons fish sauce
- 2 tablespoons distilled white vinegar
- 3 tablespoons vegetable oil
- 1/4 pound chicken thighs, cut into bite-size slices (or extra-firm or pressed tofu or large peeled shrimp)
- 1 egg
- 1 cup bean sprouts
- 2 green onions, cut thinly on an angle into 2-inch-long slices
- 2 tablespoons crushed roasted peanuts
- 1 teaspoon roasted chile powder
- 1 lime wedge

Direction

- Soak the noodles in warm water for 30 minutes, until pliable enough to bend around a finger. (If you're not using them immediately, you can drain the noodles and keep them in the fridge until ready to use.)
- In a small bowl, stir together the sugar, fish sauce, and vinegar to make a sauce.
- Heat an empty wok over high heat until it begins to smoke, then swirl in the oil. Once the oil is shimmering, add the chicken or tofu and stir-fry until the meat turns opaque but isn't fully cooked, which should take about a minute (less time for shrimp — they will cook a little more quickly). Add the noodles and sauce, then continue to stir-fry, constantly stirring, until the noodles absorb the sauce, about another minute.
- Use your spatula to push aside the noodles and leave them there, making an empty space in the center of the wok. Crack the egg into the empty space and let it cook until the edges start to set, 15 to 20 seconds. Use the edge of your spatula to break up and roughly scramble the egg, then toss it back in with the noodles while the egg is still soft. Once the egg looks mostly cooked, remove from the heat and throw in the bean sprouts and green onions, tossing thoroughly to combine. Transfer to a plate and garnish with the peanuts, chile powder, and lime wedge.

244. Pad Thai With Chicken

Serving: Serves 2 | Prep: | Cook: | Ready in:

Ingredients

- Sauce:
- 2 T tamarind paste (available on Amazon)
- 3 T Asian fish sauce (available on Amazon)
- 3 T palm sugar (available on Amazon)
- sriracha hot chile sauce: 1 ½ t for mild; 2 ¼ t for spicy --- Our choice; 3 t = 1 T for HOT!

- Next Ingredients:
- 1 large boneless, skinless chicken breast (about 8 ounces), cut into bite size pieces
- 6 oz of rice noodles, cut into 6 inch lengths
- 1 large shallot, chopped fine
- 8 oz bag of mung bean sprouts
- 2 large cloves garlic, minced
- 2 green onions, sliced diagonally
- 2 T cilantro, chopped coarse
- 1 T sesame oil
- 1 egg, lightly beaten
- 1 lime cut into 4 wedges
- 3 T dry roasted peanuts, chopped coarse
- 1-2 dozen flat leaf chives, trimmed to equal lengths about 4 inches

Direction

- Mix the sauce ingredients and let stand until used. Soak the rice noodles in hot water for 4 minutes or so until tender. Then dry the noodles and reserve at room temperature.
- Heat the oil in a wok over medium high heat while swishing around to cover the sides. Add the chicken and cook while stirring for about 5 minutes or until the chicken is starting to get brown. About 1 minute into this add the chives and stir in. About 2 minutes after the chives add the garlic and continue stirring for 2 minutes.
- Add the sauce and the rice noodles and stir until everything is coated with the sauce; about 1 to 2 minutes
- Move these ingredients to one side and pour the egg into the empty side of the wok. Stir the egg until mostly cooked (about 1 minute) then mix with the noodles and chicken.
- Add half of the mung bean sprouts and stir into the mix for about 1 to 2 minutes.
- Add the sliced green onion and cilantro, remove from the heat and stir into mixture.
- SERVING: Spoon some of the cooked mixture onto a warmed plate. Arrange some of the raw bean sprouts on the plate next to the mixture. Place a small mound of the chopped peanuts next to the mixture. Arrange some flat leaf chives on the plate along with one or two lime

wedges. (Optional) Place a small mound of red pepper flakes on the plate.

245. Paella

Serving: Serves 3-4 | Prep: 0hours0mins | Cook: 0hours0mins | Ready in:

Ingredients

- 2/3 quart chicken stock from cube or fresh
- a few strands of saffron
- 1 chicken breast
- 1 chicken thigh, skin on, bone out (or just thighs or breasts)
- 1 tablespoon vegetable oil
- salt and pepper
- 1 medium onion, diced
- 2 garlic cloves, chopped finely
- 1 teaspoon (heaped) tomato purée
- 1 red pepper, cored and roughly chopped
- 1 teaspoon smoked hot paprika
- 2-3 ounces sliced chorizo
- 1 cup paella rice (Bomba or Calasparra)
- 1/2 cup dry white wine
- 8-12 raw large shrimp, shelled, shell-on or a mix
- 1/2 cup frozen peas, thawed

Direction

- Heat up the stock or dissolve the cube in boiling water; add the saffron and stir.
- Chop each chicken thigh and breast into 4 or 5 pieces and season them with salt and pepper.
- Heat up the oil in the largest pan you have (25cm will be good) and brown the chicken pieces on all sides.
- Push them to the sides and add the onion and garlic into the middle of the pan.
- Fry it hard for a couple of minutes, then stir in the tomato puree, keeping it away from the chicken.
- Add the red pepper; fry it together with the onion and garlic for a minute.
- Turn down the heat a little and mix the chicken pieces in. Sprinkle over the smoked paprika and add the chorizo pieces.
- Pour the stock into the pan, all at once and turn up the heat. Let it bubble vigorously for two-three minutes.
- Sprinkle the rice evenly over the surface of the stock – DO NOT STIR from now on.
- Cook it for 10 minutes until the rice appears through the liquid. Gently displace any dry grains sticking to the chicken but DO NOT STIR. If it looks too dry too soon, add the white wine.
- Sprinkle the peas over the surface and arrange the prawns on top.
- Turn the heat down and simmer the paella for 10 minutes until the rice has absorbed all the liquid; you may cover the pan at this stage so the prawns cook through. If you don't have a lid to fit the pan, cover it with a large baking sheet.
- After the 10 minutes turn the heat right up for 1 minute until you can hear the rice start to pop and crackle. Keep it on for 30 seconds and take the pan off the heat.
- Cover it with a clean dry tea towel to absorb the steam, keep it like that for 10 minutes and serve in the pan placed in the middle of the table.
- If you're lucky, the mixture has stuck to the bottom of the pan; crispy and almost-burnt. This is socarrat, a characteristic of good paella. Well done – the socarrat is truly scrumptious.

246. Pan Roasted Chicken With Bacon, Rosemary And Lemon

Serving: Serves 2 | Prep: | Cook: | Ready in:

Ingredients

- 1 tablespoon olive oil
- 2 slices bacon, diced

- 1 sprig fresh rosemary, minced
- 2 chicken legs
- 2 chicken thighs
- 1 teaspoon salt
- 1/2 teaspoon pepper
- 1/3 cup chicken broth
- 3 tablespoons lemon juice

Direction

- Preheat oven to 350 degrees F.
- In an oven proof skillet heat oil over medium heat and add bacon and rosemary.
- Cook until crisp, about 5 to 7 minutes.
- Remove and drain on paper towel; set aside.
- Season both sides of chicken with salt and pepper and add to same skillet skin side down.
- Cook until skin begins to set and crisp, about 5 minutes. Turn and cook another 3 minutes.
- Return chicken to skin side down in pan and place in oven.
- Cook 25 to 30 minutes until chicken is cooked through.
- Return pan to stove top over medium heat and remove chicken to a warm plate.
- With only one tablespoon of rendered fat remaining in pan stir in broth and lemon juice again scraping any bits from bottom.
- Return bacon and rosemary to pan and cook until sauce reduces and thickens slightly, about 3 to 5 minutes.
- Season with more salt and pepper to taste if needed and serve sauce spooned over chicken pieces.

247. Pancit

Serving: Serves 6 | Prep: | Cook: | Ready in:

Ingredients

- 8 ounces rice sticks
- 8 ounces large shrimps
- 3 pieces chicken with bones
- 2 cups shredded cabbage
- 2 cups shredded carrots
- 2 cups shredded snow peas
- 2 cups chopped onion
- 1 tablespoon mashed garlic
- 3 tablespoons soy sauce (or to taste)
- 2 tablespoons sesame oil
- 1 tablespoon Aleppo pepper or chili powder
- 1 teaspoon Black pepper
- 2 pieces limes, quartered
- 1 bunch scallions

Direction

- Make the chicken stock by browning the chicken in sesame oil and covering it with water and some seasonings.
- Let the chicken simmer for one hour; cool and strain the stock.
- Shred the chicken into pieces and set aside.
- Peel the shrimps and cut off the heads and place in the stock.
- Simmer the shrimp heads and skin in the stock for 30 minutes and strain.
- Sprinkle the pepper on the shrimp and set aside.
- Heat some oil in a pot and fry the shrimp for 3 minutes till pink.
- Remove the shrimp and add the onions and shredded veggies and fry for 3 minutes.
- Add the mashed garlic and soy sauce and stir one minute.
- Remove the veggies and add the stock and bring it to a simmer.
- Add the rice sticks and cook in the stock for about 5 minutes.
- Add the veggies, shrimp, shredded chicken to the noodles and adjust seasonings.
- Serve with chopped scallions and limes.

248. Panko Crusted Chicken With Chanterelle Gruyere Sauce

Serving: Serves 4 | Prep: | Cook: | Ready in:

Ingredients

- For the chicken
- 4 six to eight ounce boneless, skinless chicken breasts, pounded a bit to even them out
- 1 cup flour
- 2 eggs lightly beaten with a few tablespoons of water
- 2 cups panko bread crumbs
- Salt and pepper
- Vegetable oil for frying
- For the sauce
- 2 tablespoons butter
- 2 tablespoons extra virgin olive oil
- 1 medium shallot, minced
- A pinch of dried thyme, crushed between your fingers
- 1 pound chanterelle mushrooms, cleaned and cut into good size chunks (or substitute another mushroom)
- 1 teaspoon instant flour (plus more if needed)
- 1/2 teaspoon salt
- 1/4 teaspoon white pepper
- 1/4 cup dry white wine
- 1 1/2 cups half and half (plus a little more if needed to thin out the sauce)
- 2 ounces shredded Gruyere cheese

Direction

- For the chicken
- Begin by heating enough vegetable oil in a large skillet to come up about a half inch in the pan. Get the oil nice and hot while you're breading the chicken.
- Season the chicken well with salt and pepper. Set up a breading station and dredge the chicken first in the flour, then the beaten egg and finally the panko.
- Brown the chicken on both sides until golden and then place them in a shallow baking dish. While you make the sauce, bake the breasts in a 350F oven for 15 to 20 minutes.
- For the sauce
- In a large sauté pan, heat the oil and butter, add the shallot and sauté until it softens. Add the mushrooms and thyme and continue to sauté until the mushrooms give off their liquid. Continue to sauté to let the liquid almost evaporate. Stir in the instant flour.
- Add the salt, pepper and wine. Simmer for about one minute.
- Stir in the half and half, bring up to a simmer and cook to thicken the sauce. If you like a thinner sauce, add a little more of the half and half. You can always sprinkle in a little more instant flour to find the right consistency. You want to simmer until the sauce coats the back of a spoon.
- Turn off the heat and stir in the shredded cheese. Ladle the sauce over the chicken and enjoy!

249. Parmesan Crusted Chicken With Herby Potatoes

Serving: Serves 4 | Prep: 0hours10mins | Cook: 0hours40mins | Ready in:

Ingredients

- Potato salad
- 3/4 pound fingerling potatoes, cut in half horizontally (about 2 cups)
- 1/2 red onion, thinly sliced (about 1/2 cup)
- 1/2 cup parsley leaves, packed
- 1/2 cup roughly chopped dill, packed
- 2 tablespoons olive oil
- 1 lemon, juiced
- 1/2 teaspoon coarsely ground black pepper
- 1/2 teaspoon Dijon mustard
- 1/4 teaspoon kosher salt
- Chicken cutlets
- 2 large boneless, skinless chicken breasts (about 2 pounds total)
- 1 cup all-purpose flour
- 1 teaspoon kosher salt
- 1 teaspoon ground paprika
- 1/2 teaspoon coarsely ground black pepper
- 3 large eggs
- 1 1/2 cups panko breadcrumbs

- 1 cup grated Parmesan cheese
- 3 tablespoons olive oil, plus more as needed
- 1 lemon, cut into wedges
- Flaky sea salt, for garnish

Direction

- Prep the potato salad: Place potatoes and a generous pinch of salt in a large pot and cover with 1 inch of water. Bring to a boil over medium-high heat and cook until potatoes are fork tender, about 20 minutes. Strain potatoes and let cool at room temperature for at least 20 minutes.
- In a large bowl, combine the cooled potatoes with the sliced onion, parsley, and dill. Set aside.
- Make the dressing: In a small bowl combine the olive oil, lemon juice, pepper, Dijon mustard, and salt. Whisk until emulsified and set aside.
- Make the chicken cutlets: Carefully slice each chicken breast in half horizontally so you end up with four thin cutlets. Place each of the four cutlets between two pieces of wax paper and gently pound them with a mallet until they are roughly 1/4-inch thick. Set aside.
- In a large shallow bowl, combine the flour, salt, paprika, and black pepper. In a second large shallow bowl, beat the eggs. In a third large shallow bowl, combine the breadcrumbs and Parmesan cheese.
- Working with one chicken cutlet at a time, dredge them in the flour mixture, then the eggs, and coat each side in the breadcrumbs. Place breaded cutlets onto a plate.
- Heat olive oil in a large cast-iron skillet over medium heat. Fry the cutlets, one at a time, until golden brown, about 4 minutes per side. Repeat with remaining chicken cutlets, adding additional olive oil to the skillet as needed, and transfer onto four serving plates.
- Serve: Toss prepared potato salad mixture with dressing. Distribute salad on top of each of the four chicken cutlets, garnish with flaky sea salt, and serve with lemon wedges.

250. Pasta Puttanesca W/ Chicken & Basil

Serving: Serves 6 | Prep: | Cook: | Ready in:

Ingredients

- For the Pasta Puttanesca
- 1 pound linguine fini or brown rice pasta (I like Pastariso)
- 6 large garlic cloves – crushed
- 3 teaspoons smashed anchovies packed in oil – chopped then smashed to make rough paste
- 3/4 teaspoon hot red pepper flakes
- 1-14 ounces can whole tomatoes
- 14 ounces "candied" tomatoes (see recipe below)
- ¾ cup pitted olives (we used a mix of green, Kalamata & Morrocan)
- 3 tablespoons capers drained – or capers packed in salt (rinsed – or if you like salty – not rinsed...)
- 1/4 teaspoon raw sugar or agave
- ½ cup white wine
- 1/3 cup olive oil
- 1 cup organic basil – chopped
- 4 chicken breasts – chopped into 2" chunks
- For the Candied Tomatoes (Adapted from Suzane Somers cookbook):
- 10-12 tomatoes (any kind but cherry)
- olive oil
- salt

Direction

- For the Pasta Puttanesca
- In large pot, put the can of whole tomatoes and their juice and smash tomatoes with your hand or a potato smasher until chunky and pulpy. Turn heat to medium and add garlic, anchovy paste, red pepper flakes, candied tomatoes, olives, sugar and white wine. Bring to boil then simmer for 35-45 minutes. Adding more wine if needs liquid.

- Meanwhile, heat olive oil over medium high heat, add chicken chunks and sear until browned but still quite juicy. Add to sauce.
- When sauce is almost done, cook pasta according to package directions. Drain.
- After sauce has cooked for 35-45 minutes add capers and basil and stir in. Let cook for 5-10 minutes more. Then serve over pasta.
- For the Candied Tomatoes:
- Slice tomatoes in half lengthwise. Place on cookie sheet. Drizzle with olive oil and sprinkle with sea salt.
- Bake in 325-degree oven until outsides are dry and wrinkly and insides are still juicy (about two hours). This will cause tomatoes to sweeten up and become absolutely delicious. (These are especially good with just picked tomatoes from the garden – if you can spare them.) Can be stored in oil in the refrigerator for one to two months. Great for when tomato season is over and you're craving that succulent sweet tomato of the summer...

251. Peachy BBQ Chicken

Serving: Serves 4-6 | Prep: | Cook: | Ready in:

Ingredients

- 250 milliliters bbq sauce
- 1/4 cup peach jam
- 1 clove garlic, minced
- 12 boneless, skinless chicken thighs

Direction

- Preheat the BBQ and set to medium high heat
- In a bowl combine the BBQ sauce, jam and garlic. Stir to combine.
- Place the chicken in an aluminum foil dish
- Pour the sauce evenly over the chicken.
- Close the lid and cook the chicken uncovered for 30-40 minutes until the internal temperature has reached 180 degrees

252. Peachy Sweet Wings

Serving: Serves 10-15 | Prep: | Cook: | Ready in:

Ingredients

- 3 pounds chicken wing drummettes
- 2/3 cup soy sauce or tamari
- 1 large jar strained peach baby food
- 2/3 cup brown sugar
- 1-2 cloves minced garlic

Direction

- Mix all ingredients except the chicken. Place wings in a 9 by 13 pan, and pour the sauce over them. Cover tightly with foil.
- Bake at 350 degrees for one hour.
- Uncover, and bake ½ to 1 hour more until wings are tender and very brown. Stir from time to time to distribute sauce.
- Remove from pan, place on platter and serve. Watch out for sticky fingers!

253. Pepita Crusted Chicken Cutlets

Serving: Serves 4 | Prep: | Cook: | Ready in:

Ingredients

- 1 1/4 cups pumpkin seeds
- 2 chicken breasts
- 3 tablespoons mayonnaise
- 1 tablespoon Dijon mustard
- 1 teaspoon ancho chile powder or smoked paprika
- 1/2 teaspoon cumin
- Pinch cayenne
- Kosher salt and pepper, to taste
- Neutral oil, for frying
- Lemon wedges or orange salsa (see notes above), for serving

Direction

- Preheat the oven to 375°F. Place pumpkin seeds on rimmed sheet pan. Transfer to oven and cook for 5 minutes — seeds should barely take on any color. Set pan aside to cool.
- Meanwhile, prepare the chicken breasts: If the tenderloin is still intact, slice it off and set it aside. At this point, you can either pound the chicken breasts to a 1/2-inch thickness, or you could cut each breast in half crosswise, to create 4 thin pieces — this is my preference.
- In a medium bowl, stir together the mayonnaise and mustard. Place the chicken breasts and tenders in the bowl and rub the mixture all over them to coat them evenly.
- Place the cooled pepitas, smoked paprika, cumin, and cayenne in a resealable bag. Seal the bag, pressing to release air before you close it completely. Holding a wine bottle by the neck, gently tap the bottom of the bottle against the seeds until they are crushed, but not uniformly fine like bread crumbs. I like a mix of full seeds, coarsely crushed seeds and finely crushed seeds. Transfer the seeds to a small rimmed sheet pan or other similar vessel.
- Transfer the breasts and tenders one by one to the vessel with the seeds, turning each to coat until each is evenly coated in seeds. Season both sides of each breast with salt and pepper to taste.
- Heat a large sauté pan over medium-high heat. Add 3 to 4 tablespoons of oil — you want a thin layer. When it shimmers, lower each breast into the pan and turn the heat down to medium. Cook for 2 to 3 minutes, flip, and cook for 2 to 3 minutes more or until evenly golden.
- Transfer breasts to a platter to rest. Let rest 5 minutes before slicing and serving.

254. Peppy Chicken Liver Toasts

Serving: Makes about 24 toasts | Prep: | Cook: | Ready in:

Ingredients

- 1 baguette, cut into 1/3 inch slices (leftover baguette expected)
- 2 tablespoons olive oil
- 1 1/2 tablespoons unsalted butter
- 3 large shallots, thinly sliced
- 1/8 teaspoon salt
- 2 slices bacon
- 4 ounces chicken livers, rinsed and patted dry
- 1 1/2 tablespoons fresh sage, minced
- Dijon mustard
- hot red jalapeño jelly

Direction

- Preheat oven to 350 degrees F. Arrange bread slices on a cookie sheet and brush with olive oil. Bake until golden, about 15 minutes.
- In a medium heavy skillet, melt butter over low heat. Add shallots and salt and cook, stirring occasionally, over low heat until evenly caramelized and fairly tacky, about 20 - 25 minutes.
- In a separate medium skillet, cook bacon over medium-high heat, turning once, until crispy. Adjust heat while cooking to prevent smoking. Remove from heat and reserve bacon for another purpose. Leave rendered fat in the pan.
- With a very sharp knife, cut chicken livers into thin, 1/8 - 3/16 inch slices. Return skillet with bacon fat to medium-high heat until just shy of smoking. Add minced sage and cook, stirring, until very aromatic and darkened, about 30 seconds. Add liver slices. Cook on each side until just browned, about 2 minutes per side, then remove to drain on a paper towel.
- Assemble the toasts. Spread about 1/4 teaspoon of Dijon mustard on each toast. Place a slice or two, depending on size, of liver on each toast. Add a dollop of caramelized

shallots. Finally, top with about 1/4 teaspoon, or more for extra pep, of hot red jalapeño jelly and serve.

255. Perfect Pear Fall Salad

Serving: Serves 4 | Prep: | Cook: |Ready in:

Ingredients

- 1/2 cup walnuts, coarsely chopped
- 1 cup granulated sugar
- 2 bosc pears
- 3 1/5 tablespoons olive oil
- 1 teaspoon whole grain mustard
- 1 tablespoon cider vinegar
- 1/4 cup dry white wine
- 1 bunch red lettuce leaves, cut into bite-size pieces
- 1 bunch baby arugula leaves
- 2 Belgian endive, thinly sliced
- 1/2 red onion, thinly sliced
- 2 ounces crumbled blue cheese
- Kosher salt
- fresh ground pepper
- 2 cooked chicken breasts, sliced (optional but suggested)

Direction

- Preheat the oven to 425 degrees.
- To make the candied walnuts, combine walnuts and sugar in a pan over medium heat. Stir constantly until all of the sugar has melted onto the walnuts and the sugar has become a clear glaze. Pour the candied nuts onto a sheet of waxed paper to cool.
- Halve and core the pears and cut into 1/2 inch slices. Heat 1/2 tablespoon of the olive oil in an oven-proof skillet over medium heat. Add the pears and wine and cook, stirring occasionally, until beginning to soften and turn color, about 8 minutes. Transfer the pan to the oven and continue cooking until the pears are cooked through and most of the liquid has evaporated, about 8 minutes.
- To make the salad dressing, whisk together the mustard and vinegar, then slowly incorporate the remaining 3 tablespoon of olive oil until well mixed. Set aside.
- Toss the lettuce, arugula, and endive together in a large bowl. Add the blue cheese, candied walnuts, red onion, dressing, and chicken. Season with salt and pepper and toss. Divide the salad onto salad plates, and place roasted pears in the center of each salad. This is best served while the pears are still warm.

256. Perfect Roast Chicken

Serving: Serves 6 | Prep: | Cook: |Ready in:

Ingredients

- 1 organic, free-range roasting chicken, 5 to 6 pounds
- 2 tablespoons exra virgin olive oil
- 1 tablespoon coarse sea salt
- 2 teaspoons freshly ground black pepper
- 2 whole heads plump fresh garlic, cut in half horizontally
- several sprigs each fresh rosemary, thyme, marjoram, lavender leaves
- 1 cup cold water or white wine (to baste the chicken)

Direction

- Heat the oven to 375 degrees F. Start by rinsing the chicken inside and out with cold running water. Drain it well and dry inside and out with paper towels. Make a mixture of about 2 teaspoons freshly ground pepper and 1 tablespoon of coarse sea salt in a small bowl. Place the bowl alongside a shallow 9 x 14-inch roasting pan. Put the olive oil in the pan and distribute evenly. You will also need a 3-foot length of kitchen string.

- Put the chicken into the pan and turn to coat well with the olive oil. Season it generously, inside and out with salt and pepper. Put about half of the herbs inside the cavity. Truss with string.
- Place the chicken on its side in the pan. Put the halved garlic heads (cut side up) and the remainder of the herbs into the pan alongside the chicken. Place the pan on a rack in the center of the oven and roast, uncovered, for 20 minutes. Baste the chicken with the water and roast for another 25 minutes. Baste again – this time with the juices in the pan -- turn the chicken to the other side, and repeat the process. This will take a total of 90 minutes roasting time. By this time the skin should be a deep golden color. Test to see if the juices run clear when you pierce a thigh with the point of a knife.
- Remove the pan from the oven and transfer the chicken to a platter on which you have placed an overturned salad plate. Place the chicken at an angle against the edge of the plate with its tail in the air. (This retains moisture because the juices flow down through the breast meat.) Cover the chicken loosely with foil. Let it rest for at least 10 minutes or up to 30 minutes. The chicken will continue to cook as it rests. Reserve the roasted garlic to serve with the chicken.
- To prepare a sauce, remove the herbs from the pan and skim as much fat as possible from the pan juices. Place the roasting pan over medium heat and scrape up any brown bits that cling to the bottom. Cook for 2 to 3 minutes, scraping and stirring until the liquid is almost caramelized. Do not let it burn. Spoon off and discard any excess fat. Add several tablespoons cold water to deglaze (hot water would cloud the sauce), and bring to a boil. Reduce the heat to low and simmer until thickened, about 5 minutes.
- While the sauce is cooking, carve the chicken and arrange it on a warmed serving platter along with the garlic.
- Strain the sauce through a fine-mesh sieve and pour into a sauceboat. Serve immediately with the chicken and the halved heads of garlic

257. Perfect Thanksgiving Turkey & Gravy

Serving: Serves 6-12 depending on size of bird | Prep: | Cook: | Ready in:

Ingredients

- Simple Brined + Roasted Thanksgiving Turkey...
- 3 onions, sliced
- 2-3 fennel bulbs, sliced
- 30 cloves of fresh garlic, sliced
- 3-4 oranges, sliced
- 3 lemons, sliced and seeds discarded
- 1/2 cup olive oil
- 1 gallon water, brought to a boil
- 18 ounces kosher salt
- 12 ounces honey
- 3 tablespoons fennel seeds, toasted
- 4 bay leaves
- 3 sprigs rosemary, bruised
- 12 sprigs thyme, bruised
- 6 juniper berries, bruised
- 2 gallons ice water
- 1 12-18 pounds organic turkey
- Dash Salt and Pepper (after the brine)
- Crazy Good Gravy...
- drippings from the roasted turkey
- 1 1/2 cups dry white wine
- 1/4 cup all purpose flour
- 3-4 shallots, minced
- 3 sprigs thyme, stems removed and chopped

Direction

- Simple Brined + Roasted Thanksgiving Turkey...

- Sweat the onions, fennel and garlic in olive oil for 20 minutes over medium heat in a covered stock pot, careful to not color them.
- Cover with the boiling water and whisk in the salt and honey so that they disperse into the water. Add all the other ingredients (citrus, herbs and spices) then turn off the heat to steep for 30 minutes.
- Chill the brine by adding 2 gallons of ice water.
- Rinse your turkey under cold water and place in a large vessel or pot. Pour the chilled brine over the bird and refrigerate for two or three days.
- Remove the bird from the brine and place in a vessel covered for one hour.
- Heat your oven to convection heat at 400 degrees. If using a still oven add 50 degrees to all the temperatures for this recipe. Note: use a quality thermometer preferably with a timer to gauge internal temperature.
- To properly roast a 16 pound bird you can plan on a 5 hour time span from start to finish. One hour to temper the bird by bringing it up to room temperature after removing it from the brine, 2 1/2 - 3 hours to cook the bird and a final hour to rest the bird after roasting. Tempering, roasting, and resting are the key to a perfectly roasted turkey or poultry for that matter.
- Stuff your bird with your preferred stuffing (I use a wild rice stuffing that I'll post next), truss the bird with kitchen string. Season the bird liberally with salt and pepper. Roll out aluminum foil with parchment paper rolled out on-top of it. Then place the bird breast side down on the paper. Wrap the parchment around the bird and then the aluminum foil around that. It should look like a silver ball of sorts when done. Place the bird again breast side down into your roasting pan rack.
- Place the bird in the oven for 30 minutes only... then turn the oven down to 200 degrees for one hour.
- After one hour at 200 degrees, remove the turkey from the oven and open the foil and parchment. Flip the bird over and tightly close up the parchment and foil again. Return to the oven at 200 degrees and roast for another hour.
- After this next hour, you should be especially aware of the internal temperature before finishing the bird in the oven. Measure the temperature by piercing deep into the thigh. Look for a final temperature of 142-148 degrees. (148-160 for more doneness)
- Remove the bird after the two hours at 200 degrees and remove the parchment and foil allowing the juices to pool in the roasting pan. Crank the oven up to 375 (425 for non-convection) and return the bird (breast side up again) to the oven until well browned and cooked to your desired cooking temp of 142-148. Expect a touch of pink near the joints for these temps but if you prefer a less moist bird you can cook it further. See above.
- Note: USDA recommends 180 for poultry, sadly this will result in the dried out birds of our childhoods...
- Once the bird has reached temp remove and place the turkey on a wood cutting board or platter to rest for one hour! Don't forget to tip the bird in the roasting pan, you want to make sure to get all of those juices out for gravy... Resting for an hour will allow all the juices to disperse back into the flesh and give you the perfect crown jewel of the table this holiday, so don't skip. If you can keep the bird in a warm area while resting (90-105 degrees) it's best but if not tent it lightly with foil.
- To Carve the Bird...Make a cut along the middle of the breast bone, let your knife slice just the side of the bone releasing the breast from the carcass. Remove the entire breast and slice on the bias, plating on the platter. Repeat on the other side. Remove the legs using the tip of your knife to release it from the joint. Remove the wings and any under meat if you like or save those parts for left overs.
- Crazy Good Gravy...
- Pour the drippings from your roasting pan into a sauce pot, set aside.
- Set the roasting pan directly over medium high heat on your stove.

- Add the white wine to the pan, careful it will sizzle and pop. Scrape the pan with a wooden spoon while the wine is sizzling, this will deglaze the pan releasing all the little bits into the liquid.
- Add the shallots and thyme, keep scrapping and stirring for 5-6 minutes...
- Place the sauce pot on a medium-high heat burner. Once hot add the flour and stir until well combined and the flour is smooth.
- Continue to stir briskly while slowly adding the wine and shallots mixture. Add in 1/2 cup increments the potato water to achieve the desired consistency. Keep in mind you may need to adjust the temperature to keep the gravy gently bubbling.
- Let the gravy simmer for about 10 minutes before tasting and seasoning with salt and pepper.
- The gravy will thicken when cooled at the table but adjust thickness with flour or water for thicker or thinner gravy.
- Serve alongside of your perfectly roasted turkey and don't blame me if your guests are not much for conversation, they will be too busy enjoying your turkey!

258. Persian Saffron Roast Chicken & Barberry Rice

Serving: Serves 4 | Prep: 0hours30mins | Cook: 1hours30mins | Ready in:

Ingredients

- Roast chicken
- 1 (3 1/2 to 4–pound) whole chicken
- 1/2 teaspoon ground saffron
- 2 ice cubes
- 1/8 cup olive oil
- 2 tablespoons melted butter
- 1 fresh lemon
- 1 head garlic
- 1 1/2 teaspoons coarse kosher salt
- 1/2 cup chicken stock
- Rice & barberries
- 1 1/2 cups basmati rice
- 3 cups water (enough to cover the rice and to come 1/2 inch over it)
- 1/2 teaspoon salt
- 4 tablespoons vegetable oil, divided
- 1/4 teaspoon ground saffron
- 1 tablespoon vegetable oil
- 3/4 cup barberries
- 1/2 teaspoon kosher salt
- 1 teaspoon sugar

Direction

- Preheat the oven to 400°F.
- Sprinkle ground saffron on ice cubes and let it melt at room temperature.
- Clean the chicken and pat dry it completely, on the skin and in the cavity. Run your fingers under the skin to make sure it's separated from the meat. But don't tear it. This is to make sure the saffron flavor can get under the skin as well.
- Mix bloomed saffron, olive oil, melted butter and the juice of 1/2 lemon in a bowl and using a small spoon, slowly pour it under the skin. Massage the skin to make sure the saffron and oil are getting all over the meat.
- Place the head of garlic in the cavity. Cross the legs and tie them using a kitchen twine. Place the chicken in a roasting pan, pour in the chicken stock, and roast for about 1 hour and 20 minutes until the thighs register at 165°F. Baste the chicken only once halfway through.
- Once the chicken is cooked, let it sit for 10 minutes before carving. Serve saffron chicken with barberry rice.
- While the chicken is roasting, make the rice. Place the rice, water, salt, and 2 tablespoons oil in a large saucepan or a pot and bring to a boil. Turn the heat to low and let it simmer until the water is almost evaporated. Using a fork, bring the rice to the middle to form a mountain shape. Add the remaining 2 tablespoons oil around the edges. Wrap the lid in a clean kitchen towel and place it on top of

the pot. Let the rice cook for another 10 to 12 minutes until fully cooked. Take 1/2 cup of the cooked rice and mix it with bloomed saffron. Set aside.
- Wash and dry the barberries. In a small pan, heat the 1 tablespoon vegetable oil over medium low heat and add the barberries to the pan. Stir constantly and add the salt and sugar. Sauté for about 3 to 5 minutes over medium-low to low.
- Transfer the white rice into serving plates and top them with some saffron rice and sautéed barberries. Serve with saffron roast chicken.

259. Pesto Stuffed Chicken Parmesan

Serving: Serves 4 | Prep: | Cook: | Ready in:

Ingredients

- Chicken Breasts
- 4 boneless skinless chicken breasts
- 3/4 cup mozzarella cheese
- 1/4 cup prepared pesto
- 2 cups white rice flour - season with 2 tsp of both salt and pepper
- 3/4 cup grated parmesan cheese
- 3/4 cup coarse cornmeal
- 3/4 cup gluten-free panko breadcrumbs (Ians brand is good)
- 4 eggs
- olive oil
- Tomato Sauce
- 1 tablespoon olive oil
- 1/2 cup finely chopped sweet onion
- 3 cloves of garlic
- 1 small 6 oz can of tomato paste
- 1 28 oz can of crushed tomatoes
- 2 15 oz cans diced tomatoes (drain the excess water but reserve to thin out sauce)
- 1 tablespoon agave nectar
- 1 teaspoon salt
- 1/2 teaspoon black pepper
- 1 teaspoon dried basil
- 1 teaspoon dried oregano
- 1/2 teaspoon garlic powder
- 1/2 teaspoon red pepper flakes (optional)

Direction

- To start, begin creating the sauce. Add the olive oil and onion to the pan and saute until onion is translucent. Add the garlic cooking for about 1 min before adding the remaining ingredients. Be careful not to burn the garlic in this step. Once the garlic has cooked about a min add the remaining sauce ingredients and stir. Turn the heat to low and let simmer while you begin preparing the chicken breasts. If the sauce is too thick at water until it reaches the desired consistency.
- Preheat oven to 400 and prepare a 9x13 baking dish by lightly spraying with olive oil.
- Take each chicken breast and create a pocket by cutting into the center of the side of the breast being careful not to cut all the way through. Stuff each breast with 2 tbsps. mozzarella cheese and 1 tbsp. of pesto.
- Put the seasoned rice flour in a shallow bowl and in another shallow bowl crack the eggs and whisk lightly to break up eggs and create the egg wash. Then in a third bowl combine 1/2 cup of the parmesan cheese, the cornmeal and the gluten free panko.
- Take the first chicken breast and coat in the seasoned flour, shaking off any excess. Then dip the chicken breast in the egg wash and then in the breadcrumb mixture covering it well. Place on a plate and then repeat with the remaining 3 breasts.
- Spread the sauce in the bottom of the 9x13 pan. This should cover the bottom but you do not want the chicken to be completely submerged so if there is too much sauce you can just reserve it for later use. Add the chicken breasts and then top with the remaining 1/4 of mozzarella and 1/4 cup of parmesan cheese (about 1 tbsp. each type of cheese over each breast).

- Bake 10-15 minutes until cheese has browned and chicken has reached internal temp of 165. If the chicken has not reached 165 but cheese is browned, cover with aluminum foil for the remainder of the cooking process.

260. Pho Sho

Serving: Serves 10 people or more | Prep: | Cook: |Ready in:

Ingredients

- Chicken Stock
- 2 Organic Chickens
- Alderwood Smoked Sea Salt
- Fresh Cracked Pepper
- 2 Bay leaf
- 2 Carrots roughly chopped
- 3 Celery stalks roughly chopped
- 1 large yellow onion roughly chopped
- For the Pho
- 12-15 Star Anise Pieces
- 6 Cinnamon Sticks
- 20 Green Cardamom Pods
- 12 Cloves
- 3 Pieces of crystallized ginger
- 1 small knob fresh ginger grated
- 1 tablespoon grape seed oil
- 2 tablespoons Organic Tamarind Paste (Aunt Pattie's)
- 2 tablespoons Fish Sauce (Red Boat 40)

Direction

- Chicken Stock
- Lightly season both chickens with salt and pepper.
- Place chicken in a large roasting dish and cook at 375 for roughly 1 to 1 1/2 hours. If you have a convection oven the process may be faster.
- Allow chickens to cool. Remove meat and set aside for later use.
- Take all chicken bones, leftover skin, fat, and/or trimmings and place in a large stockpot.
- Add carrots, onions, celery and bay leaves.
- Fill with filtered water just an inch below the top.
- Bring to a boil, then drop to a simmer. Simmer for a few hours. Strain. Discard bones and save stock.
- For the Pho
- In a small saute pan over medium heat add grape seed oil. Add all the spices to oil and toast until fragrant.
- At the same time your spices are heating up; have your chicken stock in a large stockpot at a simmer. Once the spices are fragrant add to the stock.
- Next add your tamarind paste and fish sauce. Cook this mixture for another hour or so. Let cool and then strain again.
- For the final round of cooking you may add whatever your heart desires. I like to serve this broth with the roasted chicken, onions, green onions, cilantro and lime wedges. I often switch up the carb sometimes brown rice noodles, brown rice, quinoa, or black lentils. Organicville makes a really nice organic Sriracha that's worth the money.

261. Pickle Fried Chicken

Serving: Makes 30 chicken nuggets | Prep: | Cook: | Ready in:

Ingredients

- for the chicken nuggets:
- 2 pounds boneless, skinless chicken breasts (cubed)
- 1 1/2 cups dill pickle juice (I use Mt. Olive brand)
- 1 1/2 cups buttermilk
- 1 tablespoon dry dill
- 1 tablespoon green chili powder

- 3/4 cup masa harina (sub corn meal if not available)
- 1 cup flour
- 1 tablespoon paprika, granulated garlic, coriander, turmeric, ground black pepper
- 1 teaspoon cumin, cayenne powder, dried oregano
- 2 tablespoons salt
- canola oil
- for the buttermilk ranch
- 1/2 cup plain Greek yogurt
- 1/2 cup mayonnaise
- 1/4 cup buttermilk
- 2 tablespoons fresh dill (minced)
- 1 tablespoon granulated garlic
- 1 tablespoon apple cider vinegar
- 1 tablespoon Dijon mustard
- 1 tablespoon salt

Direction

- Get the chicken brined first. In a large mixing bowl, combine pickle juice, buttermilk, dried dill, green chili powder and chicken cubes. Cover with plastic wrap and let sit in fridge for 2 hours, up to 24 hours. 2 hours does the trick though as the chicken is cubed into small pieces.
- As chicken marinades, make the ranch dipping sauce. Mix Greek yogurt, mayo, buttermilk, granulated garlic, fresh dill, apple cider vinegar, Dijon mustard and salt. Cover and let the flavors come together in the fridge as chicken brines.
- Remove chicken 15 minutes prior to cooking. Drain chicken in a colander and pat all pieces dry. In a heavy bottomed, large pan, heat 1/2 inch canola oil until hot enough to make flour sizzle when dropped in. About 350 degrees.
- Preheat oven to 250 degrees. Line a baking sheet with paper towels and place wire rack on top.
- In a shallow bowl, combine masa harina, flour, spices, salt and pepper. Sift to combine. Drop in pieces of chicken to coat in flour mixture. (Don't forget to pat the chicken pieces dry first.) Once coated, shake off excess flour and drop into oil. Cook chicken on all 3 or 4 sides for a total of 6-7 minutes. The chicken will have a brown coating when done.
- Remove chicken from oil and place on wire rack. Place in oven. Repeat process until all chicken is fried, leaving all chicken pieces on wire rack until the whole batch is fried.
- Serve hot with toothpicks and homemade buttermilk ranch for easy dipping.

262. Pinaupong Manok (Chicken Steamed By A Bed Of Salt)

Serving: Serves 4 | Prep: | Cook: | Ready in:

Ingredients

- 2.2 pounds fully cleaned chicken, neck, feet & innards removed and, if possible, skin still intact
- 6 pounds rough sea salt
- 2 packets Knorr or Maggi "Sinigang Mix" (tamarind soup base)
- 1 piece small carrot-sliced
- 1 piece cucumber-sliced
- 1 bunch onion leaves or celery stalk
- 1 piece small ginger, de-skinned, grated
- 20 milliliters EVOO (Extra Virgin Olive Oil)
- 10 milliliters calamansi or lemon juice

Direction

- Covering all parts inside and outside, rub chicken with "Sinigang Mix". Set aside.
- In suitable pan, pour in salt and make at least 2 inches thick layer at the bottom.
- Sit in chicken making sure not a part of it touches the sides of pan. (Failing which, burning occurs) Use its neck or feet as "kalso" (wedge thing) under it to ensure chicken sit upwards.
- Heat pan at medium temp and "steam" chicken for no more than 20 minutes (for very juicy inside) or up to 25 minutes (for just right

medium well state)Steaming longer will render dryness to poultry.
- While waiting heat EVOO, pour in grated ginger and heat for 1 minute. Set aside.
- Your chicken "steamed via bed of salt" is done. Mix in "calamansi juice", soy sauce and "chili-garlic sauce" for dip or grated ginger with soy sauce or whatever…it's your rule…your wild…
- Slice, garnish and serve your very own style of better than Hainanese poultry.

263. Pink Bolognese

Serving: Serves 4-6 | Prep: | Cook: |Ready in:

Ingredients

- 1/2 pound ground pork
- 1/2 pound ground veal
- 1/2 pound ground dark meat turkey
- 2 tablespoons olive oil
- 1 medium carrot, finely chopped
- 1 medium yellow onion, finely chopped
- 2 cloves garlic, minced
- 2 small tomatoes, cored and finely chopped
- 1 cup red wine
- 1 quart homemade or organic chicken broth
- 1 tablespoon chopped sage plus 2 sage leaves
- 1/2 teaspoon dried thyme
- 1/2 teaspoon dried oregano
- 1/2 teaspoon dried basil
- 1/2 teaspoon dried rosemary
- 2 tablespoons double-concentrate tomato paste, plus more to taste
- 1 cup cream
- 2 tablespoons vodka
- salt
- Freshly ground pepper
- 1 pound short pasta, like penne rigate

Direction

- In a large, heavy saucepan, brown the pork, veal and turkey over medium-high heat. Keep smashing and separating the meat while cooking. Transfer the browned meat to a bowl, and reserve. Return the pan to the stove.
- Add olive oil to the pan and place over medium high heat. Add the carrots, onion and garlic, and stir to combine. Reduce the heat to medium and cook until tender, 5 to 10 minutes. Return the meat to the pan. Stir in the tomatoes. Pour in the red wine and bring to a boil. Add the chicken broth and all the herbs and simmer for 30 minutes, stirring occasionally
- Stir in the tomato paste and continue simmering for another hour, stirring every 10 minutes or so -- you don't want any sticking or burning. The sauce should reduce and thicken.
- Pour in the cream and vodka and cook until sauce is the desired consistency. Season with salt and pepper. Taste, taste, taste -- it's up to you.
- Meanwhile, bring a large pot of generously salted water to a boil. Add the pasta and cook until al dente. Drain, then toss with the Bolognese.

264. Piri Piri Chicken Meatballs With Crispy Potatoes

Serving: Serves 6 | Prep: 0hours0mins | Cook: 0hours0mins |Ready in:

Ingredients

- Piri piri sauce
- 10 tablespoons olive oil, divided
- 2 red bell peppers, finely diced
- 2 red onions, finely diced
- 1 1/4 teaspoons salt, plus more to taste
- 4 garlic cloves, smashed, peeled, and roughly chopped
- 1 piri piri chile, roughly chopped
- 6 tablespoons red wine vinegar
- Meatballs and potatoes

- 1 pound ground chicken, preferably a combo of white and dark meat
- 2 piri piri chilies, minced
- 2 large eggs
- 5 tablespoons olive oil, divided, plus more for pan-frying
- 1/2 cup potato chip crumbs
- 6 garlic cloves, minced
- 2 tablespoons minced parsley
- 2 tablespoons minced cilantro
- 1 tablespoon grated lemon zest
- 1/4 teaspoon smoked paprika
- 2 teaspoons salt, divided plus more to taste
- 6 russet potatoes, scrubbed

Direction

- Start the sauce. Add 4 tablespoons olive oil to a very wide skillet—big enough to get the peppers and onions as spread out as possible. Set the skillet over medium-high heat. When it's shimmery and hot, add the peppers and onions. Add the salt and stir to combine. Cook, stirring occasionally, for about 20 minutes until soft and caramelized.
- When the vegetables are done, transfer half to a blender and half to the freezer (to speed cooling for the meatball-mixing). Add the garlic and chile to the blender and process until mostly smooth. Add the vinegar and rest of the olive oil and process until as smooth as possible. Season with salt to taste.
- Add the ground chicken, chilies, eggs, 3 tablespoons olive oil, potato chip crumbs, garlic, parsley, cilantro, lemon zest, paprika, and 1 teaspoon salt to a big bowl. When the vegetables in the freezer are cool, add those, too. Mix until just combined. You don't want to overwork it, or you'll end up with dense meatballs. Stick the mixture in the fridge to set.
- Meanwhile, preheat the oven to 425° F. Cut each potato in half lengthwise. Cut each half in half lengthwise. Now cut each half in half lengthwise again. This will yield 8 wedges from each potato. Add to a sheet pan. Drizzle with the remaining 2 tablespoons olive oil and 1 teaspoon salt. Toss. Lay each potato flat on one side. Bake for about 30 minutes, flipping the potatoes halfway through, until both sides are very colorful and crusty.
- After the potatoes have been in the oven for 10 or so minutes, get going on those meatballs. Set a very large skillet (maybe the same one you used for the peppers and onions) over medium-high heat. Add enough olive oil to reach a 1/4-inch or so depth. When the oil is shimmery and hot, use a cookie scoop (figure about 1 1/2 tablespoons) to dollop the meatball mixture into the hot oil. If you don't have a scoop, you can use two spoons. The mixture is too wet to roll in your hands (because we don't want dry meatballs!). And you'll need to do this in batches—don't overcrowd. Cook for about 8 minutes—progressively turning as they brown on each side—until cooked through and crusty all over. Transfer to a paper towel-lined plate to drain. Repeat with the remaining meatballs.
- Serve the meatballs and potatoes together with lots of piri piri sauce.

265. Pollo E Peperoni (Chicken With Tomatoes And Red Peppers)

Serving: Serves 4 | Prep: | Cook: | Ready in:

Ingredients

- 3 tablespoons olive oil
- 1 thick slice of pancetta (about 50 grams), diced (optional)
- 3 pounds (about 1.3 kg) chicken (either a whole one, jointed, marylands or thighs)
- 1/2 cup (125 ml) white wine
- 20 ounces (550 grams) of tinned tomatoes with their juice
- 1 garlic clove, smashed
- 1 sprig rosemary, leaves picked and chopped
- 4 large sweet red peppers
- salt and freshly ground black pepper

Direction

- Heat the oil in a sauté pan or pot and cook the pancetta until golden and crisp.
- Add the chicken pieces, skin-side down if possible, and sear until golden, then turn over and brown the other side. Season with salt and pepper.
- Splash the chicken with the white wine, and let it sizzle until it's almost all evaporated.
- Add the garlic, rosemary and tomatoes (crushed in the tin beforehand, or break them up with your wooden spoon when in the pan). Cover and cook over moderate heat. Keep an eye on everything for the first 10 minutes, stirring when necessary, then half-cover the pan and continue cooking for a further 45 minutes or until the sauce has become dense and the chicken is tender and starting to pull away from the bone. If the sauce is looking too thick but the chicken not ready, you can add a splash of water and continue cooking. Season to taste.
- Meanwhile, roast the peppers in a preheated oven (200° C/390° F), turning them once or twice, until soft and charred, about 45 minutes. Remove from oven and immediately tip into a bowl. Cover the hot vegetables with cling film and let them "steam" for about 10 minutes before peeling off the skins. Discard the seeds and stems and then rip or cut the peppers into strips and add to the chicken.
- Cook a further 5 minutes then let the pan to sit for at least 15 minutes for the flavors to mingle (better an hour, or even overnight in the fridge for the next day). You can serve it at room temperature or reheat it over low until warm.

266. Portuguese Chicken Soup Aka Canja

Serving: Serves 6-8 | Prep: 0hours15mins | Cook: 2hours0mins | Ready in:

Ingredients

- 1 Yellow onion diced
- 1 Carrot sliced
- 1 Stalk of celery sliced
- 2 Bay leaves
- 1 Stewing hen or whole chicken with legs and thighs removed
- 2 teaspoons Salt
- 1 cup Rice or soup pasta
- 2 Lemons
- Salt and black pepper to taste
- 2 sprigs thyme (optional)

Direction

- Place onion, carrot, celery, bay leaves and salt in a large pot. Add the whole stewing hen. If using a regular chicken, remove the legs and thighs for another use and place the remaining chicken, bones and all, in the pot. Add enough water to cover the chicken (about 8 cups). Bring to a boil then simmer for 1.5 - 2 hours.
- Remove chicken from pot and set aside. Add rice or soup pasta to pot and stir. Cook until rice or pasta is done to your liking. Meanwhile, shred chicken, disposing of skin and bones. If using a stewing hen, you may only want to shred the white meat.
- When rice or pasta is to your liking, add shredded chicken back to pot along with the juice of 1 lemon. Season with salt and pepper. Sprinkle thyme leaves on top (optional). Serve with remaining lemon cut into wedges.

267. Post Thanksgiving Turkey Ragu

Serving: Serves 6-8 | Prep: | Cook: |Ready in:

Ingredients

- 2 tablespoons olive oil
- 1 sweet onion, finely chopped
- 5-6 small garlic cloves, peeled and minced

- 3 carrots, peeled, finely chopped
- 2 stalks celery, sliced
- 1 green pepper, seeded, chopped
- 1/2 teaspoon dried basil
- 4-5 cups dark turkey meat, chopped
- 1/2 cup dry red wine
- Pinch of sugar
- 3 cans diced tomatoes (14.5 ounces)
- 1 can tomato paste
- Sea salt to taste
- Freshly ground black pepper to taste
- 6-8 fresh basil leaves cut into chiffonade

Direction

- Heat oil in a Dutch oven over medium heat until it shimmers. Add onion, stirring to cook and prevent onion from sticking or burning. Cook until onion begins to soften, about two minutes.
- Add carrots, stirring occasionally. Cook until carrots begin to soften, about five minutes.
- Add garlic, celery and green pepper. Stir and cook for two minutes more. Stir in dried basil.
- Add dark turkey meat. Stir to combine.
- Add red wine and sugar.
- Add cans of diced tomato, with juice. Stir mixture and bring to a simmer. Cover and turn down to low. Let ragu simmer for at least 2 1/2 hours to allow flavors to develop.
- Stir in one can of tomato paste and continue to simmer for 30 minutes more. Taste for salt and pepper, adding if necessary or desired. Add fresh basil and give ragu a stir. Serve with pasta, leftover mashed potatoes or other starch of choice; sprinkle with parmesan cheese if desired.

268. Poulet À L'Estragon (Tarragon Chicken)

Serving: Serves 4 to 6 | Prep: | Cook: | Ready in:

Ingredients

- 1 chicken, 3 1/2 to 4 pounds, cut into 8 pieces
- Olive oil
- 1 tablespoon unsalted butter
- 2 cups chicken stock or water
- 2 tablespoons tomato paste
- 4 shallots, trimmed, peeled and julienned
- 1/3 cup heavy cream
- 2 tablespoons tarragon, minced, plus four sprigs
- 1/2 cup dry white wine

Direction

- Season the chicken with salt and white pepper. Place a heavy bottom 12" skillet over medium high heat. When the pan is hot add enough olive oil to form a thin film on the bottom of the pan. Add the chicken skin side down. Brown the chicken to your liking.
- When the chicken is brown quickly remove it to a plate. Add the butter and the shallots to the sauté pan. Sauté the shallots until golden.
- Deglaze the pan with the white wine and let the wine reduce to a tablespoon or so. Add the chicken stock, tomato paste and the sprigs of tarragon. Place the chicken back into the pan and let the sauce come to a boil. Reduce the heat to a simmer.
- Place a lid on the pan and simmer the chicken until tender. About thirty minutes. Meanwhile heat the oven broiler.
- When the chicken is tender remove the lid from the pan. Carefully place the pan into the oven under the broiler and broil it for 3 to 5 minutes or however much time it takes to crisp up the skin. Remove from the oven.
- Remove the chicken to a platter. Place the pan over high heat. Add the cream and stir it in. Add the chopped tarragon. Taste the sauce and adjust the seasoning. Stir and bring to a boil.
- Sauce the chicken and serve over rice with extra sauce on the side.

269. Pozole Blanco Con Pollo

Serving: Serves 4 | Prep: | Cook: |Ready in:

Ingredients

- Pozole Blanco con Pollo
- 1 1/2 pounds boneless, skinless chicken breasts/10 full wings/10 drumsticks
- 1 can white hominy kernels
- 1 can yellow hominy kernels
- 1 can chickpeas (garbanzo beans)
- 1/2 cup uncooked rice
- 2 tablespoons peanut oil
- 1 onion, peeled and sliced
- 6 cloves fresh garlic, sliced
- 2 stalks celery and leaves, chopped
- 1 tablespoon cumin
- 1 tablespoon oregano
- 1 teaspoon white pepper
- 1 packet chicken bouillon
- salt to taste
- Garnish Plates
- 1 bunch fresh cilantro, chopped
- 1 avocado, peeled and sliced
- 2 stalks green onion, sliced green and white parts
- 6 radishes, sliced
- 3/4 cup thinly sliced raw cabbage
- 2 fresh limes, sliced
- 1/2 cup low-fat sour cream
- 12 corn tortillas or crispy tostadas

Direction

- Start 4 quarts of water boiling, on medium-high, in a large soup pot and add the chicken bouillon, Pour the peanut oil in a large sauce pan, heat until sizzling and toss in the onions, garlic, celery, cumin, oregano and salt and white pepper. Stir-fry all until light golden, and half-way done, then add them to soup pot.
- Add the 2 cans of hominy, rice and the chickpeas, cover and bring back to a boil, then simmer for 40 minutes on medium low heat. Watch the soup and stir every 10 minutes or so to prevent sticking. Place the pot on a heating pad or trivet in the middle of the table, along with soup bowls and spoons.
- Arrange the garnishes on separate dishes and set them around the pot of soup. Heat up your tortillas in an oiled, iron skillet or Teflon pan, wrap in a soft cloth to keep warm and serve them with the soup; if you prefer crispy tostadas, heat them in a 350 degree oven for 10 minutes, serve in a bowl by the soup.

270. Provençal Style Chicken In The Pot

Serving: Makes 4 to 6+ servings – depends on what else you're serving, and how hungry your guests are | Prep: | Cook: |Ready in:

Ingredients

- 1 4-pound free-range, organic chicken, whole
- sea salt and freshly ground black pepper
- Bouquet garni (include thyme, parsley stems, rosemary, marjoram, bay leaf)
- 1 cup fruity extra-virgin olive oil
- 40 unpeeled cloves of garlic
- bed of fresh herbs for the pot (should include: 1 bay leaf, the leafy top of a whole bunch of celery, a whole bunch of flat-leaf parsley, several sprigs each of marjoram, rosemary, sage and thyme (and lavender greens and summer savory, if you can find th
- 1 cup dry white wine (Loire Valley whites are great for this)
- 12 small all-purpose potatoes (about the size of a silver dollar) (WFM sells bags of multi-colored potatoes that add pizzaz)
- 12-16 small white onions, peeled
- 4 carrots, peeled and cut into chunks
- 1 pound fresh peas, shelled (or 1 10-ounce package frozen)
- 2 tablespoons flour and 1 tablespoon water for paste to seal the lid
- toasted French bread slices (for serving)

Direction

- Preheat oven to 350 degrees F. Make a mixture of salt and pepper in a small bowl. Use this to generously season the interior and exterior of a 4-pound fryer. Tie a bouquet garni together with string and put it inside.
- Pour 1 cup of olive oil into a large (about 9 quarts) Dutch oven with a lid. Add the bed of herbs and all of the garlic.
- Set the cleaned and trussed chicken on this bed and turn it over and over in the already perfumed oil. Add the dry white wine. Scatter the vegetables around on top of the bed of herbs.
- Then with all the oil, wine and aromatics below and the chicken and vegetables on top, put the lid on and seal it "hermetically" with a band of flour and water paste. Bake 1 hour and 30 minutes in the preheated oven.
- Remove from oven and allow the Dutch oven to sit undisturbed for 15 to 20 minutes. Do not lift the lid!
- In preparation for serving, put a small serving bowl (for the garlic) and a slotted spoon on the table. A pair of poultry shears is the easiest tool to use for cutting the hot chicken into serving pieces. A sturdy wooden spoon will help you hold the chicken still for cutting without burning your fingers.
- Carry the Dutch oven to the table and lift off the lid at the moment of serving, and take a deep breath. The aroma is incredible!
- Serve with toasted slices of bread which each diner will spread with the incomparable garlic purée. Don't be surprised. The chicken will not be browned.
- Teacher's Tip: When you have eaten all the chicken, vegetables and garlic, you will find yourself with a large pot of herbs and a chicken, garlicky wine-y stock. You can make a wonderful soup the next day (or several days hence) using this as a base. Here's how: Remove the herbs to a small bowl, cover with plastic wrap and refrigerate. Pour the wine/olive oil stock into a storage container, cover tightly and refrigerate overnight. When you are ready to make the soup, remove most of the oil that has risen to the top. Also overnight, soak 1 pound of small white beans in enough cold water to cover by 2 inches. The next day, drain the beans and put them back in the pot with enough water to cover by 2 inches, 6 black peppercorns and 1 bay leaf. Bring the beans to a boil and simmer for about 1 hour, until the beans are not quite tender. Drain the beans and reserve the water.
- Return the beans to the pot and now add the reserved wine/olive oil stock from the chicken to the beans. Also add the reserved herbs from last night's pot, and at least five of the following: ½ pound lima beans or fava beans, shelled and peeled; 6 potatoes, scrubbed and cut into ¾-inch chunks; ½ pound green beans, ends trimmed; 5 carrots, peeled and cut into ¾-inch chunks; 5 red onions, peeled and thickly sliced; 5 zucchini, cut into ¾-inch chunks; 3 white turnips, cut into ¾-inch chunks; 2 leeks, well washed, dried and sliced.
- Add 1 teaspoon sea salt and stir the mixture. Bring the soup to a boil and simmer for 40 to 50 minutes more. Some tubular pasta added during the last 15 minutes of cooking will add substance to this second one-dish meal. Serve the soup in large bowls with freshly grated Parmesan cheese on top and crusty bread on the side.

271. Pulled Chicken Tacos With Pineapple Salsa

Serving: Serves 4 | Prep: | Cook: | Ready in:

Ingredients

- For the tacos:
- 1 tablespoon olive oil
- 1 bell pepper, seeds and stem removed
- 3/4 red onion, sliced (keep the rest for the salsa)
- 2 teaspoons ground cinnamon

- 1 teaspoon ground cumin
- 1/2 teaspoon ground cayenne pepper
- 2 teaspoons sweet smoked paprika
- 2 cloves of garlic, minced
- 15 ounces can of chopped tomatoes
- 2 teaspoons granulated sugar
- 1 tablespoon Worcestershire sauce
- 1 tablespoon apple cider vinegar or lime juice
- 2 skinless, boneless chicken breasts
- sour cream, to serve
- tortillas, to serve
- For the salsa
- 1 cup fresh pineapple cubes
- 8 or 9 cherry tomatoes, chopped
- 1/4 cup chopped cilantro
- 1/4 red onion
- 2 teaspoons lime juice or apple cider vinegar
- 1/2 teaspoon sriracha or other hot sauce
- 1/4 teaspoon sea salt

Direction

- For the tacos: In a large pot, heat the olive oil over a medium flame.
- Cut the bell pepper into roughly 1/2-inch squares and add to the pot along with the onion.
- Add in the cumin, cinnamon, cayenne and paprika. Stir together until coated then cook, stirring until the onions are translucent and soft.
- Mix in the garlic then cook for a further minute. Pour in the tomatoes and add the granulated sugar, Worcestershire sauce and vinegar. Stir together well, scraping the bottom of the pot to make sure nothing has stuck and bring to the boil.
- Cut the chicken breasts in half then add into the pot. Submerge them in the sauce and leave to simmer on a medium-low heat, stirring occasionally, for 30 minutes.
- Remove the chicken breasts from the sauce to a cutting board, leave the sauce on the stove to stay hot. Using two forks (one to hold the meat still, the other to pull) shred the chicken. Stir the shredded chicken back in and take off the heat.
- To make the salsa: Chop the pineapple into small dice. Place into a small bowl with the tomato, cilantro, red onion, lime juice, sriracha and salt. Stir together then chill until needed.
- Warm the tortillas over the low flame of the hob then serve with the pineapple salsa, shredded chicken and sour cream.

272. Pulled Chicken On Pan Fried Corn Cakes

Serving: Serves 2 | Prep: | Cook: | Ready in:

Ingredients

- To make the chicken:
- 1/4 medium yellow onion, thinly sliced
- 2 cloves garlic, minced
- 1 teaspoon olive oil
- 1 boneless chicken breast
- 1 cup plain tomato puree
- 1 1/2 cups full sodium chicken stock
- 1/4 cup barbeque sauce
- 1-2 teaspoons Tabasco Sauce (optional)
- 5-6 dashes red wine vinegar
- 1 teaspoon salt
- Freshly ground black pepper, to taste
- To make the corn cakes:
- 1/2 cup Masarepa yellow corn meal (make sure package says "Precooked"!)
- 1/4 teaspoon coarse salt
- 3/4 cup warm water
- Butter or olive oil for pan frying

Direction

- To make the chicken:
- Heat the olive oil in a small pot, add the onion and cook until softened, about 2 minutes.
- Add in the garlic and cook until fragrant, about 1 minute.
- Place the chicken in the pot and add in the tomato puree, chicken stock, barbecue sauce, Tabasco Sauce, salt and a few turns of fresh cracked pepper. Cover the pot with a lid. If the

chicken is not fully submerged in the liquid, add more chicken stock or transfer contents to a smaller pot. Keep at a low simmer for about 35-40 minutes or until you can easily shred the chicken with a fork.
- Transfer chicken to a bowl and shred completely with a fork. Continue to cook down the liquid in the pot (about 20 minutes) until it thickens and pour about a cup of the sauce over the chicken (or more if desired). Add the red wine vinegar to the chicken and mix.
- To make the corn cakes:
- Mix the corn meal, salt and water together and set aside for 5 minutes.
- Form patties about 4-5 inches wide and a half an inch thick. Coat a frying pan lightly with butter or olive oil. Brown the patties on medium-high heat on both sides and transfer to paper towels to soak up excess oil.
- Serve the pulled chicken on the corn patties and top them with pickled radishes (or any other pickled vegetable) and some shredded romaine...maybe even some hot sauce or guacamole!

273. Quick Sesame Ginger Stir Fry

Serving: Serves 4 | Prep: | Cook: |Ready in:

Ingredients

- 1/4 cup soy sauce
- 1 tablespoon brown sugar
- 1 clove garlic
- 1/4 inch piece fresh ginger
- 1 teaspoon sesame oil
- 1/2 cup stock (any kind you have)
- 1/2 cup water
- 1 tablespoon cornstarch
- 6 cups chopped vegetables and cooked protein

Direction

- Note: Use any veggies and add-ins you like! For this version I used 1 shredded cooked chicken breast, 1 small can bamboo shoots, 1 large carrot, 1 chopped bell pepper, and ½ onion.
- Combine the soy sauce, sugar, sesame oil, stock, cornstarch, and water in a small dish, whisking with a small whisk or fork so the cornstarch doesn't have any lumps left. Grate the ginger and garlic directly into the sauce with a mini grater.
- Preheat a large skillet to medium-high heat with a drizzle of olive oil. Add the vegetables and cook for about 5 minutes until they have softened and charred just slightly.
- Pour in the sauce and add the shredded chicken or any protein you're using. The sauce should bubble and thicken immediately. Taste the sauce and adjust the seasoning to your preference with more soy sauce.
- If the sauce seems too thick, splash in a little bit of water to thin it out, about 2 tablespoons at a time. Serve over cooked rice.

274. RIVERBOAT LEMON LIME CHICKEN

Serving: Serves 8 | Prep: | Cook: |Ready in:

Ingredients

- LEMON-LIME CHICKEN
- 4   small chickens, skinned and cut into eighths
- 2   medium-sized sweet Vidalia onions, minced
- 1.5 tablespoons olive oil, preferably organic extra-virgin
- LEMON-LIME MARINADE
- 3 lemons, juicy
- 5 limes, juicy
- 1 tablespoon olive oil, preferably organic extra-virgin

- 1/2 teaspoon freshly ground black pepper, "fine" setting

Direction

- LEMON-LIME CHICKEN
- Place the chicken eighths into a stainless steel bowl, and thoroughly combine with the lemon-lime marinade.
- Cover the bowl, and refrigerate overnight, or 12 hours.
- Take a heavy-bottomed frying pan, and over a medium flame, heat the olive oil. In batches brown the onions.
- Remove the onions, and in batches, brown the chicken eighths on both sides.
- When all of the chicken eighths have been thoroughly browned, return them to the pan and add the browned onions. Cover the pan and let it simmer until the chicken parts are completely cooked, adding oil as necessary. It's very important to make sure that the chicken eighths are completely cooked through.
- Remove the pan from the flame and place the chicken parts on a platter.
- LEMON-LIME MARINADE
- Combine all of the ingredients and thoroughly whisk them into an emulsion.

275. Rachel Khoo's Sticky Malaysian Chicken With Pineapple Salad

Serving: Serves 6 to 8 | Prep: 0hours15mins | Cook: 0hours45mins | Ready in:

Ingredients

- For the glaze and chicken:
- 3 cloves garlic, peeled
- 1 1 1/4-inch piece ginger, peeled and coarsely chopped
- 1/3 cup cup runny honey
- 1/3 cup light soy sauce or tamari
- 1 red chile, with seeds
- 2 tablespoons sesame oil
- 2 tablespoons fish sauce
- 2 pounds chicken drumsticks and thighs (4 of each)
- 1 tablespoon sesame seeds, toasted
- For the Malaysian salad:
- 1 cucumber
- 1/2 small pineapple
- 1 small red onion
- 1 lime, juiced
- 1 pinch Sea salt

Direction

- Preheat the oven to 400° F. To make the glaze: In a food processor, blend all the ingredients up to the chicken together until fairly smooth. Place the chicken pieces in a large roasting pan with the glaze, tossing them well to coat. Bake for 45 minutes, remove from the oven, and sprinkle with the toasted sesame seeds.
- To make the Malaysian salad: Halve the cucumber lengthwise, then seed with a spoon and discard the seeds. Cut in half again, then slice on an angle and put in a large bowl. Peel the pineapple, cut into small cubes, and add to the bowl. Peel and thinly slice the onion. Add to the bowl, along with the lime juice. Taste and season the salad with salt just before serving alongside the chicken.

276. Radish And Sausage Quiche

Serving: Serves 4 | Prep: | Cook: | Ready in:

Ingredients

- 1/2 cup All Purpose Flour
- 3 Eggs
- 1 Radish Diced
- 3 tablespoons Butter Softened
- 1.5 cups Cheese grated(any hard cheese like parmesan or gouda)

- 4 Sausage of your choice
- 1 Onion Sliced
- 1.5 cups Milk
- 1/2 teaspoon Powdered Pepper
- 1 tablespoon Olive Oil

Direction

- In a frying pan heat olive oil and 1 tbsp. of butter. Sauté the sliced onion till soft.
- Add sliced sausage to the sautéed onion, cook for a while, when sausage starts turning light brown add the diced radish. Add salt and pepper. Cook till radish turns a little soft. Keep aside to cool down.
- In a bowl whisk together eggs, milk, butter and flour. Mix well till a smooth consistency is achieved.
- Now add the grated cheese to the batter and mix well.
- To the quiche mix add the earlier prepared sausage and radish filling. Mix thoroughly so that all the ingredients are combined.
- Pour the mixture into a quiche pan or a pie tin.
- Bake in a preheated oven at 338F or 170C for 20 minutes or till a golden brown crust is formed. Enjoy Hot along with a green salad.
- Nutritional Value - Calories- 585 Fat 19 g, Carbohydrates- 21g, Protein- 29 g

277. Rainbow Chard Barley Risotto With Chicken Sausage

Serving: Serves 4 | Prep: | Cook: | Ready in:

Ingredients

- 2 bunches rainbow chard, chopped
- 2 garlic cloves, chopped
- 1 medium onion, chopped
- 3 tablespoons olive oil
- 1 cup pearl barley
- 5-6 cups chicken stock, heated
- 1/2 cup white wine
- 4 pre-cooked, favorite chicken sausages
- salt/pepper to taste
- 1/2 cup parmesan, grated

Direction

- Heat a large pot over medium heat, and add 1 1/2 tablespoons of olive oil.
- Add the onions and cook until translucent, about 5 minutes.
- Add the pearl barley, stirring to coat the grains with the olive oil. Sauté for a minute, until the grains are slightly toasted in color.
- Add the wine, and cook until most of the liquid has been absorbed.
- Add a couple ladles of the warm chicken stock, stirring occasionally and allowing the barley to cook until most of the liquid has been absorbed. Continue to follow this same process, until you see that the barley takes on a creamy consistency and there is still a slight bite to the grains.
- Sauté the chopped garlic until soft, about 1 minute
- Add the chopped rainbow chard, stirring the leaves with the sautéed garlic, and making sure the garlic does not burn. Sprinkle with salt and continue to cook until wilted.
- Heat the oven to 400 degrees. Place chicken sausages on an aluminum foil-lined sheet pan. Cook until full heated through. Cut on the bias.
- Combine the wilted rainbow chard and garlic in with the risotto.
- Add the parmesan and stir until fully blended.
- Pour into bowls and top with chicken sausage. Add more parmesan, salt and pepper, if desired.

278. Ramen Redux

Serving: Serves 2 | Prep: | Cook: | Ready in:

Ingredients

- 2 packets Ramen Noodle Soup (Chicken flavor)
- 1 small onion (or half a large)
- 1 celery stalk
- 4 green onions
- 1 cup frozen peas
- 1 leftover chicken breast
- 1/2 cup carrot, julienne or shred
- 4 fresh garden basil leaves (optional)
- 1 lime, cut in wedges (optional)
- 1 cup bean sprouts (optional)

Direction

- Boil or roast the chicken until just done (no pink juices when poked). You can save the water, just strain any fat out of it first, set chicken on plate to rest and save cooking juices in bowl or measuring cup. If you are using a cooked leftover breast, simply set it aside.
- Slice the onion into thin strips. Shred the carrot. Chop the green onion, cut the lime in to sections for squirting, roll up the basil like a burrito and slice into thin strips, wash and drain the bean sprouts.
- In the pot where the soup will live, heat on medium and add a little oil and the onions, celery, carrots, salt and pepper to taste. Stir as these cook until a bit tender, about 4 minutes. Then add the flavor packets from the noodles just at the end.
- Pour in the reserved cooking water if you boiled the chicken in step 1, otherwise add 4 to 5 cups of water.
- Slice the chicken breast very thinly against the grain. Add to the pot. Add the peas as well.
- Add the noodles and let them simmer until tender. Pour the soup into two serving bowls and garnish with basil, lime and sprouts, if you wish.

279. Real Deal Buffalo Wings

Serving: Makes 20 wings | Prep: | Cook: | Ready in:

Ingredients

- 1 quart vegetable oil
- 2 pounds chicken wings
- 1/2 cup ketchup
- 3 tablespoons butter
- 1/2 cup white vinegar
- 2 tablespoons dark brown sugar
- 1/2 teaspoon ground cloves
- 2 dashes tabasco

Direction

- Wash chicken wings, cut in two pieces at drumette, and pat dry with paper towel.
- Heat vegetable oil in a heavy 8-quart pot or fryer until a bread cube dropped in the oil quickly browns.
- Carefully place the wings in the hot oil.
- While the wings are frying, melt butter in a large saucepan.
- Add the remaining ingredients and stir over low heat until blended. Add extra tabasco to taste.
- When the wings are thoroughly browned and appear crispy at the edges, lift them out of the oil with a slotted spoon, carefully strain the excess oil, and add the wings to the sauce.
- Turn up the heat on the sauce and stir the wings until they are coated.
- Immediately place on a platter and serve with blue cheese and crisp celery spears.

280. Roast Chicken Legs With Grapes And Shallots

Serving: Serves 4 | Prep: | Cook: | Ready in:

Ingredients

- 1/2 pound red seedless grapes (you can also use green or a combination of the two)
- 4 large shallots
- 2 tablespoons chopped fresh thyme
- 1 tablespoon olive oil
- 4 chicken legs
- 3-4 tablespoons butter, softened
- 1 teaspoon honey
- Salt and freshly-ground black pepper, to taste

Direction

- Preheat the oven to 400°F. Cut the grapes into small clusters and thinly slice the shallots. In a large bowl, combine the grape clusters, half of the chopped thyme, and olive oil, gently mixing so that the grapes are well coated.
- In a small bowl, combine the rest of the chopped thyme, butter, honey, salt, and pepper. Loosen the skin from the chicken legs by working your fingers between the skin and meat, making sure not to tear the skin in the process. Rub generous amounts of the butter mixture under the skin, and rub the remainder all over the top and bottom of the legs. Reposition the skin if necessary.
- Place the chicken in a large casserole dish (most oven safe pans will work) and tuck grape clusters into the spaces between the chicken legs. Sprinkle shallots on top. Roast until the juices run clear, around 30 minutes. Allow to rest for 5-10 minutes.

281. Roast Chicken Salad With Arugula And Pomegranate Seeds

Serving: Serves 4 | Prep: | Cook: | Ready in:

Ingredients

- 2 boneless, skinless chicken breasts
- 2 teaspoons olive oil
- salt and pepper to taste
- 2 tablespoons white wine vinegar
- 1 tablespoon non-fat plain yogurt
- 2 tablespoons whole-grain Dijon mustard
- 1/4 teaspoon maple syrup
- dash of cinnamon
- 1/2 cup pomegranate seeds
- 2/3 cup packed arugula

Direction

- Preheat oven to 425 °F. Rub chicken breasts with olive oil and sprinkle with salt and pepper. Place breasts in a foil-lined baking dish or roasting pan and bake for 10 minutes. Reduce the heat to 400°F and bake for another 15 to 20 minutes, until the juices run clear.
- Preheat oven to 425 °F. Rub chicken breasts with olive oil and sprinkle with salt and pepper. Place breasts in a foil-lined baking dish or roasting pan and bake for 10 minutes. Reduce the heat to 400°F and bake for another 15 to 20 minutes, until the juices run clear.
- Once chicken is cool, chop or shred into bite-sized pieces. Add the vinegar mixture to the chicken and stir well so that the chicken pieces are evenly coated. Stir in pomegranate seeds and arugula. Season again with salt and pepper to taste.

282. Roast Chicken With Garlic Croutons

Serving: Serves 6 | Prep: 0hours20mins | Cook: 1hours15mins | Ready in:

Ingredients

- 1 whole chicken (about 4 pounds)
- Kosher salt and freshly ground black pepper
- 5 carrots, peeled and cut into 3-inch lengths
- 3 shallots, peeled and halved lengthwise
- 1 head garlic, halved
- 1 lemon, halved
- 3 tablespoons extra-virgin olive oil
- 6 ounces crusty bread torn into 1-inch pieces
- Chopped parsley, for serving

Direction

- Season chicken generously with salt and pepper. Chill, covered, overnight.
- Let chicken stand at room temperature for 1 hour. Preheat oven to 450°F. Toss carrots and shallots with 2 tablespoons oil and season with salt and pepper; arrange in an even layer in the center of a large roasting pan to create a rack for the chicken. Pat chicken dry; rub with remaining 1 tablespoon oil, tie legs with twine, and place over vegetables in roasting pan. Add garlic and lemon halves to pan. Roast 25 minutes.
- Reduce oven temperature to 375°F; cook, flipping vegetables once, until vegetables are tender and chicken is golden brown and a meat thermometer inserted into the thickest part of the breast registers 155°F, 30 to 40 minutes. Transfer carrots and shallots to a serving platter; squeeze with lemon juice. Transfer chicken to a cutting board to rest.
- Squeeze garlic cloves from skins and mash into a paste. Toss with bread cubes in pan juices and season lightly with salt and pepper; spread into an even layer. Bake, tossing once, until golden and crisp, 9 to 12 minutes.
- To serve, carve chicken and arrange on platter. Scatter croutons around chicken and serve sprinkled with parsley.

283. Roast Chicken With Oranges And Olives

Serving: Serves 6 | Prep: | Cook: | Ready in:

Ingredients

- 3 pounds bone-in, skin-on chicken pieces (drumsticks, thighs, legs)
- 4 oranges, 2 sliced into half-inch circles and 2 juiced
- 2 tablespoons honey
- 4 garlic cloves, peeled
- 1.5 cups dry white wine
- 1 cup Castelvetrano olives

Direction

- Preheat oven to 400 degrees
- Pat chicken dry and arrange in large baking dish in a single layer; season generously with salt and pepper
- Slice two oranges into 1/2 inch thick rounds and nestle in and around chicken
- Peel garlic cloves and place in baking dish whole
- Combine orange juice and wine, and whisk in honey
- Pour orange juice and honey mixture and wine all around chicken
- Bake for 1 hour and 15 minutes, or until meat is opaque and juice runs clear when cut (as opposed to pink)
- Serve chicken over rice, quinoa, couscous or other cooked grain with pan sauce ladled on top

284. Roasted Garlic Chicken

Serving: Serves 4 | Prep: | Cook: | Ready in:

Ingredients

- 1 small chicken (free range or organic is always preferable)
- 7-8 young carrots, save the stems
- 3-4 heads of garlic
- 1 lemon
- Olive oil
- Sea salt and freshly ground black pepper

Direction

- Preheat the oven to 200°C.
- Cut the very top of each garlic head to open the garlic cloves. Cut the lemon in halves and place one half together with garlic in a small baking dish, generously add good quality olive oil and sprinkle with sea salt. Bake for

half an hour until garlic becomes soft and tender. Remove the dish from the oven and let the garlic and lemon cool.
- While the garlic is in the oven prepare the carrots. Wash the carrots and peel them if needed. Wash the stems, pick the leaves and chop them finely.
- When the garlic is cool enough to handle it slide the softened cloves out into a bowl. Then squeeze the roasted lemon juice into the same bowl and add the chopped carrot leaves (you can optionally save some to sprinkle the chicken before roasting). Mix it all together in a puree and season with salt and freshly ground black pepper to taste.
- Preheat the oven to 180°C.
- Cover the chicken and carrots with the garlic mixture. If you cook chicken with skin you can also place some of the puree between the skin and the breast. We usually remove the skin to reduce the quantity of fat in the dish. Cut the remaining half of lemon into 5-6 pieces and place it together with the chicken and carrots in the backing dish which you used to cook garlic. If you have some garlic puree left this is the time to add it to the baking dish. Sprinkle with a little bit of olive oil, remaining carrot leaves, salt and freshly ground black pepper.
- Place the dish in the oven and roast chicken for 35-40 min, then turn the heat up to 220°C and roast another 20 min or until your chicken becomes as golden as you wish it to be.
- Remove the dish from the oven and serve the chicken with carrots and a peace of roasted lemon. Bon Appétit!

285. Roasted Fennel And Red Quinoa Salad, Chicken, Arugula, tomato, Sherry Vinaigrette.

Serving: Serves 4 | Prep: | Cook: | Ready in:

Ingredients

- 1 Fennel bulb
- 1 pound Skinless chicken breast
- 2 cups Red quinoa
- 2 handfuls Baby arugula
- 1 cup Medium diced tomatoes
- 1 tablespoon Sherry wine vinegar
- 1 teaspoon Extra virgin olive oil
- 1 tablespoon Cannoli oil
- 3 cups Low sodium chicken stock
- 1 pinch Salt
- 1 pinch Fresh ground pepper

Direction

- Thinly slice fennel bulb and toss with extra virgin olive oil, salt and pepper. Place on sheet pan and spread evenly. Roast in oven for approximately 15 minutes
- Meanwhile in a heavy gauge sauce pan add quinoa, chicken stock, salt and pepper and cook for about 15 minutes
- Preheat grill pan on medium high heat, season chicken breast with salt and pepper and grill both sides until internal temperature reaches 160 degrees
- When quinoa, fennel and chicken are complete, place in a non-reactive metal bowl and add baby arugula, chopped tomatoes, sherry vinegar.
- Toss with extra virgin olive oil, salt and pepper.
- Place in 4 separate serving bowls and garnish with fennel fronds. Enjoy!

286. Salad With Pear, Magret De Canard, Jerusalem Artichokes And Hazelnut

Serving: Serves 4 | Prep: | Cook: | Ready in:

Ingredients

- 250g Jerusalem artichokes
- Mixed lettuce leaves

- 12 slices of magret de canard/ Sliced and smoked fillets of duck breast (dry)
- 1 pear
- 2 tablespoons walnut oil
- 1 tablespoon balsamic vinegar
- 1 handful chopped hazelnuts

Direction

- Wash and peel the Jerusalem artichokes. Steam them for 15 minutes.
- Once Jerusalem artichokes are cooked, cut them into dices. Season with pepper and salt. Heat some canola oil in a pan and fry for 5 minutes.
- To assemble the salad, put lettuce, orange, slices of duck breasts and Jerusalem artichokes in a bowl and sprinkle with walnut oil, creamy balsamic vinegar and hazelnuts. Season some more if needed but smoked duck is quite salty.

287. Saliva Chicken Meatballs

Serving: Serves 4 as an appetizer | Prep: 1hours45mins | Cook: 0hours14mins | Ready in:

Ingredients

- Meatballs
- 1 pound (450 grams) boneless skin-on chicken thighs
- 1/4 pound (105 grams) chicken knuckles/cartilage (if unavailable, omit)
- 1 1/2 tablespoons grated ginger
- 1 1/2 tablespoons sake
- 2 1/2 teaspoons toasted sesame oil
- 2 teaspoons fish sauce
- 1 1/4 teaspoons ground white pepper
- Canola oil, for shaping the meatballs
- Sesame Sauce (below)
- Ultimate Sichuan Chile Oil
- Finely ground Sichuan peppercorns, for dusting
- Sesame Sauce
- 1/2 cup (127 grams) tahini
- 3 garlic cloves, smashed
- 1 1/2 tablespoons soy sauce
- 1 tablespoon toasted sesame oil
- 2 teaspoons balsamic vinegar
- 1/2 teaspoon sugar
- 1/2 cup crushed ice, plus more if needed
- 2 tablespoons finely chopped cilantro or scallions

Direction

- Meatballs
- Keep 50 percent of the skin on the chicken thighs (discard the rest or use it to make schmaltz for another recipe), then cut the thighs into small chunks. Scatter on a sheet pan and flash-freeze for 1 hour, until hardened. Meanwhile, season the chicken knuckles, if using, with a little bit of salt and pepper, then cook in a skillet over medium-high heat until evenly browned on all sides. Finely mince them until they resemble coarse breadcrumbs, then set aside in a large bowl.
- Transfer the frozen chicken chunks to a food processor and pulse several times (you might have to scrape the bottom a few times) until coarsely ground. Add the ginger, sake, sesame oil, fish sauce, and white pepper and run the processor until the mixture is even and smoothly ground. Transfer to the bowl with the chicken knuckles and mix everything together evenly.
- Rub your hands with a bit of oil, then shape the mixture into 15 small meatballs. My tool for cooking the roundest and most evenly browned meatballs is—a takoyaki pan (the specially designed pan with large holes that makes Takoyaki, Japanese octopus balls)! I place each meatball into each hole on the takoyaki pan brushed with a bit of oil, then I cook them over medium heat, turning each meatball frequently with a wooden skewer, until evenly dark brown and cooked through, about 10 minutes. If you don't have a takoyaki pan, you can do this in a skillet, or bake the meatballs on a sheet pan under the broiler for 12 to 14 minutes.

- Generously douse the meatballs with sesame sauce, then smother again with My Ultimate Chile Oil. Dust with more finely ground Sichuan peppercorns.
- Sesame Sauce
- In either a blender or a food processor, combine the tahini, garlic, soy sauce, sesame oil, vinegar, sugar, and ¼ cup of crushed ice. Blend until the mixture is smooth, then add 2 more tablespoons of the crushed ice at a time and continue to blend for 30 seconds, adding ice until the sauce is the texture of loose mayonnaise. Set aside (or refrigerate for up to 3 days). Just before using, mix in the cilantro or scallions.

288. Sangria Chicken

Serving: Serves 8 | Prep: | Cook: | Ready in:

Ingredients

- 8 pieces bone-in, skin-on chicken thighs
- 1 piece small yellow onion
- 1 cup sliced or pre-cut carrots
- 3 pieces garlic, chopped
- 2 tablespoons olive oil
- 2 sprigs rosemary
- 1/4 teaspoon red pepper flakes
- 1 1/14 cups red wine
- 1 cup orange juice
- 3 tablespoons brown sugar
- 2 pinches salt
- 2 pinches pepper

Direction

- Preheat oven to 425 degrees F.
- Season chicken with salt and pepper.
- Place the onions, carrots, and garlic in a roasting pan or casserole/baking dish. Toss with salt, pepper, red pepper flakes, rosemary, and olive oil. Spread around the bottom of the dish and place chicken on top, skin side down.
- Mix red wine and orange juice together, then pour mixture over chicken and vegetables. Roast the chicken for 40 minutes, flipping halfway so you'll finish with the skin side up.
- Remove dish from oven, take out chicken pieces and set aside in a separate dish, covered in foil. Pour wine and vegetable mixture in a saucepan and add brown sugar. Cook over medium high heat to reduce sauce, about 20-30 minutes.
- Place chicken back in baking dish, add the reduced sauce and vegetables, and place back in oven for 5 minutes before serving.

289. Sausage, Sauerkraut, And Spicy Mustard Potato Bowl

Serving: Serves 4 | Prep: | Cook: | Ready in:

Ingredients

- 4 large golden potatoes
- Olive oil
- 2 yellow onions
- 2 pounds kielbasa
- 1 can of beer (I used Genesee Cream Ale)
- 1 16 oz bag of sauerkraut, drained
- celery salt, to taste
- freshly ground black pepper
- 1 heaping tablespoon of dijon mustard
- 1 heaping tablespoon of whole grain mustard
- 1 heaping tablespoon of mayonnaise (or as much as you like, to taste)
- 1 drizzle of heavy cream (to taste)
- Cayenne powder, to taste
- 1/4 cup freshly chopped parsley, divided
- Fried egg (optional)

Direction

- Prep your ingredients: Bring a large pot of salted water to a boil. Roughly cube the potatoes into 1-2 inch pieces (leave the skins on, if desired). Thickly slice the yellow onions.

- Boil the potatoes until fork tender, but not overcooked. Drain and set aside. Keep warm.
- Meanwhile, sauté sliced onions over pretty high heat in olive oil until browning and crisping up in spots. Remove from pan. Add whole kielbasa and cook on kind of high heat without moving until during dark brown and splitting open in spots on both sides (flip once). Add sliced onions back to pan. Add beer. Add sauerkraut. Season with celery salt and pepper. Bring to a boil and then reduce to simmer for about 30-40 minutes or until the liquid has reduced and all alcohol has cooked off. Season to taste with more salt. Stir in half the parsley. Cut the sausage into larger pieces.
- While the sausage is cooking, make the potatoes by adding heaping tablespoon of Dijon mustard, heaping tablespoon of whole grain mustard, a bit of mayo (to your liking) and a drizzle of heavy cream. Season with celery salt and pepper. Mix well to combine, mashing the potatoes just lightly. Season with a bit of cayenne powder. Keep warm.
- To serve: divide potatoes between bowls, top with sauerkraut and sausage. Top with parsley and a fried egg (optional but delicious)

290. Savory Duck Buns Aka Kalua Manapua

Serving: Makes 16 baked buns | Prep: | Cook: | Ready in:

Ingredients

- For Filling
- 2-2 1/4 pounds duck legs (4)
- 1 teaspoon whole white peppercorns
- 2 teaspoons coarse sea salt
- 1 1/2 teaspoons liquid smoke
- 1 whole chipotle in adobo, seeds removed and chopped
- 2 tablespoons sherry vinegar
- 3 tablespoons distilled white vinegar
- 2 teaspoons maple syrup
- Additional fillings for buns (added when stuffing): 1/3 cup chopped cilantro (including stems), 3 generous tablespoons apricot preserves
- For Buns
- 1 packet active dry yeast
- 1/3 cup warm tap water (90-115 degrees – warm but comfortable against your skin – too high a temperature will kill your yeast)
- 2 tablespoons sugar
- 3 1/2 cups all purpose flour
- 1/2 teaspoon kosher salt
- 2 teaspoons baking powder
- 1 cup coconut milk (I use Chao Koh brand – be sure to shake before opening)
- 1/4 cup whole milk
- 1/4 cup all vegetable shortening, such as Spectrum, melted
- Sesame oil for greasing the bowl
- 1 large egg
- Splash of water
- pinch of salt

Direction

- For Filling
- Dry duck legs with a paper towel. Combine white peppercorns and salt in a mortar and pestle; mash until pepper is fragrant and coarsely ground. Sprinkle both sides of duck legs with mixture, pressing salt and pepper into the bird.
- Heat a deep wide pot or Dutch oven until almost smoking. Add duck legs, skin side down and cook until skin is golden and has crisped a bit, about 7 minutes. Transfer legs, skin side up into bottom of slow cooker. Pour rendered fat over duck.
- Add liquid smoke, chopped chipotle, vinegars and maple syrup to the slow cooker, drizzling each over all four legs. Close and cook for four hours on high. Transfer cooked duck legs to another bowl and remove skin and bones. Shred meat and place in a bowl, allowing it to cool slightly. Cover and refrigerate until ready to fill buns. While meat is chilling, get your buns going.

- For Buns
- In a small bowl or Pyrex measure, dissolve yeast in warm water. Add sugar and gently stir. Let mixture soften for 5 minutes. Mixture should foam and double in volume. This means your yeast is alive and ready to make your buns. If it does not double in volume, discard and start again.
- Measure out flour into a large bowl. Add salt and baking powder, stirring to combine.
- Add yeast mixture, scraping the container with a spatula to get it all out. Add coconut milk (I use the same measuring cup that had the yeast mixture), milk and melted vegetable shortening. Stir mixture until it becomes a shaggy mass. Turn dough out onto a cool, lightly floured surface and knead until smooth and elastic, about 5-8 minutes.
- Grease a large bowl with sesame oil. Place dough in bowl and turn to coat. Cover bowl with plastic wrap and let the dough rise in a warm, draft free place for about an hour, or until doubled in bulk. I have had good results by heating one cup of water in a microwave for one minute and then placing the covered bowl in the microwave with the heated water.
- When you are about 15 minutes away from filling buns, remove filling from refrigerator. Add the chopped cilantro to the shredded duck and place it near wherever you are going to fill your buns. Place apricot preserves into a small bowl and set it next to the duck filling. Cut 16 pieces of parchment, about 2" x 2" and lay out on a large rimmed baking sheet. Set aside.
- When dough has doubled, punch down and divide into 16 portions. Gently flatten each dough ball into a circle by pulling out the sides of the circle with the tips of your fingers. You want the very center of the circle to be thicker than the edges – imagine a sunny side up egg. Place a heaping tablespoon of duck filling onto the center (the thickest part of your circle). Top with ½ teaspoon of apricot preserves. Carefully gather up the edges around the filling and pinch and twist to seal the bun. Gently transfer bun to prepared baking sheet with parchment paper, pinched side down. Repeat with remaining dough and filling. Let the buns rise for 30 minutes.
- While filled buns are rising, preheat oven to 350 degrees. Make an egg wash by combining egg, a splash of water and pinch of salt. Gently brush bun tops with egg wash and bake for 18-20 minutes. Enjoy immediately or allow buns to cool completely and then freeze. I have had good results reheating manapua in the microwave, on the defrost setting for 30 seconds and then an additional 10 seconds. NOTE: All 16 will fit on one baking sheet, although most likely the manapua will puff up and fuse to the one next to it. While I thought they might leak, I used a knife to separate them without any problem.

291. Scallion, Dijon And Chicken Ham Cake Salé

Serving: Makes 1 loaf | Prep: | Cook: | Ready in:

Ingredients

- Salé Batter
- 3.5 ounces unsalted butter, at room temperature
- 1 teaspoon whole grain dijon mustard
- 1 teaspoon kosher salt
- 1/4 teaspoon cracked black pepper
- 2 eggs, at room temperature
- 4.2 ounces all purpose flour, sifted
- 2/3 teaspoon baking powder
- Add Ins
- 3.5 ounces chicken ham or other cold cut of your liking, diced
- 3 tablespoons chopped scallions
- 4.4 ounces shredded mozzarella cheese

Direction

- Preheat the oven to 340 degrees Fahrenheit (170 degrees Celsius.)

- Beat the butter, mustard, salt, and black pepper until light and fluffy. Add in the eggs one at a time, beating well. Sift in the flour and baking powder and stir all together with a rubber spatula until 80% combined. Lastly, add the ham, scallions and shredded cheese into the batter and mix well.
- Pour into a parchment-lined loaf tin, (approximately 7.9? L x 2.3? W x 2.1? H) And, using the rubber spatula, press down on the middle of the batter to create a concave shape. This allows the salé to rise evenly and limits the chances of a dome forming.
- Bake for 35-40 minutes or until the top becomes firm to the touch and turns a light brown. Cool for 10 minutes before releasing the salé from the tin. Slice and serve immediately.
- Note 1: if you prefer to check for doneness using the skewer or toothpick method, there should be no wet crumb clinging to the stick when you pull it out but there may be some melted cheese on it.
- Note 2: serve with a sparkling wine such as Champagne or my favorite and less expensive alternative Yellow Tail Bubbles. Chilled light red wines such as Cabernet Franc or Pinot Noir, and light whites such as Chardonnay also pair well with this cake salé.
- Note 3: for leftovers, slice the salé into cubes and spear with black olives and roasted cherry tomatoes to serve like tapas.
- Note 4: alternatively, leftovers can also be baked under a broiler until crispy (think crostini) and topped with creamy ricotta mixed with roasted garlic.

292. Sesame Chicken With Radicchio & Orange Salad

Serving: Serves 2 | Prep: 0hours0mins | Cook: 0hours0mins | Ready in:

Ingredients

- 2 navel oranges
- 1 head radicchio
- 2 boneless, skinless chicken breasts
- 3/4 cup sesame seeds
- 1 teaspoon kosher salt, plus more to taste
- 1/2 cup peanut oil, depending on the size of your pan
- 1/2 tablespoon toasted sesame oil

Direction

- Assemble the salad. Halve the radicchio lengthwise. Cut out the core, then roughly chop. Add to a bowl. Peel the orange—either with your hands or a knife. To do with a knife: cut the top and bottom off each orange. Stand on one end, then guide your knife from top to bottom, removing as little flesh as possible. Cut into thick rounds, then chop into chunks. Add to the radicchio. Stick in the fridge while you make the chicken.
- Halve the chicken breasts horizontally. Freezing them for about 15 minutes beforehand make this easier (a trick I learned from Cooks Illustrated). Place these between plastic film or parchment and pound to an even 1/4- to 1/2-inch thickness.
- Add the sesame seeds to a mortar. Use a pestle to roughly crush until some seeds are powdery, others whole. Stir in the salt. Dump this onto a plate and spread into an even layer.
- Add the peanut oil to a straight-sided cast-iron skillet—you want about 1/4-inch depth, so adjust as needed. Set on the stove over medium-high heat. Dredge the chicken pieces in the sesame mixture, pressing firmly to fully coat. Check if the oil is hot: If you drop in a few seeds, they should instantly sizzle, not drop to the bottom or burn. When it's hot, add the sesame-coated chicken. Depending on the size of your pan, you might have to do this in batches. If they're overcrowded, they'll steam versus brown.
- Cook for 3 to 4 minutes per side, until the outside is browned and the inside is cooked through. Transfer to a cooling rack to drain.

- Cook the remaining chicken if necessary, adding more oil to the pan if necessary.
- While those rest for a moment, dress the salad. Season with a pinch of salt and add the sesame oil. Toss. Taste and adjust the salt and oil to taste.
- Serve the sesame chicken immediately with the salad on top or alongside.

293. Shaken (not Stirred) Corn Dogs

Serving: Makes 8 corn dogs | Prep: | Cook: | Ready in:

Ingredients

- 1 1/4 cups corn meal
- 3/4 cup whole wheat pastry flour
- 1 1/2 teaspoons aluminum-free baking powder
- 1/2 teaspoon sea salt
- 2 tablespoons honey
- 2 eggs
- 3/4 cup whole milk
- 8 uncured turkey hot dogs
- 8 wood skewers
- 1/2 cup whole wheat pastry flour, for dredging
- 2 quarts canola oil for frying

Direction

- Preheat 1-2" oil in large pot to 375 degrees.
- Skewer hot dogs.
- Place cornmeal, flour, baking powder and salt into the quart jar. Secure lid and shake until ingredients are combined.
- Add eggs, milk and honey. Shake again until mixed thoroughly. Open jar and give batter a few stirs with a spoon to make sure all ingredients are incorporated.
- Pour reserved 1/2 C flour onto plate and roll skewered hot dogs in flour to coat.
- Dip hot dogs into jar several times to coat with batter making sure all parts of floured hot dog are coated. Let excess batter drip off.
- Place corn dog in 375 degree oil and cook until golden brown.
- Remove to paper towel lined plate.
- Corn dogs can be eaten immediately or brought to room temperature and frozen. Reheat frozen corn dogs in 350 degree oven for 10-15 minutes or until hot.

294. Showstopper Stuffed Squash

Serving: Serves 6 | Prep: | Cook: | Ready in:

Ingredients

- 3 whole acorn squashes
- 2 cups plain yogurt (Greek or whole milk recommended)
- 35-40 ounces bulk sausage (I prefer Italian Chicken Sausage from Whole Foods)
- a few cloves of garlic
- half an onion
- 2 large handfuls roughly chopped hearty greens (kale, chard, spinach, etc)
- a small handful chopped fresh parsley, cilantro, basil or scallions
- any extra veggies of your choosing, chopped (bell peppers, leeks, carrots, etc)
- several glugs of cooking oil (grapeseed, canola, or olive oil)
- salt and pepper to taste

Direction

- OPTIONAL but recommended prep step: Ideally the evening or a few hours before you want to serve this, wipe/clean the outsides of your squashes. Cut them in half, sticking your knife in at the top, going through or right next to the stem. Using your fingers, pick out the seeds and place directly on a baking sheet, trying to get as few stringy-parts as you can (a few are ok). Once you've pulled out all the seeds, place a dry paper towel on top of them and press it down all around them to absorb as much moisture as you can. The seeds will be sticky and will stick to the paper towel - that's ok. When the paper towel is mostly saturated, pick off the seeds sticking to it and discard the paper towel. Spread seeds evenly on the sheet and place in oven (turned off) overnight or for several hours to help dry out the seeds. If you are doing this the night before, at this point I recommend scooping out the stringy insides of the squash and discard. You can then put the squash halves back together, using a rubber band to keep them in place, and put in the fridge until the next day. When you check the seeds (the next morning or after a few hours), they should be noticeably dry and slightly stuck to the sheet, but will come off easily when scraped with a spatula or your fingers. Loosen them up and spread evenly again. Roast in a 250 degree oven for 5-10 minutes. Be careful - these are VERY easy to burn. I recommend continuously setting a timer for 3-min intervals and checking that often. Seeds are done when they are crispy to the bite. When finished, toss with a little oil and salt/pepper/spices of your choice.

- If you skipped step one, wipe/clean the outsides of your squashes. Cut them in half, sticking your knife in at the top, going through or right next to the stem. Scoop out the stringy insides of the squash with a spoon or grapefruit spoon if you have it. If you did not do step one, you can save the insides to pick out the seeds later, or just discard.
- Place squash halves on a roasting pan with the skin side touching the pan. Sprinkle each one with a little oil, using your fingers to spread the oil around each half, then sprinkle each with salt and pepper. Roast for about 35-50 minutes at 400 degrees, until they are golden and a fork goes in easily. When done, turn the oven off but keep squash inside to stay warm.
- While squash are roasting, place about 2 cups of yogurt into a small and pretty serving bowl. Wash, dry, and finely chop your handful of herbs (or scallions), then stir into the yogurt. Wash your lemon and zest it directly into the bowl. Cut lemon and squeeze half of it into the bowl, catching seeds with a small sieve. Stir and taste. Add more lemon juice if you like. Put yogurt sauce in the fridge until serving time.
- Wash and cut your kale or other greens into roughly bite-size pieces. If using greens with a thick stalk (like kale), I remove the stalks and chop them into small pieces to add to the stir-fry as well. Chop/dice your onion and any other veggies you're adding. Crush garlic, peel it and then roughly mince.
- Heat your sauté pan on medium heat. Add a good glug of oil and your garlic, onions, chopped kale stalks, and any other hearty veggies (save greens for the end). Sauté until fragrant and mostly softened. Turn heat down if it's going too fast. Cut open your sausage packages and add directly to the pan. Using a spatula or wooden spoon, break up the sausage into bite size pieces. Allow to brown and cook thoroughly, flipping and mixing after a few minutes on each side. When you're pretty sure the sausage is cooked, place all the greens on top. Add about a quarter cup of water, then cover with a lid to let the greens steam. After about a minute or two, remove the lid. Greens should be brightly colored. Mix in thoroughly and turn off the heat.
- At this point your squash should be ready. Place squash halves on plates, one half per person. Carefully spoon sausage mixture into each squash to make a heaping portion. Top with a few spoons of yogurt sauce, and (optionally) some toasted squash seeds. (If you did not make the seeds, you could also top with a few nuts, breadcrumbs, or other crunchy topper of your choice. OR it's also perfectly delicious without a topper!) Serve with spoons and remind guests to scoop bites of squash along with bites of sausage mixture! Keep yogurt sauce on the table in case folks want extra.

295. Shoyu Chicken Over Rice

Serving: Serves 3 | Prep: | Cook: |Ready in:

Ingredients

- 6 Chicken thighs
- 2 tablespoons Chopped fresh ginger
- 2 cups Soy sauce
- 1 cup Water
- 4 tablespoons Chopped garlic
- 1 bunch Green scallions
- 1/3 cup Sugar

Direction

- Put water, soy sauce, sugar, garlic, and ginger in a Dutch oven.
- Add chicken thighs and cover and refrigerate for 4-6 hours.
- Put Dutch oven in oven and bake at 375 for 30-40 minutes depending on size and whether bone in or bone out chicken.
- Remove chicken and serve with white rice. Use sauce as desired for amazing rice drizzle. Top with chopped scallions for some vegetable, jk it's pretty and taste good.

296. Shredded Chicken Gorditas

Serving: Serves 4 | Prep: | Cook: |Ready in:

Ingredients

- Gorditas
- 2 cups masa harina
- 1 1/4 cups water
- 1/4 cup vegetable oil
- Shredded Chicken
- 4-5 chicken breasts
- 1/4 cup tequila
- 3 tablespoons honey
- 1 jalapeno, chopped
- 1 onion, chopped
- salt and pepper to taste
- 1 tablespoon cayenne pepper
- 1 cup chicken broth

Direction

- You definitely need to start the chicken first. I put all the ingredients in my slow cooker (love that thing!) and let sit on the high setting for a few hours. As the chicken cooks, start to shred it and let it simmer in the juices. WARNING: it's going to make your house smell AWESOME!
- Ok, when the chicken is at or near done, you can start making your gorditas. In a large bowl, mix the masa harina, water, and 1/4 cup of oil. Wrap the dough in plastic wrap and roll into a thick log. How thick? Well that just depends on how big you want your gorditas to be. Mine were about 3-4 inches in diameter (after flattening, so about 2-3-inch-thick log). Divide the log into 1 inch slices. I got about 12 gorditas with this, and this was plenty for 3 people.
- Flatten each gordita either with a rolling pin, or you could be more rustic and use your hands like I did. Be careful though, the dough will be VERY fragile so you kind of have to be gentle and loving with it.
- Heat a large skillet or griddle under high heat and cook gorditas in batches (I found that 3 at a time fit in the pan nicely) for about 2 minutes per side. Set aside on plate as each one is done. When all gorditas are cooked, either wait until skillet gets cool or get out new skillet if you can't wait. Place enough oil in the skillet to bring it about 1/4 inch up the pan. If you do this with the hot skillet, you'll probably burn yourself, so that's why I said to either get a new skillet or wait until the other one cools. It's all about safety first, right? Right.
- When oil is hot enough for frying, add the gorditas, in batches again, and fry for about 2 minutes per side, when they're nice and golden. When each is done, press the center

with a spoon to kind of make a little indentation. Dry on paper towel-lined plate.
- Top the indentations with the shredded chicken, sour cream, salsa, cheese, and whatever else you'd like to top it with. The toppings are really endless.

297. Shredded Red Chile Chicken Tacos

Serving: Serves 6 | Prep: | Cook: | Ready in:

Ingredients

- 4 boneless, skinless chicken breasts
- 2 cans El Pato red chile sauce
- 3 cups Canola oil for frying tortillas
- 20 corn tortillas
- 1 yellow onion, diced

Direction

- Throw chicken breasts into a hot pressure cooker, secure lid and bring to 2nd ring. Reduce heat to low and cook 10 minutes if frozen, 7 if thawed. Let pressure come down by removing from heat. Boil chicken for 15-18 minutes if you don't have a pressure cooker. Remove chicken breasts and place in a Kitchen Aide Mixer (or similar) with the cookie dough attachment.
- Pour chicken broth from pressure cooker into a bowl and set aside. Wipe out the pot with a paper towel and return to medium-high heat. Add 3 tablespoons oil to pot, let heat for a few minutes then add chopped onion. Cook for 5 minutes until golden brown and translucent. Add shredded chicken to pot and toss to coat. Let sit for 5 minutes, toss and cook a few minutes more. Pour in El Pato chile sauce and toss to coat. Cook a few minutes till heated through.
- Meanwhile, in a small sauce pot, heat 1/2 of the oil over medium high heat. Using tongs and a fork, carefully place tortillas, one at a time into the pot of oil. Using the tong and fork shape them into tacos. Remove from oil when golden brown and crispy. Place on a pile of paper towels to drain. Scoop chicken into taco shells, garnish as you please.

298. Smoked Chicken Salad With Peanuts And Apples

Serving: Serves 4 to 6 | Prep: | Cook: | Ready in:

Ingredients

- Dressing:
- 1/2 cup fresh raspberries
- 1/4 cup extra-virgin olive oil
- 2 tablespoons fresh lemon juice
- 1 tablespoon honey
- Kosher salt
- Freshly ground black pepper
- Salad:
- 4 cups mache leaves
- 1 cup shredded smoked chicken
- 2 Roma tomatoes, seeded and diced
- 1 Granny Smith apple, cored and diced
- 1/2 cup crumbled feta cheese
- 1/2 cup peanuts
- 1/4 cup pitted green olives, thinly sliced
- 3 scallions, thinly sliced

Direction

- Dressing:
- Combine the raspberries, olive oil, lemon juice, and honey in a blender and mix until smooth. Season with salt and pepper, to taste.
- Salad:
- Toss together the mache, chicken, tomatoes, apples, feta, peanuts, olives, and scallions in a large serving bowl. Drizzle the dressing over the top and toss to coat.

299. Smoked Corn Chowder With Crispy Duck Skin

Serving: Serves 4 | Prep: | Cook: | Ready in:

Ingredients

- Dry Rub
- 2 tablespoons kosher salt
- 1 tablespoon paprika
- 1 tablespoon black pepper, ground
- 1 teaspoon cumin, toasted and ground
- 1/2 teaspoon coriander, toasted and ground
- 1/2 teaspoon chipotle chili powder
- 1/2 teaspoon dried thyme
- 1/2 teaspoon Mexican oregano
- Corn Chowder
- 1 boneless duck breast, split
- dry rub
- 6 ears corn, cleaned
- 1 tablespoon butter
- 1 medium onion, chopped
- 1/2 bell pepper, chopped
- 1/2 celery stalk, chopped
- 4 cups water or chicken broth
- 1 cup milk
- 1 sprig thyme
- 1 sage leaf
- 1 bay leaf
- 1 small russet potato, peeled and cubed
- 3/4 cup heavy cream or half-and-half
- salt and pepper to taste

Direction

- Dry Rub
- Mix ingredients well and use to season any dark meat before smoking. Store leftovers in a tightly sealed container.
- Corn Chowder
- Wash and dry duck breasts. With a sharp knife, score skin and fat, being careful not to cut into the meat. Coat both sides of breasts with dry rub and refrigerate uncovered up to one day.
- Prepare your smoker according to manufacturer's instructions, using your preferred smoking wood. Place two ears of corn on the lower rack just above the water pan. Place duck skin side up on the top rack over the corn. Smoke until duck is cooked through, about 40-50 minutes. Remove duck and corn from smoker.
- Once corn has cooled enough to handle, cut the kernels from the ears into a large bowl and discard cobs. Cut kernels from the four remaining ears into same bowl and reserve cobs for the stock.
- Remove skin from one duck breast half and chop. In a large, heavy pot over low heat, render fat from the skin. Remove crisped skin from pot with a slotted spoon and place on paper towel-lined plate to cool. Discard any fat over 1 tablespoon that remains in the pot. Add 1 tablespoon butter to the duck fat and increase heat to medium-high.
- Sauté onion, bell pepper and celery in duck fat and butter until wilted. Do not brown. Add corn cobs and remaining ingredients through potatoes. Bring to a simmer and cook until potatoes are tender, about 15 minutes. Discard corn cobs, thyme sprig, sage and bay leaf.
- Transfer soup to blender in batches and purée until smooth. (For a velvety consistency, strain soup through a fine mesh strainer and press on solids to extract as much liquid as possible, then discard solids.) Stir in heavy cream or half-and-half and adjust seasoning to taste. To serve, ladle soup into bowls and top with crispy duck skin.

300. Smoked Duck Breast With Creamy Wasabi Green Onion Dipping Sauce

Serving: Serves 4 to 6 | Prep: | Cook: | Ready in:

Ingredients

- 4 medium (about 3/4-inch/2 cm thick) duck breast halves, excess skin trimmed

- Sea salt
- Freshly ground black pepper
- Handful of smoke chips (your choice of wood)
- 1/2 cup (120 ml) crème fraîche
- 1 to 1 1/2 teaspoons wasabi paste
- 2 teaspoons usukuchi shoyu (light-colored soy sauce)
- 1 green onion, thinly sliced
- 1 to 1 1/2 teaspoons freshly squeezed lemon juice

Direction

- Using a sharp paring knife, score the skin of the duck breasts at 1/3-inch (8 mm) intervals crosswise. Score it again at about 1/2 inch (1 cm) intervals lengthwise. Be careful not to penetrate the meat. Lightly season both sides of the duck breast with salt. Set the breasts skin-side up on a plate, uncovered, and let rest in the refrigerator for 12 to 24 hours. Remove from the refrigerator about 30 minutes prior to smoking to bring them close to room temperature. Pat dry with a paper towel.
- Set the smoke chips in the donabe. Set up the bottom and middle grates with the duck breasts skin-side up on each. The thicker pieces should go on the bottom tier. Set the donabe, uncovered, over high heat. Wait until the smoke chips start to release smoke, about 7 to 8 minutes. Cover, and fill the reservoir in the rim of the base a little over half full with water. Smoke for 9 to 10 minutes over high heat, and then turn off the heat. Let rest undisturbed for 20 minutes.
- Meanwhile, make the sauce. Whisk together the crème fraîche and wasabi paste in a medium bowl until smooth. Add the usukuchi shoyu and green onion and stir. Gradually stir in the lemon juice. Adjust the seasoning with a pinch of salt, if desired.
- Transfer the duck breast to a cutting board and slice crosswise along the scored lines (or thinner if you like). Serve with the dipping sauce on the side.

301. Smokey Chicken, Rainbow Vegetable Saute And Cruncy Almonds

Serving: Serves 2-3 | Prep: | Cook: | Ready in:

Ingredients

- 1/2 pound Boneless, skinless chicken breast
- 1 Large beetroot, diced
- 2-3 Small turnips, diced
- 1 Large carrot, diced
- 1 Zucchini, diced
- 1 Onion
- 4-5 Green collard leaves
- 1 teaspoon Smoked paprika
- 1 teaspoon Ras-el-Hanout Morrocan Spice Blend
- 1 Clove of garlic
- A handful of raw almonds
- Olive oil for cooking
- Salt and pepper to taste

Direction

- Chop the onion in half-moons and dice the beetroot, carrot, zucchini and turnips in small 1/2?x1/2? cubes.
- Cut the chicken breast in strips. Drizzle olive oil in a pan on high heat, add the chicken pieces and cook for 6-8 minutes, turning the heat down to medium halfway through and stirring frequently. Add the smoked paprika, stir to coat, then remove the chicken from the heat and transfer to a plate.
- Return the pan to the heat, add in some more olive oil and cook the onion for 4-5 minutes. Add in the diced root vegetables, the minced garlic and the ras-el-hanout and continue cooking until the vegetables are tender, about 10-15 minutes. This is when you meditate on what's happening in front of you.
- Chop the collard greens into strips. I remove the end of the stem, roll the leaves into a bundle and slice them with a knife cross-wise.

When the vegetables are almost done, add the collard greens and stir constantly until they have reduced.
- Add the chicken back in, stir to combine and top with a handful of coarsely chopped almonds. Serve immediately.

302. South Station Bourbon Chicken

Serving: Serves 4 | Prep: | Cook: | Ready in:

Ingredients

- 8 boneless skineless chicken thighs sliced 1/2 inch strips
- 8 scallions sliced thin
- 1/4 cup Jack Daniels or other good bourbon
- 2 tablespoons honey
- 2 tablespoons cornstarch
- 2-4 tablespoons grapeseed oil
- salt & pepper to taste
- 1/2 teaspoon garlic powder
- 1 chicken liver minced fine

Direction

- Coat the chicken with a mixture of the corn starch, salt & pepper, garlic powder, and saute in hot grapeseed oil in a wok or saute pan, add the minced fine livers at the very end for flash frying.
- Add Jack mixed with honey to the pan to deglaze and immediately remove from heat, top with scallions and serve on rice or on lettuce shredded fine.

303. Southern Chicken Dressing

Serving: Serves 15 | Prep: | Cook: | Ready in:

Ingredients

- Cornbread
- 2 cups yellow cornmeal
- 1 cup self rising flour
- 2 cups milk
- 1 cup vegetable oil
- 1 tablespoon sugar
- 2 teaspoons salt
- 1 tablespoon baking powder
- 1 egg
- 3-4 tablespoons bacon grease to oil the bottom of skillet
- Southern Chicken Dressing
- 1 pan of cornbread
- 1 loaf of stale Italian bread
- 2 hard boiled eggs
- 1 raw egg
- 4 cups cooked chicken thighs cut into rough cubes
- 1 cup chopped celery
- 1 cup chopped onions
- 3-5 teaspoons ground sage
- 2 teaspoons ground black pepper
- 1/2 teaspoon ground salt
- 3-4 14 ounce cans of chicken broth

Direction

- Cornbread
- Preheat oven to 350°F.
- Grease bottom of a cast iron skillet with the bacon grease. Set aside.
- Mix dry ingredients together.
- Add the oil, egg and milk to the dry ingredients in the bowl. With a hand mixer, combine all ingredients until the batter is smooth.
- Spoon the batter in the cast iron skillet.
- Place the skillet in the oven and bake for 45 minutes.
- Southern Chicken Dressing
- Preheat oven to 350°F.
- Boil 1 cup onions and celery until soft and translucent. Strain the water and set the celery and onions aside in a small bowl.

- Boil 2 eggs. After boiling, cool and peel. Slice the eggs into 1/4" slices.
- Cut the pan of cornbread into 1/4 pieces. You might not use all of the pieces. Crumble enough cornbread where it will fill half of a 12" by 9" small roasting pan.
- Tear apart pieces of the stale Italian bread so they are roughly the size of peas. Full the rest of the roasting pan with the bread. Mix thoroughly with your hands or a large spoon.
- Add the chicken meat, celery, onions, and sliced eggs to the cornbread/bread mixture. Mix thoroughly.
- Add 1 can of chicken broth, stir and add another can of chicken broth. If the dressing isn't as moist as you'd like, add more chicken broth.
- Add rage sage, salt and black pepper. Stir well.
- Stir in 1 raw egg into the dressing and stir.
- Place the pan in the preheated oven.
- Take out the dressing every 30 minutes and scrape the dry sides, so that all areas are cooked. If you like your dressing moist, cook 45-60 minutes or dry for 1 hour to 2 hours.

304. Southwestern Chicken Salad

Serving: Serves 2 | Prep: | Cook: | Ready in:

Ingredients

- 5 ounces Spring Green Salad mix
- 1 large boneless, skinless chicken breast
- 1/4 red onion, chopped medium
- 1 Pasilla pepper, chopped medium
- 2 green onions, chopped medium
- A few sprigs of fresh cilantro, chopped (optional)
- 16 cherry tomatoes, cut in half
- 1 avocado, cut in slices
- 16-18 small corn chips
- 1/2 cup Light Ranch Dressing
- 1 teaspoon Hot Chili Sauce
- 1 teaspoon fresh ground black pepper to taste
- 1 pinch red pepper flakes

Direction

- Rub chicken with Kirkland Sweet Mesquite Seasoning (Amazon or COSTCO) and put in the refrigerator for an hour or two to marinate. Remove 30 minutes before cooking.
- Cook chicken in a small cast iron skillet about 5-8 minutes. Shred and chop with a stainless steel spatula while cooking. Set aside.
- Prepare dressing and set aside to allow flavors to blend.
- Cut up the onion, pasilla pepper, green onions, tomatoes and cilantro. Mix all ingredients together then toss the salad with the dressing. Sprinkle with the corn chips and serve.

305. Special Stuffing

Serving: Serves 10-12 | Prep: | Cook: | Ready in:

Ingredients

- giblets and neck meat from turkey
- 16 ounces cubed dried herbed cornbread (I like rosemary sage)
- 1 1/4 cups butter
- 2 medium onions
- 5 large stalks celery (chopped)
- 1 1/2 cups chicken broth (preferably organic)
- 1/4 cup white onion (chopped)
- Splash white wine

Direction

- First: (about 2 hours ahead) boil giblets and neck for two hours in salted water. Let cool. When cool shred neck meat and chop giblets into small pieces. Set aside
- Melt butter and sauté onions and celery until almost translucent. Add to herbed cornbread

- cubes in large bowl along with the melted butter and mix well.
- Add chopped giblets and shredded neck meat and mix well. Drizzle chicken broth and a splash of white wine overall and mix well until just moistened (if stuffing in bird -- stuffing will continue to get moister as it cooks in bird).
- Salt and pepper stuffing to taste -- but do not over-salt-- juices from bird will flavor as well.
- Stuff in bird and bake. Or if baking separately -- place in casserole dish and bake at 375 degrees for 20-30 minutes.
- Note: You can also use the water from the turkey/giblets boiling/and or in place of stock.

306. Spiced Smoked Tea Shortbread With Gingered Orange

Serving: Makes 36 treats | Prep: | Cook: | Ready in:

Ingredients

- Lacquered Black Bean Duck Confit
- 1/2 cup water
- 1 teaspoon lapsang souchong (or 1 teabag)
- 2 tablespoons shallots, minced
- 1 tablespoon garlic, minced
- 2 teaspoons ginger, minced
- 1 tablespoon fermented black beans, rinsed, chopped
- 1 tablespoon soy sauce
- 1 teaspoon maple syrup
- 1/2 orange (zested, juiced)
- 5 ounces confit duck meat
- cilantro for garnish
- Smoked Tea Shortbread with Gingered Orange
- 1 1/4 cups AP flour
- 1/4 cup brown sugar
- 1 1/2 teaspoons lapsang souchong tea
- 1/2 teaspoon salt
- 4 peppercorns
- 1/4 teaspoon szechuan peppercorns
- 1/4 teaspoon whole coriander
- 2 cloves
- 8 ounces unsalted butter
- 1 cup fresh orange juice (zest first and reserve)
- 2 teaspoons grated ginger
- 2 teaspoons orange zest
- 1 teaspoon lemon zest
- 1/2 cup sugar
- 1 teaspoon lapsang souchong (or 1 teabag)
- 3 eggs
- 1/2 teaspoon baking powder
- 2 tablespoons flour
- 1/4 teaspoon salt

Direction

- Lacquered Black Bean Duck Confit
- Boil water and steep teabag for about 5 minutes. If using confit duck legs, remove skins and render with any fat you can scrape off in a pan. You can save the crispy skin for garnish (or snacking). Cook shallots, ginger, garlic and black beans in fat for a few minutes until beginning to brown and very fragrant. Add tea, soy, syrup, juice and zest and simmer a bit while you pull meat off the bone into 1" or so chunks. Add meat to sauce and cook, stirring until sauce has just turned into a glaze. Remove from heat.
- Place a small piece of duck on an orange square and garnish with cilantro. These are best served right away while they are still warm or room temperature and still a bit crispy, but can also be gently warmed the next day.
- Smoked Tea Shortbread with Gingered Orange
- Heat oven to 350. Line an 8" baking dish with foil and grease with butter or cooking spray. Mix flour, sugar, tea and salt in a bowl. Toast spices briefly in a pan until fragrant then grind to a powder. Stir into flour. Cut butter into flour and mix until it resembles a medium crumb. Press into baking dish and bake about 18 minutes or until brown.

- Meanwhile, heat orange juice and ginger in a small pot and reduce to 1/4 c. Mix flour, baking powder, sugar, tea, salt and zest, then stir in eggs. Strain juice into egg mixture and mix until smooth. Pour over hot crust and return to oven until set and lightly browned, about 20 minutes. Remove and cool. Gently peel off foil and cut into small squares.

307. Spiced Turkey Breast With Balsamic Grilled Peaches

Serving: Serves 4 | Prep: | Cook: | Ready in:

Ingredients

- 1 tablespoon minced garlic
- 1 bay leaf, crumbled
- 1 tablespoon brown sugar
- ½ teaspoons black pepper
- 1 teaspoon ground allspice, cinnamon or cloves
- 2 tablespoons olive oil
- ¼ cups low-sodium soy sauce
- 1 cup finely chopped onion
- 1 ½ pounds boneless, skinless turkey breast (about half of a whole turkey breast)
- 1 tablespoon balsamic vinegar
- 4 peach halves (preferably fresh) or pineapple spears

Direction

- Combine first 7 ingredients and set aside 3 tablespoons of the mixture.
- Add onions and turkey breast to remaining mixture, place in a shallow bowl or zip lock bag, and marinate 1 to 4 hours, turning several times.
- To grill: Remove turkey breast from marinade and grill over medium high heat 12 to 15 minutes per side or until internal temperature reaches 165°F.
- Add balsamic vinegar to reserved marinade and place 1 tablespoon in the hollow of each peach half. Grill over medium heat for last 10 minutes.
- To roast: Preheat oven to 400°F.
- Place turkey on broiler pan in center of oven and roast for 20 minutes or until internal temperature reaches 165°F.
- Add balsamic vinegar to reserved marinade and place 1 tablespoon in the hollow of each peach half. Put in oven with turkey the last 10 minutes.
- Serving: Remove turkey breast from heat and let rest 5 minutes before slicing.
- Per 4-oz. Serving: 224 calories, 30 gm protein, 14 carbohydrate, 6 gm fat, 1 gm sat fat, 4 gm mono fat, 70 mg cholesterol, 2 gm fiber, 457 mg sodium.

308. Spiced Yogurt Baked Chicken On Roasted Broccoli

Serving: Serves 4 | Prep: | Cook: | Ready in:

Ingredients

- Baked Chicken in Spiced Yogurt
- 2 large chicken breasts (ca. 1.75 lbs total)
- 10 ounces plain Greek low sugar yogurt
- 1 teaspoon black or white pepper
- 1/2 teaspoon ground cumin
- 1/2 teaspoon ground coriander
- 1 tablespoon red pepper flakes
- 1/4 teaspoon cinnamon
- 2 teaspoons lemon zest
- 2 tablespoons lemon juice
- 3/4 cup parmesan cheese (divided)
- 1/4 cup EVOO
- 4 cups chopped broccoli
- 4 large garlic cloves, sliced thin
- 1 teaspoon black pepper
- 1/4 cup EVOO
- 2 teaspoons lemon juice
- 6 tablespoons pine nuts (divided)
- 1/2 cup parmesan cheese

Direction

- Toss the broccoli with the garlic, 5T pine nuts, EVOO and pepper
- Lay out the mixture on a parchment covered sheet pan
- Bake at 425F during the last 20 minutes of preparing the chicken
- Remove and toss with lemon zest, lemon juice, cheese, and 1T pine nuts; use as a bed for the chicken (below)
- In a mixing bowl, combine the yogurt with all of the other ingredients, reserving 1/4 c of cheese
- Spread a thin layer of the yogurt mixture on the bottom of an 8x8 baking dish
- Place the chicken breasts into the baking dish, and coat with the remaining yogurt mixture
- Bake at 375 for 45 minutes (internal temperature at the thickest part should be 165-170F); top with the cheese about 10 minutes before the end
- Remove, slice, and serve over the broccoli

309. Spicy Chicken Vegetable Soup

Serving: Serves 6 | Prep: | Cook: | Ready in:

Ingredients

- 2 whole chicken breasts, bone in and skin on
- 1 onion, quartered
- 1 cup chopped celery leaves and ribs
- 4 cups chicken stock
- 1/2 head cabbage, thinly shredded
- 1 large jar salsa
- 1 teaspoon salt
- 4-5 cups frozen vegetables
- 2 teaspoons cumin, or more to taste
- 3 splashes Cholula, or more to taste
- 1/4 cup chopped cilantro

Direction

- Cover the chicken with water, add onion, celery and leaves, pinch of salt, peppercorns if desired, and a pat of butter (don't ask me why, my mom always did). Stew chicken until done.
- Allow to cool and remove skin. Shred chicken.
- Add chicken and stock to large pot. Add salsa and seasoning.
- Add thawed vegetables. I usually use corn, green beans, and peas that I've frozen from the farmer's market, but you can use supermarket frozen or even canned vegetables. Use any combination of veggies you like. It's adaptable!
- Add shredded cabbage and simmer soup for at least 30 min. Taste and add Cholula or other hot sauce as desired.
- If I'm not dieting, it's good with tortilla strips on top. I also stir in some fresh cilantro before serving.

310. Spicy Lemongrass Coconut Tacos

Serving: Serves 4 | Prep: | Cook: | Ready in:

Ingredients

- Marinade
- 1.5 pounds Chicken Breast
- 1 tablespoon Fresh Ginger- Diced
- 1 tablespoon Fresh Garlic- Minced
- 1 cup Gluten-Free Soy Sauce
- 16 ounces Unsweetned Canned Coconut Milk
- 1 sprig Fresh Lemongrass
- 3 tablespoons Fresh Thai Basil Leaves
- Sauce and Tacos
- 8 Corn Tortillas
- 1.5 cups Shredded Purple Cabbage
- 4 tablespoons Chili Garlic Sauce
- 4 tablespoons Unsweetened Canned Coconut Milk
- 1 teaspoon Lime Juice

Direction

- Mix together all ingredients in marinade. Let sit for 3-12 hours.
- Cook chicken in marinade at 350 degrees for 20 minutes until cooked throughout.
- Sauce: mix together chili garlic paste, coconut milk, and lime juice.
- Warm tortillas (either on stove top or microwave for 30 seconds)
- Top tortillas with purple cabbage, chicken, and sauce.
- Enjoy!

311. Spicy Thai Chicken And Sweet Potato Stew

Serving: Serves 10 | Prep: | Cook: | Ready in:

Ingredients

- 2 tablespoons Olive Oil
- 3 Yellow Onions, roughly diced
- 1 Head of Garlic, finely chopped
- 2 tablespoons Ginger, finely chopped
- 1-3 Hot Green Peppers, finely chopped
- 1 teaspoon Tumeric
- 4 teaspoons Cumin
- 5 Sweet Potatoes (medium), peeled and cut into large cubes
- 4 Chicken Breasts, cleaned and cut into large pieces
- 28 ounces Coconut Milk (regular or low fat)
- 7 cups Chicken Stock
- 2 cups Frozen Green Peas
- 2 cups Bulgur Wheat
- 1 Lemon

Direction

- On medium heat, add 2 tbsp. of olive oil to a large soup pot.
- Once the oil is hot, add the onions and cook for 5 minutes, stirring often.
- Add the garlic, ginger and chili peppers and cook together for another 2 minutes, stirring often so that the garlic does not burn.
- Add the turmeric and cumin, stirring them together with the aromatics for 1 minute.
- Add the sweet potatoes, chicken, coconut milk and chicken broth. Bring to a boil, and then cover and let simmer for 20 minutes until the chicken is cooked and the potatoes are soft.
- Mash about half of the sweet potatoes against the side of the pot with a fork.
- Add the peas and bulgur wheat, and simmer for another 15-20 minutes uncovered until the bulgur is cooked and has soaked up most of the liquid.
- Before serving, give the soup a final stir so that all of the ingredients are combined. Once in a bowl, squeeze half of a lemon over the soup for a final burst of freshness, and then enjoy!

312. Spinach Chicken Feta Thin Crust Pizza + Variations

Serving: Serves 4 | Prep: | Cook: | Ready in:

Ingredients

- Creamy Garlic Pizza/Pasta Sauce
- 1 1/3 cup heavy cream
- 2 TBSP butter/magrarine
- 2 TBSP minced garlic
- 1/4 cup corn starch
- 1 chicken bouillon cube
- pinch white pepper & salt
- 1/3 cup Parmesan cheese
- Pizza Toppings
- 1 14 oz bag frozen chopped spinach
- 1 medium jar of mushroom stems & pieces (or fresh mushrooms if you have them)
- 4 oz feta cheese, crumbled
- 1/4 purple onion, halved, then sliced thin
- 1 14 oz can of white meat chicken
- 4 oz cheddar cheese shredded (for 2nd variation)
- 1/4 green bell pepper, sliced thin
- dried oregano, pepper, salt

Direction

- SAUCE: Melt the butter in a heavy saucepan along with the minced garlic. Sautee for 3 minutes over medium heat. Pour cold cream into the pan and follow with the cornstarch, chicken bouillon (crushed), parmesan cheese, salt and white pepper. Stir over medium heat with a whisk until smooth and thickened--add a little water if it thickens too much, but be sure to stir it all in. The consistency should be about that of mayonnaise... Set aside.
- Preheat your oven to 425 degrees. Since the pizzas are thin crust they won't work well sitting directly on the rack--place them on dark metal pans or a pizza stone.
- Spread half the garlic cream sauce on the pizzas. Squeeze out the thawed spinach and sprinkle over the pizzas, then sprinkle the chicken pieces over both pizzas (break the pieces up with your fingers). Drain and squeeze the liquid from the mushrooms and distribute pieces over both pizzas. On one pizza add the shredded cheddar and green pepper slices. On the other pizza add the crumbled feta and the purple onion slices.
- Sprinkle both pizzas with oregano, salt and pepper, then slide into the oven for 14 minutes. Use a pizza cutter to cut 6 slices, and serve with fresh salad. NOTE: you can also cut the pizzas into square slices and serve as hor d'oeuvres.
- Variation: Use the same white sauce, but pick up a pack of Pepperoni, usually by Hormel, at the Dollar Tree, and add green bell pepper slices, purple onion, mushrooms and Mozzarella cheese.

313. Spinach Mushroom Pasta & Meatballs In Garlic Wine Sauce

Serving: Serves 4 | Prep: | Cook: | Ready in:

Ingredients

- 22 turkey meatballs, cut in half
- 1 white onion, sliced thin
- 1/2 bag of red and green peppers, frozen (or 1/2 fresh pepper, red & green)
- 1 1/2 tablespoons finely minced garlic
- carton large white whole mushrooms, cut each in half
- Butter-flavored PAM
- 1 teaspoon olive oil
- 1 bag of frozen, chopped spinach
- 1/2 cup Parmesan cheese
- 1 wine glass of white wine
- 1 teaspoon California Garlic powder w/parsley
- large cube of chicken bouillon
- 8 oz. flat egg noodles

Direction

- Spray a wide saucepan with the PAM, then pour in the teaspoon of oil (this recipe is low-fat--if that is not a concern, use 3 TBSP butter), then sauté the sliced onion, minced garlic and peppers.
- When the vegies begin to soften a little, put in the meatballs (thawed) that have been cut in half, sprinkle on 1/2 the Parmesan cheese and mix well. Stir-fry the mixture for 5 minutes, uncovered.
- Microwave the frozen spinach for two minutes only, then place on top of the mix in the pan; sprinkle on the rest of the Parmesan cheese, crumble the cube of chicken bouillon over it, and sprinkle the garlic powder + 1/4 cup water, then put the cover on the pan and cook on low heat for 5 minutes. Stir gently, turn off the heat, then pour the wine over the mixture and put the cover on until you are ready to serve. Plate the dish within 10 minutes and top with a little Parmesan. Serve with white wine!

314. Split Breast Of Chicken With Roasted Carrots And Potatoes

Serving: Serves 3 - 4 | Prep: | Cook: | Ready in:

Ingredients

- 3 - 4 chicken breasts (with skin, on the bone)
- 4 - 5 cloves of garlic, minced
- 2 tablespoons olive oil
- 1 1/2 teaspoons salt
- 1 sprig rosemary (free from my garden!)
- fresh cracked black pepper
- 4 red potatoes, quartered
- 8 carrots, peeled
- 2 one inch wide slices of onion

Direction

- Pre-heat the oven to 425°F. Wash and pat dry the chicken breasts. Separate the skin from the meat to create a pocket.
- Mince the rosemary. Add the rosemary to a small bowl along with the garlic, salt, pepper and olive oil. Stir to combine.
- Use about 1/6th of the olive oil mixture under the skin of each breast. Rub another 1/6th on the outside of the skin. Sprinkle with additional salt and pepper if you wish.
- Arrange the vegetables in the bottom of a roasting pan or casserole dish. Season with salt and pepper to taste. Place the chicken, skin side up, on top of the vegetables.
- Roast for 30 minutes at 425°F. Cover with foil and return to a 375°F oven for another 20 - 30 minutes. (Always check the temperature of your chicken at the thickest part, it should read at least 180°F)
- Serve each person a breast, two carrots and four potato wedges. The liquid in the pan can be reduced and thickened slightly to be served as a gravy.

315. Spring Hill Ranch's New Mexico Green Chile Sauce

Serving: Makes 4 cups | Prep: | Cook: | Ready in:

Ingredients

- 2 tablespoons lard (use shortening or oil if you must, but it's not the same)
- 1/4 medium white onion, finely chopped
- 3 medium cloves of garlic, chopped
- 2 tablespoons all-purpose flour
- 4 medium new mexico #6 or big jim chiles, roasted, peeled and finely chopped (about 1 pound or 2 cups) (or a 13-ounce container frozen diced green chiles) (or 3 4-ounce cans of diced green chiles)
- 1 1/2 cups good water or low-sodium chicken broth
- 1/2 teaspoon kosher salt (omit if your broth is not low-sodium)
- 1/2 - 1 pounds shredded prok or beef (optional)

Direction

- In a heavy bottomed skillet over medium heat, heat the lard until it is shimmering but not yet smoking. Sauté the onion until it has softened and become translucent, about 4 minutes. Add the garlic and stir until it is nice and fragrant, about 1 minute. Add the flour and mix it in well, stirring constantly for at least 2 minutes to cook out the flour-y taste.
- Add in the green chiles, water (or stock), and salt and simmer the sauce uncovered, stirring often for 20 minutes, until most of the liquid has evaporated and the sauce has thickened slightly.
- Serve the sauce hot over or under your southwestern meal. Kept in an air tight container, this sauce should last a week or more in the refrigerator. It freezes well.

316. Sriracha Hot Wings

Serving: Serves 2-4 | Prep: | Cook: |Ready in:

Ingredients

- 1 tablespoon neutral oil
- 2 teaspoons sesame oil
- 1/8 - 1/2 cups sriracha, depending on spice tolerance
- 2 tablespoons honey
- 2 tablespoons soy sauce
- 1 tablespoon rice vinegar
- 2 pounds chicken wings
- 1 tablespoon oil

Direction

- In a large bowl, mix together the oil, sesame oil, sriracha, honey, soy sauce, rice vinegar, and minced garlic. Add the chicken wings and mix well. Marinate in the fridge for an hour.
- When ready to cook, remove the wings from the bowl being sure to reserve the marinade. Heat up the tablespoon of oil in a wok or large non-stick frying pan over medium-high heat. Add the wings and cook, flipping every so often until cooked through, about 10-15 minutes, depending on wing size.
- Add the reserved marinade to the pan and turn heat to high to reduce the sauce until glossy and sticky, about 3-4 minutes. Enjoy immediately.

317. Sticky Blackberry Honey Hot Wings

Serving: Serves 24 wings | Prep: | Cook: |Ready in:

Ingredients

- 24 chicken wings
- 2.5 cups blackberries
- 1/2 cup honey
- 1 tablespoon ketchup
- 1/4 cup orange juice
- 1.5 tablespoons chipotle tabasco (or more to your liking..and you can use hot sauce of your choice plus a sprinkle of chipotle powder)
- 1 tablespoon brown sugar
- 1 teaspoon balsamic vinegar
- 1 pinch ground black pepper
- 1/4 cup melted butter
- zest from 1 orange

Direction

- Preheat oven to 400 degrees, and put wings in for 40-50 minutes (until cooked through).
- While wings are baking, make sauce: puree berries, honey, ketchup, orange juice, hot sauce, brown sugar, and balsamic until smooth. If you dislike the seeds, strain (I like to leave them in). Mix puree with melted butter. Set aside.
- After wings have cooked for 40-50 minutes, drain juices. Pour sauce over wings and coat evenly (you might have sauce leftover). Stick back in the 400 degree oven for 10 more minutes, turning often. About half way through, sprinkle a little more brown sugar on top, and mix in, sprinkle orange zest on top. For last few minutes of cooking, turn on broiler.
- Reserve remaining sauce for dipping, or for another use (like eating with a spoon or dipping tortilla chips into or basting on salmon.)
- Enjoy!

318. Straight Up, Down Home Southern Fried Chicken With Honey

Serving: Serves 4 | Prep: | Cook: |Ready in:

Ingredients

- 1 broiler/fryer chicken, cut into 8 pieces
- 1 quart buttermilk

- 1 tablespoon garlic powder
- 1 1/2 tablespoons onion powder
- 2 tablespoons paprika
- 1/4 cup hot sauce, Louisiana style
- 1 teaspoon cayenne
- flour, for dredging
- peanut oil, for frying
- 1 tablespoon Good quality bacon fat
- 1 large cast-iron skillet, at least 12in.
- 1 fry/candy thermometer
- Honey

Direction

- Marinate chicken in buttermilk and hot sauce overnight, or at least 12 hours.
- Make a rub with garlic and onion powders, paprika, cayenne, 1 Tablespoon salt & 1 teaspoon black pepper.
- Heat bacon fat and enough peanut oil to come up 1/8 inch up the side of the skillet. Heat oil to 325.
- Remove chicken from marinade, season with rub.
- Dredge in flour.
- Fry. Maintain oil temp, about 10-12 min per side depending on thickness of the chicken. 180 internal temp.
- Drain on brown paper bags or paper towels. Serve with honey.

319. Stuffed & Seared Chicken Thighs With Refrigerator Door Mustard

Serving: Serves 4 | Prep: 0hours40mins | Cook: 0hours20mins | Ready in:

Ingredients

- 4 boneless* (see note below), skin-on chicken thighs (about 1 1/3 pounds)
- 2 teaspoons coarse sea salt
- 4 tablespoons Refrigerator-Door Mustard, recipe follows
- 1 teaspoon grapeseed or canola oil
- 1 sprig fresh thyme or oregano (optional)
- 2 tablespoons cold unsalted butter (optional)
- Refridgerator-Door Mustard
- 1/2 cup capers, drained
- 2 tablespoons green peppercorns in brine, drained and rinsed
- 2 anchovy fillets, drained
- 1 1/2 tablespoons whole-grain mustard
- 1 1/2 teaspoons Dijon mustard

Direction

- First, make the Refrigerator-Door Mustard: Finely chop the capers, peppercorns, and anchovy fillets by hand or in a food processor and combine well. Mix with both mustards. Store in the refrigerator for up to 1 month.
- Season the skin side of the chicken with 1 teaspoon of the salt. Flip over and season the flesh side with the remaining salt. Let cure for 30 minutes before stuffing.
- Preheat the oven to 400°F. Place 1 tablespoon of the mustard down the center of each thigh. Bring one side of the thigh over the other to enclose the filling. Stretch the skin so it covers all the meat and secure the seam with a toothpick.
- Heat an ovenproof medium pan over medium-high heat for 30 seconds. Add the oil and tilt the pan to coat the surface. Add the thighs, seams facing to one side. Turn the heat down to medium; cook until the skin is deeply golden and crisp, 6 to 7 minutes. Turn to sear the other side, about 5 minutes more.
- Once both sides are seared, carefully pour the excess fat out of the pan. Place the pan in the oven and roast until the chicken is fully cooked, 5 to 7 minutes. Place the thighs on a serving plate. Add the thyme and cold butter, if using, to the still-hot pan. Swirl to infuse the butter and combine it I with the other bits in the pan. As soon as the butter melts, spoon it liberally over the chicken. If you want, discard the thyme spring. Serve immediately.

- *BONING A CHICKEN THIGH: Lay the thigh skin side down on your cutting board. With a thin, sharp knife, trace the full length of the bone to expose it fully. Next, scrape along one side of the bone, from joint to joint, to release the meat. If you focus on carefully cleaning the bone, rather than cutting at the meat, you'll leave the chicken nicely intact. As you continue to scrape and loosen the bone from the meat—don't forget to cut around the joints—you'll be able to roll it over and cut it out.

320. Stuffed Tomato Chicken

Serving: Serves 6 | Prep: | Cook: | Ready in:

Ingredients

- 4 cups cooked red Quinoa
- 8 large tomatoes
- 2 chicken thighs
- 1/2 cup sweet barbecue sauce
- 2 cups spinach leaves
- 1/4 cup Italian bread crumbs

Direction

- Pre heat oven to 350 degrees
- Place chicken thighs in a baking pan. Pour barbecue sauce over chicken, and let marinate until oven is heated to 350 degrees.
- Bake chicken for 30 minutes.
- Once chicken removed from the oven, let cool off for 10 minutes.
- Chop chicken into 1/4th inch or bite size pieces and set aside.
- Make sure oven still remains on 350 degrees, in order to bake the stuffed tomatoes.
- In a large pot, add your cooked quinoa with the chopped chicken. Turn stove onto a medium-low heat and stir quinoa mixture. Add spinach, and continuously stir until well mixed, and then set aside.
- Cut the top of each tomato and remove the inside in order to create space for the quinoa mixture.
- Add the filling into the tomatoes.
- Sprinkle bread crumbs on top of the tomatoes, making sure that the mixture is well covered.
- Take a baking tray and spray with cooking oil
- Place tomatoes on the baking tray and into the oven for 10-12 minutes or until the tomato skin begins to crack.

321. Sumac Chicken With Cauliflower And Brussels Sprouts

Serving: Serves 4 | Prep: | Cook: | Ready in:

Ingredients

- 3 tablespoons olive or avocado oil, divided
- 1 tablespoon Sumac
- 1 teaspoon kosher salt, divided
- 1 teaspoon light brown sugar
- 1 teaspoon paprika
- 1/4 tsp red pepper flakes
- 1 pound cauliflower florets
- 1 pound Brussels sprouts, halved lengthwise
- 2 pounds chicken thighs/drumsticks/bone-in, skin-on breast
- 1 small lemon, halved lengthwise and thinly sliced
- 1 small red onion, cut into ¾ inch wedges
- 1 cup cup finely chopped fresh flat-leaf parsley or cilantro; preferably, a mix
- 1 tablespoon fresh lemon juice
- 1 small garlic clove

Direction

- Preheat oven to 425°F.
- Combine 2 Tbsp. oil with sumac, ¾ tsp salt, brown sugar, paprika, and red pepper in a medium bowl. Place cauliflower and Brussels

sprouts on a foil-lined baking sheet. Add half of oil mixture; toss to coat.
- Add chicken pieces and lemon slices to pan. Rub remaining oil mixture over chicken. Bake for 20 minutes. Stir vegetables. Sprinkle onion wedges over pan. Bake for 20 more minutes, or until chicken is done.
- Combine remaining 1 Tbsp. oil, parsley, and remaining ingredients in a small bowl. Spoon parsley mixture evenly over chicken and vegetables. Serve with warm whole-wheat couscous, if desired.

322. Summer Grilled Chicken Cacciatore

Serving: Serves 6-8 | Prep: | Cook: | Ready in:

Ingredients

- Grilled chicken
- 1 whole chicken cut up and seasoned with salt pepper and a touch of ground red chile flakes
- Cacciatore sauce ingredients
- 2 tablespoons EVOO
- 1 tablespoon unsalted butter
- 6 cloves garlic, peeled and halved, chopped
- 1 sweet onion, quartered and cliced
- 10 ounces baby bella mushrooms, sliced
- 3 tablespoons capers
- 1 green bell peppers, cored, seeded, and sliced into strips
- 1 red bell pepper, cored, seeded, and sliced into strips
- 1 yellow pepper cored, seeded, and sliced into strips
- 1 cup dry white wine (I use red if there is some open)
- 2-3 cups chicken broth or stock
- Juice of 1 grilled lemon and a bit of lemon zest
- 1 (28-ounce) can whole tomatoes, with their juice, crushed or and equal amount of fresh plum tomatoes
- 6 ounces fresh tomato sauce
- salt and pepper, for seasoning
- pinch of red pepper flakes
- 2 sprigs fresh oregano leaves, chopped or a teaspoon of dried
- 1/4 cup fresh basil leaves, torn
- 1/4 cup Italian parsley, minced
- 1 teaspoon fresh rosemary, minced
- 1 Bay leaf
- Garnish with a little more parsley before serving
- grated cheese for garnish

Direction

- Grilled chicken
- Season a whole cut up patted dry chicken with EVOO salt, pepper and a touch of ground red pepper flakes, grill over medium high heat until well browned, but not completely done.*Cut the chicken into 8 pieces. Everything can be prepped and the cacciatore can be prepared completely on the grill for a fantastic dinner Al Fresco
- Cacciatore sauce ingredients
- The pepper assortment is a guideline, today I picked more peppers so I have quite a variety. In a large sauté pan over medium high heat add the oil and butter, sauté mushrooms until they have a little crispness to them remove them from the pan. Add the peppers and onions sauté until soft add garlic and sauté for a minute or two. Add the wine, stirring to pick up any pan goodies, add the chicken and simmer until almost all of the wine has evaporated. Stir in capers, the tomatoes, 2 cups of the chicken stock or broth, lemon juice and zest, tomato sauce, herbs and season with salt and pepper. Simmer for about 45. Add mushrooms and simmer 10 minutes. Remove bay leaf. Garnish with additional minced parsley a little freshly grated Parmesan or Romano cheese, serve with pasta of your choice, for the summer version I make saffron orzo.

323. Sunday Chicken Ragu

Serving: Serves 4 | Prep: | Cook: | Ready in:

Ingredients

- 2 pounds chicken thighs, boneless, skinless, cut into 1-1 1/2 pieces
- 3/4 inch piece of pancetta, small dice
- 3 tablespoons EVOO
- 1 tablespoon butter
- 1 sprig thyme leaves removed and minced
- 1 tablespoon fresh sage, minced
- 1 1/2 teaspoons rosemary, minced
- 2 large shallots, minced
- 1-2 garlic cloves, minced
- 1 carrot, peeled and finely diced
- 1/4 cup celery, finely diced
- 3/4-1 cups light dry red wine
- 1 pint cherry or grape tomato assortment, halved
- 1 15 ounce can diced tomatoes, drained (save juice)
- Salt and pepper to taste
- Final tablespoon of butter to finish

Direction

- Cook pancetta in 2 tablespoons EVOO and a tablespoon butter, stirring occasionally, 2 minutes. Add thyme, sage and rosemary, cook stirring, 30 seconds. Add chicken and cook, stirring until chicken is no longer pink on the outside, 3-4 minutes. Add shallots, garlic, carrot, celery, cook, stirring occasionally, 5 minutes.
- Add drained tomato juice and wine and simmer, uncovered, stirring occasionally until liquid is reduced to about 1 cup, about 10 minutes. Add tomatoes, salt, and pepper, simmer, stirring occasionally, until sauce is thickened, 10 minutes. Season with salt and pepper. Stir in a tablespoon of butter and check seasonings. Can be made a day ahead, cooled chilled covered.

324. Sunday Chicken With Roasted Vegetables And Garlic Breadcrumbs

Serving: Serves 4-6 people and can easily be doubled | Prep: | Cook: | Ready in:

Ingredients

- 5 slices of day-old bread
- 2 cloves garlic, finely chopped
- ¾ cup Pecorino Romano cheese, grated with a box grater
- ¾ cup fresh parsley, finely chopped
- 2 sprigs fresh rosemary, stemmed and finely chopped
- 1 lemon, zested and juiced
- 6-7 tablespoons extra virgin olive oil (divided)
- 4 bone-in, skin-on chicken legs with thighs attached
- 1 bone-in, skin-on chicken breast, split (for diners like my husband, who prefer white meat)
- 1 ½ tablespoons vegetable or grapeseed oil
- 1 purple onion, cut into six wedges
- 1/2 large bulb of fennel, cut into six wedges (keep some of the core attached so that the fennel retains a wedge shape)
- 4 small Yukon Gold potatoes (or other thin skinned potatoes) cut into 2-inch pieces (roughly 5 ounces)
- 1 sweet potato, pared, and cut into 2-inch pieces
- 1 red bell pepper, stem and seeds removed, sliced into 2 inch pieces
- 6-7 tablespoons extra virgin olive oil (divided)
- ¼ cup plus 1 tablespoon dry white wine or vermouth
- Salt and freshly ground black pepper to taste

Direction

- First, make the breadcrumbs. Tear bread into large pieces and add to food processor. Whir for about 30 seconds or until bread is consistency of thick cornmeal. It's okay if some of the pieces are not completely uniform in size. Remove from food processor and add to medium size bowl. Add garlic, cheese, parsley, rosemary, and lemon zest. Add two three finger pinches of salt (about ¼ teaspoon) and stir (I use my hands) until combined. Drizzle in 2 tablespoons olive oil and continue stirring until mixture feels slightly moistened but not wet. Add more olive oil if needed. Set aside.

- Preheat oven to 350 degrees. In large, heavy casserole (I like cast iron) or a rimmed baking pan, add vegetables (onion, fennel, red pepper, potato and sweet potato) in one layer. It's okay if vegetables are slightly crowded, but you don't want them on top of each other. Drizzle 3 tablespoons olive oil over vegetables and 1 tablespoon white wine. Add about ½ teaspoon of salt (or to taste) to vegetables and some freshly ground pepper. Mix with your hands until combined. Cover casserole (use foil if you don't have a lid that will fit) and place casserole or baking pan in oven and let roast for 25 minutes uninterrupted.
- While vegetables are roasting, start cooking the chicken. Heat large sauté pan over medium heat and add vegetable oil. Season chicken on both sides with salt and pepper. When oil is hot, add chicken pieces to pan. Do not crowd the pan. You may need to sauté the chicken in batches. Let chicken cook for at least 8-10 minutes per side. When the underside is a lovely golden brown, turn chicken and cook on the other side. After chicken has browned and is crisp looking, put on a platter. Remove pan from heat, and add wine to pan. Put pan back on the heat and turn heat to low. Scrape up all the lovely brown bits from the pan and let liquid simmer for about a minute.
- Remove roasted vegetables from the oven and give everything a good stir with a spoon. Nestle chicken pieces in between vegetables. Pour any juices that have accumulated from the chicken over the vegetables. Drizzle the wine and fond from the sauté pan over the vegetables. Add breadcrumb mixture in a generous and even layer over vegetables and chicken, making sure to tuck bread crumb mixture into any crevices between vegetables and chicken. You may not use all of the bread crumbs. Cover casserole again and put back into the oven. Roast for about 40 minutes. Your kitchen will start to smell delicious.
- Remove casserole from oven and take off lid. Turn up heat on the oven to 400 degrees. Drizzle lemon juice and a tablespoon or so of olive oil over chicken and vegetables. Put pan back into oven uncovered for about 10-15 minutes or until breadcrumbs are a beautiful burnished golden color and chicken is completely cooked.
- Lift casserole out of oven. When plating this dish, give each diner a piece of chicken and a nice array of vegetables. Drizzle some of the pan juices over the vegetables and chicken and serve. This dish is delicious with a dry white wine, some crusty Ciabatta bread and a salad with an acidic dressing. I like mixing orange or tangerine supremes, meaty black olives, arugula and razor thin slices of fennel with a red wine vinegar and olive oil vinaigrette.

325. Super Easy Slow Cooker Chicken And Dumplings (with Gnocchi!)

Serving: Serves 6 | Prep: | Cook: | Ready in:

Ingredients

- 3 stalks celery, diced
- 3 medium carrots, trimmed and diced
- 1 medium onion, peeled, trimmed, and diced
- 2 cloves garlic, minced
- 2 1/2 pounds bone-in, skin-on chicken pieces, preferably dark meat
- 1/2 cup flour
- 1/2 teaspoon pepper, plus more for seasoning
- 1 teaspoon salt, plus more for seasoning
- 1 cup chicken stock

- 2 teaspoons fresh thyme leaves
- 1 pound packaged gnocchi

Direction

- Layer the celery, carrot, onion, and garlic in the bottom of a slow cooker.
- In a dish, combine the flour, salt, and pepper. Dredge the chicken on all sides in the flour mixture, then place on top of the veggies in the slow cooker. Pour in the stock and sprinkle with the thyme leaves.
- Cover the slow cooker and cook on HIGH for 3 hours or LOW for 6-8 hours depending on your schedule. When the cooking time is over, the chicken should shred very easily. Remove the chicken from the slow cooker and add the gnocchi. Stir the gnocchi into the vegetable mixture and cover; cook on high for 30 minutes. While the gnocchi is cooking, remove the skin and bones from the chicken and tear into bite-sized chunks.
- After 30 minutes, taste a gnocchi to be sure it is cooked through. If it is too chewy in the center, cook for 15 minutes or until cooked through. Add the chicken back to the slow cooker and taste; add salt and pepper to your preference until the dish is very flavorful.
- If at any point the soup becomes very thick, splash in more stock to thin to your liking. Serve with extra thyme on top, if desired. Enjoy!

326. Super Gingery Chicken And Herb Soup

Serving: Serves 2 | Prep: 0hours15mins | Cook: 1hours0mins | Ready in:

Ingredients

- 1 quart chicken stock
- 12 ounces chicken breast, cut into strips or tenders or whatever part of the chicken you prefer
- 7 ounces fresh ginger
- 2 cups fresh spinach, lightly chopped
- 3/4 cup Basil and cilantro, chopped
- 4 cloves of garlic, slightly mashed with flat edge of a knife
- 2 large eggs
- 1 teaspoon fish sauce
- 1/2 lime
- white vinegar for poaching the eggs

Direction

- Peel the ginger, I use a regular spoon, and cut in to 1/8" slices. Put ginger and garlic in pot with the chicken stock. Bring to a boil and then let simmer covered for an hour.
- Poach the chicken in the stock. I used chicken tenders, because that's what I was allowed to order from Publix the week I first made this, but any chicken will do. The chicken breast strips will cook in roughly 10 minutes, remove from the broth. When cool enough to handle shred by hand.
- At this point you finish the recipe or stop and hold it for a later date. I usually turn the broth off so it does not evaporate anymore and let the garlic and ginger continue to infuse for another hour or so.
- Return the broth to a boil. In a separate shallow pan add water and white vinegar for egg poaching.
- Divide the fresh herbs and chicken in half and place in two soup bowls.
- Poach the eggs in the shallow pan with simmering water and roughly tablespoons for white vinegar. If you do not know how to poach an egg, fear not! But I would recommend mastering one prior to this point in the recipe.
- Strain the ginger chunks and garlic cloves from the broth. Add the spinach to the broth until it is wilted but still green, no more than a minute. Finish with the fish sauce and juice from the lime and stir in.
- Pour broth with spinach into the prepared bowls and top each with a poached egg.

- You can add rice or rice noodles for heartier meal.

327. Sweet Corn Chicken Stew With Mushroom

Serving: Serves 4 people | Prep: | Cook: | Ready in:

Ingredients

- Sweet Corn and Chicken Pieces
- half cup Sweet Corn
- half cup Muchroom
- two tablespoons Chicken Soup
- half piece Red Onion
- pinch teaspoons Salt
- Not Any

Direction

- Rinse your Chicken and put it in a pot. Add your Sweet Corn, Mushrooms (cut in halves), Red Onion cut in small block and one tablespoon of Parsley Herbs. Then mix and cook for 20-25 minutes on medium heat. After 20-25 minutes, add half Chicken soup in a cup mixed with water and stir to mix. Then leave chicken soup to cook for 10 minutes, while continuously stirring to mix with the chicken. If the saltiness is not enough, put some little salt to taste.

328. Tamale Pie

Serving: Serves 6-8 | Prep: | Cook: | Ready in:

Ingredients

- Filling
- 1 pound ground turkey
- 1 large yellow onion, chopped
- 1 poblano pepper, chopped
- 1 jalapeno, minced
- 1 green pepper
- 1 tablespoon olive oil
- 1 cup canned whole tomatoes
- 1 cup frozen sweet corn
- 3 cloves garlic, minced
- 1.5 cups shredded mexican cheese blend
- 1.5 teaspoons cumin
- 1.5 teaspoons chili powder
- 1/4 teaspoon salt
- Dash nutmeg
- Topping & Garnish
- 3 cups water
- 1.5 cups cornmeal
- 1/2 teaspoon salt
- 1.5 tablespoons butter
- 2 jalapenos
- sour cream

Direction

- Preheat oven to 375 degrees
- Begin to sauté the onion and peppers in the olive oil. Once onions are translucent (about 3-5 minutes), add the garlic, turkey, and spices. Cook for 5 minutes and add tomatoes and frozen corn. Cook 5 more minutes. Add cheese.
- While cooking the filling, bring water and salt to boil in a small saucepan. Once boiling slowly whisk in cornmeal. Once thickened remove from heat and stir in butter.
- With a slotted spoon, move turkey mixture into a 9x13 inch pan. Carefully smooth cornmeal topping over the turkey mixture.
- Cut jalapenos into rings and remove seeds in the middle of the rings. Place on top of the cornmeal topping.
- Bake for 40 minutes. Serve with a dollop of sour cream.

329. Tandoori Chicken Wraps

Serving: Serves 4 | Prep: | Cook: | Ready in:

Ingredients

- 2 cloves garlic, peeled
- 1 (3-inch) piece fresh ginger, peeled and roughly chopped
- 1/2 small red onion, roughly chopped, plus 1/4 of the onion, thinly sliced
- 1/2 cup plus 2 tablespoons 2% Greek yogurt
- 1 tablespoon olive oil
- 4 teaspoons tomato paste
- 2 teaspoons hot paprika, divided
- 1-1/2 teaspoons ground coriander
- 1-1/2 teaspoons ground cumin
- 1 pound boneless, skinless chicken thighs
- 2 tablespoons chopped fresh cilantro
- 1/4 teaspoon kosher salt
- 4 whole wheat flatbread wraps
- 4 large pieces Romaine lettuce
- 1/2 cup grape tomatoes, halved

Direction

- In blender or food processor, process garlic, ginger, chopped onion, 2 tablespoons yogurt, oil, tomato paste, 1-3/4 teaspoons paprika, coriander and cumin until it forms a mostly smooth paste (there will be a few chunks, that's OK). Place chicken in large zip-top bag; pour marinade over chicken. Seal bag and refrigerate at least 2 hours or up to overnight.
- Preheat oven to 400 degrees F. Remove chicken from marinade; discard marinade. Place chicken on rimmed baking pan and bake 18 to 20 minutes or until internal temperature reaches 165 degrees F, turning once. Transfer chicken to cutting board; let stand 5 minutes. Slice chicken crosswise into 1/2-inch pieces.
- Meanwhile, in small bowl, stir together cilantro, salt, and remaining 1/2 cup yogurt and 1/4 teaspoon paprika.
- Build wraps using flatbread, lettuce, tomatoes, sliced onion, chicken and yogurt mixture.

330. Tangine Gravy

Serving: Serves 8 | Prep: | Cook: | Ready in:

Ingredients

- 2 cups turkey brown bits / drippings
- 2 cups turkey stock
- 1/2 cup olive oil
- 1 cube butter
- 2 yellow onions (finely chopped)
- 1 head of garlic (finely minced)
- 1 cup Muscat Wine
- cups 1/4 to 1/2 cup of flour (to preferred thickness)
- 1 cup dried apricots (pre-soaked in warm water)
- 1 cup dried cranberries
- 1 cup pitted prunes
- 1 cup raisons (yellow, sultana, currents)
- 1 teaspoon safron
- 2 tablespoons ginger (fresh fine grated)
- salt and white pepper to taste
- 2 cups olives- mix of green & black

Direction

- In a large skillet heat olive oil and 1/2 cube of butter. Add onions & garlic, slow sweat, adding in brown bits & drippings caramelize, deglazing intermittently with the Muscat, then add in small amounts of flour at a time, alternating with the turkey stock continue stirring (to avoid lumps) to your preferred thickness. Add in all the other ingredients including the saffron, ginger, salt, and white pepper - cook till raisons, cranberries, apricots, and prunes are plumped. Use additional stock & remaining 1/2 cube of butter as needed to maintain preferred consistency. Serve over Thanksgiving turkey, stuffing (Awesome) & mashed potatoes.
- Then bring on the Belly Dancers & dessert!

331. Thai Curry Noodle Soup

Serving: Serves 2 | Prep: | Cook: | Ready in:

Ingredients

- 4 Cloves of Garlic (for taste)
- 1 cup Shallots (for taste)
- 2 Small Potatoes
- 2 cups Coconut Milk
- 4 tablespoons Curry Powder
- 1-3 tablespoons Thai Red Curry Paste
- 1 cup Vegetable Stock or chicken broth
- 2 Chicken Thighs with Bone (If vegan leave out)
- 1 Large Carrot

Direction

- Peel and dice the potatoes (about 2cm squares) and chop the carrot into half-moons. De-skin the garlic cloves and shallots (keep them whole if low FODMAP). In a deep saucepan fry the potatoes, garlic, carrot, and shallots with the curry powder for 3 minutes (stir continuously making sure the veggies are coated in the curry powder).
- Now add the coconut milk, curry paste, chicken broth, bring to a boil (stir continuously).
- Now add the chicken and bring the curry to a light simmer and cook for 30 minutes. While waiting soften the noodles by placing them in a large bowl emerging them in cool/warm water (not hot) for 15-20 minutes.
- By now the noodles should be soft so place them in serving bowls. Make sure the chicken is cooked all the way through; if it's ok place the chicken onto of the noodles and then pour the curry soup over the noodles making sure to get the vegetables (Low FODMAPers, avoid the shallots and garlic)
- Garnish with some coriander and enjoy!

332. Thai Inspired Chicken Coconut Soup

Serving: Serves 2 | Prep: | Cook: | Ready in:

Ingredients

- For the marinade
- 1 Lime, zested and 1/2 juiced
- 1 Red chili pepper, grated (The pepper's skin will be left over, which should be diced and saved for later)
- 1 teaspoon Ginger, grated
- 2-3 Cloves garlic, grated
- 1 tablespoon Vegetable or coconut oil
- 1 teaspoon Honey
- 1 bunch Basil leaves, chopped (chopped Reserve half to use in the soup later)
- 1 pinch Salt
- For the soup
- 2 Chicken thighs with legs attached OR 2 diced chicken breasts
- 1/2 Onion, diced
- 1 tablespoon Ginger, diced
- 2 Cloves garlic, diced
- 1 teaspoon Fish sauce
- 1 teaspoon Tamarind paste
- 12 ounces Coconut milk, fresh or canned
- 1/4 Lemon, juiced
- Salt, to taste
- Dried chili flakes, to taste

Direction

- Combine all the ingredients of the marinade together in a small bowl and whisk with a fork to combine. Place the chicken in a plastic bag and pour over the chicken. Let stand for 20-30 minutes at room temperature or up to 2 hours in the fridge. (Be sure to remove 15-20 minutes before cooking to bring the chicken to room temperature)
- Heat a soup pot over medium-high heat and add vegetable oil. Add the chicken and sear until golden brown on the outside, then remove.

- Add some more oil, then add the onions and a pinch of dried chili flakes, then fry until translucent (about 5 minutes).
- Add the ginger, garlic, and red pepper skins (left over from the marinade) and fry for 1-2 minutes until the garlic is fragrant. Then add the fish sauce and tamarind paste, then give everything a good stir to combine the flavors. (Don't forget to scrape the bottom of the pot to remove all the charred bits of pure flavor left over from the chicken ☐)
- Re-add the chicken to the pot, followed by the coconut milk. Let simmer over medium-low heat for 10-20 minutes, or until the chicken is cooked and beginning to flake apart. (Check back relatively frequently since coconut milk has the tendency to boil over!)
- Add a pinch of healthy salt, red chili flakes, remaining lime juice, a dash of lemon juice, and some more chopped basil. Taste and adjust accordingly. Plate, garnish with some chopped fresh cilantro, and enjoy out in the sun with a side of freshly-made rice ☐ ☐

333. Thanksgiving Osso Buco

Serving: Serves 4 | Prep: | Cook: | Ready in:

Ingredients

- 2 pounds turkey drumsticks, cut crosswise into 1 1/2 inch thick pieces (ask your butcher to do it unless you have a chain saw, or like to suffer)
- 1 finely chopped yellow onion
- 2 diced carrots
- 2 minced garlic cloves
- 8 diced Turkish apricots
- 16 dried cranberries, halved
- 1 cup hard cider
- 1/4 teaspoon allspice
- 1/4 teaspoon cinnamon
- 1/4 teaspoon nutmeg
- Salt and freshly ground black pepper

Direction

- Preheat oven to 325°F.
- In a large cast iron casserole or Dutch oven, heat the oil over medium-high heat. Season the turkey pieces with salt and pepper and brown them nicely, about two minutes per side.
- Remove the turkey from the pan. Add the onion and cook over medium heat, until the onion is very soft and slightly caramelized, for about five minutes. Add the garlic, and cook for another minute. Add the carrots and cook for another five minutes. Stir in the apricots, cranberries, allspice, cinnamon, nutmeg and cider. Place the turkey pieces back into the casserole, coat with the sauce, and bring to simmer.
- Cover the casserole with a lid and put it in the oven. Cook until the meat is very tender and begins to fall of the bones, for about 2 to 2 1/2 hours. (If it becomes dry during cooking, feel free to add a bit more liquid.)
- Adjust the seasoning if needed. Serve warm with mashed potatoes and the sauce spooned on top.

334. The Alchemist's Chicken (Chicken Roasted With Seville Oranges, Onions And Bay)

Serving: Makes up to 2 chickens, enough for 6-10 | Prep: | Cook: | Ready in:

Ingredients

- 1 - 2 3-1/2 half pound whole chickens, pin feathers removed, cavity cleaned and the bird rinsed and patted dry
- 1 lemon, halved crosswise, and one of the halves cut in half again
- 2 Seville (sour) oranges
- 1 Vidalia-type onion, diced (about 1-1/2 cups)
- 2 shallots, diced

- 3 cloves garlic, minced
- 3 fresh bay leaves, rinsed, central vein removed and the leaves broken up a bit
- freshly-ground pepper to taste
- 1/3 to 1/2 cups olive oil

Direction

- Pre-heat oven to 375°.
- Sprinkle chicken lightly with salt. Stuff cavity with a lemon quarter, and truss.
- Grate zest of the two oranges, and add to the bowl of a food processor. Halve the oranges crosswise, and, holding the halves over a bowl to catch any juices, remove the seeds with a longish knife or the point of a swivel peeler (they can be very stubborn). Cut the orange halves in half again to make it easier to remove the flesh from the peel. Add the flesh to the bowl of the food processor, pulling apart into smaller sections. If any juices were collected in the bowl, strain out the seeds and add juices to the food processor bowl as well.
- Juice one of the lemon halves, strain and add to the food processor bowl.
- Add next 5 ingredients, cover the food processor bowl, and pulse the motor to puree a bit. Through the feed tube and with the motor running, add the oil in a thin stream until emulsified and the paste has the consistency of sour cream. There will be flecks of green bay leaves--that's o.k.
- Set the chicken, breast side down, on a rack in a roasting pan and smear the back, thighs and legs generously with the paste. I sometimes smear some paste under the skin as well. Add about 1/2 cup of water to the bottom of the pan and roast about 20 minutes or so to color the underside.
- Flip the chicken, add more water if necessary to the bottom of the pan to keep the paste from burning, and roast until the juices run clear, about 165° on a meat thermometer. You can lift the bird with tongs, allowing some juices to drain back into the pan. If they are pinkish, roast a little longer. This may take an hour to an hour and a half or so altogether (including the initial 20 minutes), depending upon the size of your chicken. Keep an eye on the legs; they should remain plump and juicy. A shriveled, dry look or the skin separating from the end joint is a sign the chicken is getting overdone. If the bird is browning too quickly, you can reduce the heat to 350°.
- When the skin is nicely browned and the bird looks and smells done and passes all the aforementioned tests, it is done, Remove from the oven and serve.

335. The BEST Chicken Thigh Recipe You Will EVER Have!

Serving: Serves 6 | Prep: 0hours10mins | Cook: 1hours0mins | Ready in:

Ingredients

- 1 pound Chicken Thighs
- 2 tablespoons Extra Virgin Avocado Oils
- 2 teaspoons Garlic Powder
- Salt and Pepper

Direction

- Preheat oven to 400 degrees Fahrenheit and line a baking sheet with tin foil (the tin foil is optional).
- Place the chicken thighs onto the baking sheet.
- In a bowl, pour in 1 tbsp. of avocado oil and brush the chicken down.
- On the same side, season with 1 tsp garlic powder and salt and pepper for taste.
- Flip the chicken over and do the same to the other side.
- Bake in the oven for 30-minutes, flip, and cook for an additional 30-minutes.
- Remove the chicken from the oven and let rest for 5-10 minutes before serving or storing in a glass container.

336. The Crispiest Cutlets

Serving: Serves 4 | Prep: | Cook: |Ready in:

Ingredients

- 1 pound turkey, pork, or chicken cutlets, pounded to about 1/4 inch thick
- Kosher salt
- Freshly ground black pepper
- 2 cups flour
- 1-2 eggs, beaten
- 2 cups Panko breadcrumbs
- 1 cup canola or vegetable oil

Direction

- Lay meat out on a cutting board and sprinkle generously with salt and pepper on both sides.
- Dip cutlet in flour and shake off excess. Next, dip in egg mixture and let excess drip off. Lastly dip into breadcrumbs and make sure it's completely covered. Transfer back to cutting board. Repeat with remaining cutlets.
- In a large frying pan, heat oil over medium-high heat until dropping a little bit of water causes it to sizzle. Add cutlets, working in batches if needed, and fry until crispy and brown (about 3-4 minutes). Flip and repeat on other side. Add more oil if needed before next batch.
- Transfer cooked cutlets to plate with paper towel to drain out some oil. Serve immediately.

337. The Empy Nester Gourmet's Rich And Creamy Roast Turkey Gravy

Serving: Serves 8-10 | Prep: | Cook: |Ready in:

Ingredients

- Rich and Creamy Roast Turkey Gravy
- Drippings from 15 lb. - 18 lb. roast turkey
- 2 cups Chicken broth
- 3 tablespoons flour
- 1/4 cup white wine
- salt and freshly ground pepper to taste
- 3 teaspoons Gravy Master
- Hot water
- Rich and Creamy Roast Turkey Gravy
- Drippings from 15 lb. - 18 lb. roast turkey
- 2 cups chicken broth
- 3 tablespoons flour
- 1/4 cup white wine
- Salt and freshly ground pepper to taste
- 3 teaspoons Gravy Master
- Hot water

Direction

- Rich and Creamy Roast Turkey Gravy
- Drain fat from bottom of turkey roasting pan.
- Over medium heat on range top, deglaze pan with 1/4 cup wine and 2 cups chicken broth, making sure to scrape up brown bits.
- In small bowl, mix 3 tbsp. flour with hot water. Stir to dissolve flour. Add to pan drippings and broth.
- Let simmer 10 minutes over low heat, stirring continuously.
- Add Gravy Master. Stir well.
- Add salt and pepper to taste, and if desired, herbs such as bay leaf, fresh sage, fresh rosemary and fresh thyme.
- Pour through a sieve into a medium-sized saucepan, making sure not to leave any brown bits left at bottom of roasting pan, but removing herb leaves.
- Allow to simmer over low heat for another 5-10 minutes until thick and creamy, adjusting seasonings (salt and pepper) if necessary. Serve hot with roast turkey.
- Rich and Creamy Roast Turkey Gravy
- Drain fat from bottom of turkey roasting pan.
- Over medium heat on range top, deglaze pan with 1/4 cup wine and 2 cups chicken broth, making sure to scrape up brown bits.

- In small bowl, mix 3 tbsp. flour with hot water. Stir to dissolve flour. Add to pan drippings and broth.
- Let simmer 10 minutes over low heat, stirring continuously.
- Add Gravy Master. Stir well.
- Add salt and pepper to taste, and if desired, herbs such as bay leaf, fresh sage, fresh rosemary and fresh thyme.
- Pour through a sieve into a medium-sized saucepan, making sure not to leave any brown bits left at bottom of roasting pan, but removing herb leaves.
- Allow to simmer over low heat for another 5-10 minutes until thick and creamy, adjusting seasonings (salt and pepper) if necessary. Serve hot with roast turkey.

338. Tom Kha Teacups

Serving: Makes scant 5 cups | Prep: | Cook: | Ready in:

Ingredients

- 4 cups good chicken broth, preferably homemade
- 2 pieces lemongrass stalks, very roughly chopped, white and tender green parts only
- 1 piece galangal (or ginger), 2 inches in size, very roughly chopped
- 1 ounce shrimp shells (optional, but highly recommended)
- 1/2 cup coconut milk
- 1/4 cup fish sauce
- 1 tablespoon palm sugar simple syrup
- 8 kaffir lime leaves
- 1/4 cup cilantro leaves, roughly chopped and packed
- 2 thai chiles, stems removed, roughly chopped

Direction

- In a saucepan on high heat, add the chicken broth, lemongrass, galangal, shrimp shells (if you're using them), coconut milk, fish sauce, and palm sugar simple syrup. Bring to a boil, then bring the heat down to low and cover. Simmer for 15 minutes.
- Remove the lid and turn the heat off. Add the lime leaves, cilantro, and Thai chiles, then put the cover back on. Let stand for 4 minutes.
- Strain the broth and discard all the aromatics. Serve in teacups, bowls, or just leave it in the sauce pan and use a bendy straw.

339. Tomatillo Chicken Soup

Serving: Makes makes 1 big pot (6-8 servings) | Prep: | Cook: | Ready in:

Ingredients

- for the soup:
- 1 1/2 pounds boneless skinless chicken breasts (cubed)
- 10 - 12 tomatillos (paper removed and rinsed)
- 1 yellow onion (diced)
- 7 cloves garlic (sliced)
- 1 poblano
- 1 can mild or hot green chilies
- 3 teaspoons cumin
- 3 teaspoons oregano (dried)
- 3 teaspoons green chili powder
- 1 1/2 teaspoons ground coriander
- 1 lime (juice)
- 6 cups low sodium chicken broth
- salt and pepper
- olive oil
- for the toppings:
- fresh cilantro
- queso fresco
- non fat Greek yogurt
- red onion (diced)
- red cabbage (shaved on mandolin)
- lime slices
- avocado cubes

Direction

- You're going to multitask to begin. Get three things going around the same time. Turn on your broiler. Place tomatillos on foil lined baking sheet and pop under the broiler. Let one side char for about 4 minutes, then flip over and let the other side char for another 4. Remove from broiler and set to rest.
- As tomatillos char, char the poblano on a gas burner or pop into the over under the broiler with the tomatillos. Let all sides char. Let cool once charred, then remove stem and most seeds before dicing up.
- As tomatillos and poblano char, heat a soup pot or Dutch oven over medium high heat and add olive oil. Drop in chicken breast cubes and add 1 tsp cumin, oregano, green chili powder and 1/2 tsp coriander. Add some salt and pepper as well. Let cook for about 7 minutes until browned a bit. It may not be entirely cooked through, but that's okay. Remove to a plate.
- Lower heat to medium and add a bit more olive oil. Add onion and garlic, with 1 tsp cumin, oregano, green chili powder and 1/2 tsp coriander. Let cook for 5 minutes. Add in diced poblano and can of chilies. Let cook for another 3 minutes.
- Add the whole charred tomatillos with their skin and all juices. Crush a little bit with your cooking utensil and mix everything to combine. Add salt and pepper. Add the juice of 1 whole lime.
- Add all chicken broth with remaining cumin, oregano, chili powder and coriander. Add an extra dash of salt. Bring to a boil. Once boiling lower heat, cover and let simmer for 30 minutes.
- After 30 minutes, puree with an immersion blender until mostly smooth. Add chicken back in and let simmer for 45 minutes over low heat, until chicken is super tender.
- Serve in a bowl with lots of fresh cilantro, cabbage, Greek yogurt, onions, lime juice, avocados and queso fresco. Feel free to leave anything out, or add anything else that sounds yummy.

340. Turkey Andouille Chili

Serving: Serves 8-10 | Prep: | Cook: | Ready in:

Ingredients

- 2 tablespoons peanut, canola, or vegetable oil, divided
- 1 pound andouille sausages (4 links), chopped
- 1 medium yellow onion, diced
- 1 medium carrot, diced
- Salt to taste
- 2 jalapeno peppers OR 1 serrano pepper, seeded and minced
- 1 poblano (pasilla) pepper, seeded and diced
- 4-6 garlic cloves, minced
- 2 teaspoons ground cumin
- 2 teaspoons chili powder
- 1 teaspoon paprika (regular or smoked)
- 1/4 teaspoon ground cinnamon
- 1 pound ground turkey (preferably dark meat)
- 2 (14 oz) cans fire-roasted diced tomatoes
- 2 (14 oz) cans low-sodium black beans
- 1 (14 oz) can low-sodium pinto beans
- 1 (14 oz) can low-sodium red kidney beans
- Shredded cheddar or pepper jack cheese for serving (optional)

Direction

- Heat 1 tbsp. oil in your largest stockpot or Dutch oven over medium heat. Add sausage and cook, stirring occasionally, for about 5 minutes, or until the sausage starts to brown. Add onion, carrot, and a pinch of salt, and cook, stirring frequently, for another 6-7 minutes, or until the onion is translucent. Add peppers, garlic, cumin, chili powder, paprika, and cinnamon, and cook, stirring frequently, for 1-2 minutes, or until the whole mixture is fragrant.
- Add remaining 1 tbsp. oil and ground turkey. Cook, breaking up the meat with your spoon or spatula, until the last traces of pink are gone.

- Add tomatoes and beans, along with their liquid. Increase the heat to medium-high and bring to a boil, then reduce the heat to keep the liquid at a steady simmer. Simmer, uncovered, for 1 to 1 1/2 hours, or until the chili has coalesced and thickened to your liking. Taste and season with salt, if desired.
- Serve the chili warm, topped with cheese (if desired). Leftovers will keep, tightly covered, in the refrigerator for up to 3 days, or in the freezer for up to 4 months.

341. Turkey Curry Meatballs

Serving: Makes 2 dozen | Prep: | Cook: | Ready in:

Ingredients

- 1.3 pounds ground turkey
- 2.5 teaspoons curry powder (I used Penzey's Singapore Seasoning)
- 1 large egg
- 3 tablespoons panko
- 1 inch hunk of ginger minced
- 1 green onion sliced in half lengthwise and chopped
- 1 shallot, chopped fine
- juice of 1/2 a lime
- 1/2 a red jalapeno seed removed, minced
- 1 tablespoon parsley, chopped
- vegetable oil

Direction

- Heat 2 tablespoons of oil in a pan over a medium-low heat, add the shallot and ginger and sauté for 2 minutes. Add in the onion and the pepper and continue to cook for about 5 more minutes. The purpose is to get everything soft but not crispy. Remove from the heat.
- Meanwhile mix together the egg, turkey, curry powder, panko and lime juice. When the onions, pepper and ginger have cooled add them to the mixture and make 1" meat balls.
- Wipe out the pan and add another 2 tablespoons of vegetable oil over a medium-high heat. Working in batches (about 3 so you don't over crowd the pan) cook the meat balls until they are cooked through, about 7 minutes.

342. Turkey Lentil Chili

Serving: Serves 8 to 10 | Prep: | Cook: | Ready in:

Ingredients

- 1 pound ground turkey
- 1 medium onion, chopped
- 2-3 garlic cloves, finely minced
- 5 to 6 cups chicken stock
- 2 cups brown lentils, picked through, rinsed
- 1 (15 oz) can tomato sauce
- 1 (14.5 oz) can diced cut tomatotes
- 1 tablespoon chili powder
- 1 teaspoon ground cumin
- 2 to 3 teaspoons epazote
- 1 teaspoon crushed red pepper flakes
- salt and pepper to taste
- green onion, sliced
- cheddar cheese, grated

Direction

- In a heavy stock pot, saute the onion and garlic until onion is transparent. Crumble in the ground turkey and cook until turkey is cooked through, stirring frequently.
- Add from broth through epazote, stir to blend, bring to a boil; reduce heat, cover and cook on medium heat for 30 to 40 minutes or until lentils are tender. At end of the cooking time, season with salt, pepper and red pepper flakes.
- Garnish each serving with sliced green onions and grated cheddar cheese, if desired.

343. Turkey Soup

Serving: Serves 6-8 | Prep: | Cook: | Ready in:

Ingredients

- White Beans
- 2 cups dried white beans
- 2 teaspoons baking soda
- cold water
- 3 thyme sprigs
- 1/2 cup onion, finely chopped
- 1 garlic clove, finely chopped
- 1 smoked turkey wing
- Turkey Soup
- 1 medium onion, diced
- 2 garlic cloves, chopped
- 2 teaspoons cumin, ground
- 3 tablespoons grapeseed oil
- 6 cups turkey stock
- 4 cups cooked turkey, chopped
- 3 cups cooked white beans
- 1/3 cup cilantro stems, finely chopped
- 1 chipotle pepper, dried
- 2 roasted poblano peppers, chopped
- 2 chilaca chile peppers, chopped
- jalapeno salt

Direction

- To prep white beans, spread them on a large sheet tray and remove any debris.
- Transfer beans to a large, heavy pot and cover with about 3 inches of cold water. Sprinkle with baking soda.
- Drain and rinse beans and return beans to pot. Add thyme, garlic onions and smoked turkey. Add water until beans are completely submersed. Place over high heat and allow to boil. Using a skimmer, remove any foam and reduce the heat to medium-high. Cover with a lid and cook 30 minutes. Add salt to taste and cook an additional 30 minutes or until beans are tender. Transfer beans to another dish and set aside.
- Using the same pot over medium heat, add oil and onions. Allow to cook until slightly soft, about 3 minutes. Add the garlic, cumin and peppers. Cook about 2 minutes, stirring occasionally.
- Stir in the turkey stock, turkey and cilantro stems and cover with a lid. Bring to a boil and reduce the heat to medium low. Allow to simmer 10 to 12 minutes, stirring halfway through the cooking process.
- Ladle into bowls and enjoy with slices of crusty bread and a glass of white wine.

344. Turkey Veggie Meatballs With Spaghetti Squash

Serving: Serves 4 | Prep: | Cook: | Ready in:

Ingredients

- 1 pound lean ground turkey breast
- 1 spaghetti squash
- 2 14 oz cans fire roasted crushed tomatoes
- 1/2 cup fresh parsley
- 1 tablespoon extra virgin olive oil
- 1 1/4 teaspoons tsp italian seasoning
- 1/2 teaspoon garlilc
- 1/2 teaspoon crushed red chili pepper
- 2 zucchini, peeled & shredded
- 1/2 yellow onion, finley chopped
- 1 cup carrots, shredded (about 2 medium carrots)
- Top with grated parmesan cheese

Direction

- Preheat oven to 425 F degrees
- Cut spaghetti squash in half, remove seeds, then cover with tin foil & bake 40 minutes
- Meanwhile roughly shred carrots, onion, zucchini, garlic & half olive oil in a food processor
- In a medium mixing bowl, add turkey, shredded vegetables and spices
- Form into 12 meatballs
- Heat a large skillet to medium & add other half extra virgin olive oil

- Add meatballs to skillet & cook 10 minutes then flip and cook another 5 minutes
- Reduce heat to low
- Add diced tomatoes to skillet & simmer 5 minutes
- Meanwhile remove spaghetti squash from skins using a fork
- Add parsley & spaghetti squash to skillet & coat with sauce
- Serve immediately & sprinkle with parmesan

345. Turkey Green Curry

Serving: Serves 2 | Prep: | Cook: | Ready in:

Ingredients

- half white onion chopped
- 3 minced garlic cloves
- four slices of ginger

Direction

- Sauté onions, garlic, ginger, till soften. Put in the coconut milk and a splash of chicken stock. Then mix in the chile, soy sauce, rice vinegar, sugar and curry paste. Let simmer for couple of minutes.
- Put the coconut milk mixture in the blender and blend with salt, basil and mint till smooth.
- Put the sauce back into the pan and simmer then cook the ground turkey in another pan with oil till brown. After it gets brown throw it into the sauce for 10 minutes till it is cooked. Serve with rice or noodles and enjoy.

346. Turkey Meatloaf

Serving: Serves 8 | Prep: | Cook: | Ready in:

Ingredients

- 2 pounds ground turkey
- 10 ounces fronzen spinach
- 1/2 packet fairway mozarella
- 1/2 packet mushrooms
- 1 small yellow onion
- 1/2 cup seasoned breadcrumbs
- 2 teaspoons chopped garlic
- 3 tablespoons worcestershire sauce
- 2 eggs
- 1.25 cups pasta sauce
- salt
- pepper

Direction

- Pre-heat oven to 400FChop onions and mushrooms in food processor and cook with garlic
- After cooked, let cool and pour 2 tbsp. of Worcestershire sauce
- In a bowl, mix turkey, eggs, 3/4 cup of pasta sauce, bread crumbs and 1 tbsp. of Worcestershire and salt and pepper to taste
- To meat mix, add mushrooms and onion mix.
- In a foil meatloaf pan, add half of the turkey mixture. Press a 1 inch indentation, mounding in center, spoon mozzarella and spinach in and add remaining turkey mixture
- Spread remaining pasta sauce evenly on top.
- Cook in pre-heated 400 F oven for 45 and make sure meatloaf registers 170F, let stand 5 min before slicing.

347. Turkey Pot Pie With A Crispy Parmesan Crust

Serving: Serves 8 | Prep: | Cook: | Ready in:

Ingredients

- 2 tablespoons canola oil
- 1/2 cup celery, diced
- 1/2 cup carrots, diced
- 1/2 cup onion, diced
- 1/2 cup parsnips, peeled and diced

- 1 cup button mushrooms, sliced
- 1/4 cup flour
- 2 1/2 cups Turkey or chicken stock (homemade is best, but whatever you have is great)
- 2 teaspoons poultry seasoning or powdered turkey gravy mix
- 2 cups turkey, cooked and shredded
- 1 cup frozen peas, thawed
- 1 cup frozen green beans, thawed
- 1/4 cup half and half
- Salt and pepper to taste
- 6 sheets of phyllo dough
- 1/4 cup Parmesan cheese, finely grated

Direction

- Spray a 2 ½ quart casserole dish with cooking spray and set aside. Preheat oven to 350 degrees F. Heat the oil in a large skillet over medium heat. When the oil is hot, but not smoking, add in the celery, parsnips, carrots, onion and mushrooms. Cook for 5 minutes or until the onion mixture is soft, but not brown.
- Sprinkle the flour over the onion mixture and stir until the oil and flour become a paste. Cook for 2 minutes more to remove the raw flour taste. Slowly stir in the stock and bring to a boil. Add in the poultry seasoning/turkey gravy powder. Reduce the heat to medium and cook for about 5 minutes more or until the mixture is thickened. Add in the turkey, peas and green beans as well as the half and half and cook for 5 more minutes. Remove from heat and taste, adding salt and pepper to your liking. Pour into the prepared casserole and let cool for a few minutes.
- Lay one sheet of phyllo on top of the casserole and spray with cooking spray. Repeat with two more sheets of phyllo. Sprinkle ½ of the Parmesan over the casserole and then top with the remaining sheets of phyllo (again, sprayed between each sheet). Sprinkle the remaining Parmesan on top and tuck the edges of the phyllo loosely into the sides of the casserole. Cut a few vents in the phyllo with a sharp knife to let steam escape.
- Bake for 35 to 40 minutes or until the top is golden brown and the filling is bubbling up through the vents you cut into the crust. (Hint: Place a sheet of foil over the top if the phyllo and Parmesan topping appear to be getting brown too fast).
- Let cool for 10 minutes.

348. Turkey, Lentil, And Mixed Brown Rice Soup

Serving: Serves 6 | Prep: | Cook: | Ready in:

Ingredients

- 1 1/2 tablespoons unsalted butter
- 1/2 cup chopped onions
- 1/2 cup chopped carrots
- 1/2 cup chopped celery
- 1 clove peeled garlic, minced
- 4 cups low-sodium turkey stock, preferably homemade (can sub chicken stock)
- 1 bay leaf
- 2 teaspoons sprigs fresh thyme or 1/2 teaspoon dried
- 1/2 cup dried green lentils
- 1 1/2 cups chopped cooked turkey (can sub cooked chicken)
- 1 1/2 cups cooked mixed brown rice (or any cooked rice of choosing)
- 2 teaspoons dried parsley (or a handful of chopped fresh, if you have it on hand)
- 2 teaspoons balsamic vinegar
- Ground pepper and Mrs. Dash or salt, to taste

Direction

- In a Dutch oven or soup pot, melt the butter over medium high heat. Add the onions, carrots, and celery and cook until the vegetables are starting to soften, about 7 to 10 minutes. Add the garlic and cook a minute more.

- Next add in the turkey (or chicken) stock, bay leaf, thyme, and lentils. Cover and bring to a boil.
- Once boiling, reduce heat to low and simmer with cover on for 45 minutes.
- Uncover and stir in turkey and cooked rice, and continue simmering until lentils are tender, about 15 more minutes. Remove the bay leaf and thyme sprigs, then add the parsley and balsamic vinegar. Taste test, then add ground pepper and Mrs. Dash or salt, to taste. Serve with crusty bread.

349. Turmeric Yogurt Grilled Chicken

Serving: Serves 6 | Prep: 0hours3mins | Cook: 0hours12mins | Ready in:

Ingredients

- 1 1/4 cups plain whole-milk yogurt
- 1 tablespoon ground turmeric
- 1 teaspoon ground cumin
- 2 teaspoons Morton's kosher salt, divided (or 3 1/2 teaspoons Diamond Crystal, divided)
- 1 teaspoon light brown sugar
- 1 tablespoon lemon juice, or to taste
- 2 tablespoons olive oil
- 2 1/2 to 3 pounds boneless, skinless chicken thighs
- 1/2 cup chopped cilantro leaves with tender stems + lemon wedges (optional)

Direction

- In a small bowl, stir together the yogurt, turmeric, cumin, 1 teaspoon kosher salt, brown sugar, lemon juice, and olive oil into well integrated. Taste and adjust seasoning and acidity.
- In a bowl or plastic zipper-lock bag, combine chicken with 1/2 cup yogurt sauce and the remaining 1 teaspoon kosher salt, turning to evenly coat (reserve the rest of the yogurt sauce for serving). Cover and refrigerate for at least 30 minutes, or up to 24 hours.
- Heat grill to medium-high. Brush your grates clean, then brush with oil. Grill chicken until golden brown and cooked through, about 5 to 6 minutes per side, or until 165 degrees F in the thickest part. Top with cilantro and serve yogurt sauce and lemon wedges on the side (if using).

350. Ultimate Chicken Tikka Masala

Serving: Serves 8 | Prep: 9hours0mins | Cook: 1hours15mins | Ready in:

Ingredients

- Tikka Marinade
- 1 cup plain Greek or whole milk yogurt
- 1 tablespoon fresh lemon juice
- 2 teaspoons ground cumin
- 2 teaspoons garam masala
- 2 teaspoons cayenne
- 3 grinds of fresh black pepper
- 1 teaspoon salt or to taste
- 8 whole cloves
- 1 tablespoon ginger minced
- 2 cloves of garlic minced
- 3 boneless, skinless chicken breasts cut in 1.5 inch cubes
- Sauce
- 3 tablespoons sunflower oil
- 1 large onion cut into thin half wheels
- 2 cloves of garlic finely minced
- 2 serrano chilies roasted, seeded, and diced (optional)
- 1 tablespoon ground cumin
- 2 teaspoons paprika
- 1 tablespoon garam masala
- 2 pinches Salt and fresh black pepper to taste
- 1 28-ounce can San Marzano whole peeled plum tomatoes, roughly chopped
- 1 cup heavy cream

- 4 sprigs Fresh cilantro for garnish

Direction

- Mix all of the marinade ingredients in a large mixing bowl.
- Fold in the chicken, cover, and refrigerate overnight.
- Heat the oil in a large casserole.
- When the oil is hot, turn the stove to medium and add the onion. Brown the onions until they are caramelized. This takes about 20 minutes of constant stirring, and you might get lazy and want to shortchange this step. Resist the temptation and do it properly. This is the most important step for bringing rich flavor to your sauce. Also, if you want a little more onion in the dish try adding a second smaller onion and cut it into larger wedges. This adds some nice textual variation to the dish.
- Next, add the garlic and chilies, and sauté for 1 to 2 minutes.
- Now add the cumin, paprika, and garam masala. Fry these spices with the onions for a minute to release their flavor. Add salt and pepper directly prior to adding tomatoes. This helps draw the flavor of the onions, spices, and tomatoes together.
- Next, add the chopped tomatoes and mix well. It is alright to add the juice contained within the tomatoes themselves, however, be very conservative with the remaining juice in the can. You may find you want to add a little for volume, and that's fine, however, if you add too much your sauce will be very watery.
- After the tomatoes have cooked with the spices for a few minutes add the heavy cream, thoroughly mix, and bring to a simmer. Stir occasionally.
- While the sauce is simmering, take the chicken out of the refrigerator, and place on wooden skewers.
- If you feel like making the effort you can grill the chicken outside on a charcoal grill (using real wood charcoal). This is the best way. However, it adds a decent amount of time, and if you're cooking more than one dish, it can be a huge pain running in and out of the house. The other option is a stove top grill iron. Lightly coat the iron with oil, and once it is hot enough, cook the chicken skewers.
- Once the chicken is fully cooked, take it off of the grill and put it to the side to cool for 8 to 10 minutes. This seals in the flavor and ensures the tenderness of the meat.
- By now the sauce should have thickened nicely. Remove the chicken from the skewers and fold it into the sauce. Raise the heat slightly and stir for 2 to 3 minutes.
- Remove from heat, and serve over basmati rice. Garnish with some fresh cilantro. See my recipes for spicy creamy peas and vegetable korma, they make excellent side dishes.

351. Vanilla Carrot Broth

Serving: Makes 2 quarts | Prep: | Cook: | Ready in:

Ingredients

- 2 quarts Carrot Juice
- half cup Finely chopped onion
- 1 cup Chicken (or Vegetable Stock)
- 1 tablespoon Sherry Vinegar
- 2 Vanilla Beans, halved and scrapped
- 2 thyme sprigs
- 2 whole bay leaf
- quarter teaspoons smoked paprika
- 1 teaspoon whole peppercorn

Direction

- Heat chicken (or vegetable stock) to 190-200 degrees (just before boiling) and place the halved and scrapped vanilla bean seeds in the stock and allow to steep covered for 20 minutes.
- In a small amount of oil (approximately 1 TBS) cook the onions over medium heat until they start to become aromatic and translucent. Dust the onions with the paprika and stir for

approximately 30 seconds. Add the peppercorns, bay leaves, thyme sprigs. Stir a few times and add the sherry vinegar.
- Allow the vinegar to reduce quickly. Add the vanilla infused chicken (or vegetable stock) and bring the mixture to a boil.
- Add the carrot juice and remove from heat. Cover and sit undisturbed for 20 minutes. Strain through a fine-mesh strainer, cool and reserve for later use.

352. Vietnamese Classic Chicken Salad

Serving: Serves 2 | Prep: | Cook: | Ready in:

Ingredients

- For the salad
- 1/2 a medium-size onion, any color will do
- 1/2 a small cabbage, preferably savoy
- 1/2 pound chicken
- 2 tablespoons sugar
- 2 tablespoons white vinegar
- 3-5 sprigs Vietnamese coriander if available; otherwise regular cilantro will do
- 1/2 cup roasted, unsalted peanuts
- For the dressing
- 3 tablespoons sugar
- 3 tablespoons lime juice
- 1 1/2 tablespoons fish sauce
- 1 tablespoon minced garlic
- 1 tablespoon chopped chili peper (optional)

Direction

- Prepare a big bowl of ice cold water. Thinly slice the onion, place it in that bowl, and leave for 15 minutes to get rid of the sharpness of the onion, or else you'll be crying eating the salad ^^
- Strain the onion, place it in a bowl, add sugar and vinegar, then stir it all together and let it sit for at least 30 minutes.
- Place chicken in a pot, add enough cold water to cover the chicken completely, then bring to a boil. Turn off heat and leave chicken in the pot for 15 minutes. After that transfer chicken onto a plate, let it cool down, then separate chicken from the bone by hand and tear it into pieces. If you preferred grilled chicken, you can use that instead.
- Thinly slice the cabbage; chop the cilantro
- Squeeze the marinated onion with bare hands or cheese cloth
- In a small bowl, stir all the dressing ingredients together.
- In a salad bowl, place chicken, cabbage, onion, coriander, then toss the salad and add peanuts on top.

353. Vietnamese Sticky Wings

Serving: Serves 2 | Prep: | Cook: | Ready in:

Ingredients

- 2 pounds chicken wings
- 1/2 cup warm water
- 1/2 cup fish sauce (Phu Quoc brand)
- 1/2 cup sugar
- 1/2 teaspoon freshly ground pepper
- 6 cloves of garlic, minced
- 1/2 cup rice flour
- 1/4 cup cornstarch
- 2 teaspoons baking soda
- 1 quart vegetable for frying
- 1 lime for garnish
- 1 green chile pepper

Direction

- For the marinade, combine water, fish sauce, and sugar in a large bowl and whisk until sugar is completely dissolved. Add minced garlic.
- Add the wings and toss to coat. Cover and refrigerate overnight (at least 8 hours for the

- most flavor). Turn them every 4 hours to make sure the wings are marinated evenly.
- Drain the wings by leaving them in a colander for 10 minutes.
- Sift rice flour, cornstarch, and baking soda in a mixing bowl.
- In a large pot over medium heat, fill the pot to about 2 inches of oil and bring it to 350 degrees F (if you don't have a thermometer, leave it on medium heat).
- Toss the wings, a few at a time, in flour then shake off excess flour.
- Fry the floured wings for about 8-10 minutes, 4 minutes on each side (8 minutes for smaller wings and 10 minutes for larger wings) until golden brown.
- Transfer them to a tray lined with paper towel to drain off excess oil.
- Drain the garlic pieces from the marinade and deep fry them until golden brown. Reserve for later.
- In a saucepan, simmer the marinade over medium-high heat until it becomes syrupy and dark golden in color, about 10-12 minutes.
- Toss the wings in the reduced sauce. (If you don't want your wings too sticky, use a brush and glaze them as much or as little as you like.)
- Place the wings in a serving dish, sprinkle fried garlic on top, and then add lime wedges and green chiles.

354. West African Chicken Peanut Stew

Serving: Serves 4 | Prep: | Cook: | Ready in:

Ingredients

- 8 chicken thighs
- 1 teaspoon ground coriander (cilantro)
- salt to taste
- ground black pepper to taste
- 2 red bell peppers
- 1/4 scotch bonnet chillies
- 2 1/2 tablespoons vegetable oil
- 2 bay leaves
- 1 jumbo cube (optional, see notes)
- 8 tablespoons smooth peanut butter
- 3 tablespoons tomato puree
- 4 1/4 cups water (1 litre)

Direction

- Season the chicken pieces with coriander, salt and pepper and set aside.
- Peel and slice the onions and garlic.
- Deseed and chop peppers and scotch bonnet chilies.
- Heat 1.5 tbsp. of oil in a nonstick frying pot and quickly brown chicken pieces. You might have to do this in two or more batches as you don't want to crowd the pieces in the pot. Remove pieces from the pan and set aside on a plate.
- Heat the remaining oil in the pot and throw in the onions, garlic, scotch bonnet, bay leaves and 6 tbsp. of water and stir very well. Fry for about 5 minutes until the mixture very fragrant. (Take note of this fragrance as this is what I call the real salone food smell).
- Throw in the red pepper, stir it and fry the mixture covered for another 5 minutes. Then add in the peanut butter, tomato puree, jumbo cube and stir fry quickly for 30 seconds until these are both mixed in.
- Add in the browned chicken pieces and the water, bring to the boil, reduce and simmer for about 50 minutes. Stir the mix a couple of times during the 50 minutes as the peanut butter could settle at the bottom of the pot.
- Taste stew and adjust salt and pepper and then turn off.
- Serve with rice (plantains or bread) and garnish with nuts, herbs and spring onions.
- Notes -The peanut stew foams up during boiling, so you need to reduce it to a simmer as soon as it starts to boils. Jumbo cube (or maggi cube) is a stock cube used to flavor food in Sierra Leone. It can be bought in a lot of shops selling ethnic food. If you don't want to

use a jumbo cube then omit it and replace the water with some stock.

355. White Chicken Chili

Serving: Makes 10 generous bowls | Prep: | Cook: | Ready in:

Ingredients

- Chili
- 3 cooked chicken breasts (or the meat from a rotisserie chicken), cut into bite-size chunks
- 15 ounces can pinto beans, drained
- 15 ounces can cannelini beans, drained
- 7 ounces salsa verde (I use Herdez)
- 8 ounces can diced green chiles
- 4 cups quality chicken stock
- 2/3 cup heavy cream
- 1 small yellow onion, chopped
- 2 cloves garlic, minced
- 1 tablespoon olive oil
- 2 teaspoons ground cumin
- 1 teaspoon ground coriander
- 1 teaspoon dried oregano
- 1 teaspoon chili powder
- 1/2 teaspoon smoked paprika
- 1/8-1/4 teaspoons ground cayenne (to taste)
- 1/2 teaspoon freshly ground black pepper
- 2 teaspoons kosher or coarse sea salt
- Toppings
- 2 ripe avocados
- 1/2 fresh lime
- 1 teaspoon olive oil
- 1/2 teaspoon kosher or coarse sea salt
- 8 ounces sour cream
- 8 ounces shredded sharp cheddar cheese
- 1/2 bunch cilantro, coarsely chopped
- few handfuls tortilla chips (I love sweet potato tortilla chips with this)

Direction

- In large stockpot, sauté onion in oil over medium heat 3-4 minutes. Add garlic and cook one minute more, then add beans, salsa, and green chiles and stir well. Add chicken stock, cream, and all seasonings and bring to simmer. Simmer lightly for 10-15 minutes to allow flavors to come together. Add cooked chicken, stir, and simmer just till heated through. Taste once more for seasoning and add salt and pepper as desired.
- While chili is simmering, remove pit and peel from avocados and roughly chop the flesh. Place in small bowl with the juice of the half a lime, olive oil, and salt. Mix well and set aside, then prepare other toppings as needed. Serve hot bowls of chili with mix-ins as desired.
- Note: this chili finishes with a thin consistency more like chicken soup than a traditional red beef chili. The melted cheese and sour cream provide some additional texture, and that's plenty for me. However, if you prefer a thicker chili, there's an easy fix. At the start of the recipe, add an extra can of cannellini beans. Once you've added stock, cream, and seasonings, but before adding chicken, use an immersion blender to puree the beans and create a richer consistency. Continue recipe as above.

356. Whole Slow Cooker Poached Chicken

Serving: Serves 4 | Prep: 0hours15mins | Cook: 4hours0mins | Ready in:

Ingredients

- 3 bunches scallions
- 1 bunch cilantro, stems and leaves
- 1 whole chicken (about 4 pounds)
- 2 celery stalks, chopped into 2-inch pieces
- 12 shiitake mushrooms, stemmed
- 6 thin slices of ginger
- 6 star anise
- 1 teaspoon peppercorns (white, if possible)
- 1 tablespoon plus two teaspoons coarse salt

- 8 cups water

Direction

- In a 5- to 6-quart slow cooker—a smaller slow cooker will be too small—place two bunches of scallions and half the cilantro on the bottom. Then place the chicken on top, breast up. Add the celery, mushrooms, ginger, star anise, peppercorns, and salt. Then add the water, adding more if the chicken isn't covered (or almost covered). Cook on high for 2 to 3 hours (or on low for 4 or more hours), or until the chicken reaches 165 degrees.
- When the chicken is cooked, carve it into portions and divide it among the bowls. Divide the mushrooms among the bowls, too. Strain the broth and ladle it over the chicken and the mushrooms. Coarsely chop the remaining cilantro and scallions and sprinkle them over each bowl. Serve.

357. Wild Gochujang Wings

Serving: Makes 10 wings | Prep: | Cook: |Ready in:

Ingredients

- 10 chicken wings
- 1 dash salt & pepper to taste
- 1 tablespoon cooking or vegetable oil
- 5 tablespoons Bibigo's Gochujang hot sauce

Direction

- After prepping the chicken wings, season them wings salt and pepper.
- Heat the oil in a large pan or skillet to 375 degrees F. Fry the chicken wings in oil for about 10 minutes or until done. Remove chicken and drain on paper towels.
- After draining, toss the cooked chicken wings with Gochujang sauce - add as much or as little as you would like!

358. Wild Rice, Chicken And Almond Soup

Serving: Serves 4 to 6 | Prep: | Cook: |Ready in:

Ingredients

- 1 pound boneless, skinless chicken breast, cut into large strips (or chicken tenders)
- salt and pepper to taste
- 1 tablespoon poultry seasoning blend
- 2 teaspoons olive oil
- 1 medium onion, chopped
- 3 large carrots, peeled and diced
- 1/2 red bell pepper, diced
- 1 large clove garlic, minced
- 3 tablespoons butter, divided
- 3 tablespoons flour, divided
- 5-6 cups chicken stock
- 2 cups cooked wild rice
- 1 1/2 cups whole milk
- 1 cup grated sharp cheddar
- 1/2 cup slivered almonds

Direction

- Season the chicken pieces well with salt, pepper and poultry seasoning. Sauté in a stockpot with the oil over medium-high heat until they're well browned and just cooked through, about 4 minutes per side. Remove the chicken and set aside.
- Add 2 tbs. of the butter to the pan. Add the onion, carrot, bell pepper, and garlic; sauté for 5 to 7 minutes until the veggies are softened.
- Add 2 tbs. of the flour and stir until incorporated; cook for 2 minutes. Stir in 5 cups of the stock. Add the wild rice and simmer for 15 minutes or so.
- Meanwhile, melt the remaining 1 tbs. butter in a saucepan over medium heat. Stir in the remaining tbs. flour and cook for 2 minutes. While the flour cooks, heat the milk in the microwave until it's warm, about 1 minute. Whisk the warm milk into the flour-butter

roux and cook until it's smooth and thickened. Whisk in the cheddar until it's melted into the milk. Stir the cheesy sauce into the soup and heat through.
- Shred the cooked chicken and add along with the almonds just before serving. Add extra chicken stock if the soup is too thick. This soup freezes very well.

359. Yellow Mole With Chicken And Masa Dumplings

Serving: Serves 6-8 | Prep: | Cook: | Ready in:

Ingredients

- Yellow Mole with Chicken
- 2 ancho chiles, rinsed, stemmed, and seeded
- 2 guajillo chiles, rinsed, stemmed, and seeded
- 1 pound pound tomatillos (6–8), husks removed, rinsed
- 1 medium ripe tomato
- 4 garlic cloves
- 2 whole cloves
- 1 teaspoon ground cinnamon
- 1 teaspoon dried oregano, preferably Mexican
- 2 teaspoons kosher or coarse sea salt
- 1/4 teaspoon freshly ground black pepper
- 3 tablespoons vegetable oil
- 1/4 cup chopped white onion
- 5 cups chicken or vegetable broth, homemade or canned
- 3 medium fresh hoja santa leaves or 5 dried, or 2 cilantro sprigs (optional)
- 3 tablespoons vegetable oil
- 8 chicken breasts, thighs, or drumsticks, or a combination
- Kosher or coarse sea salt and freshly ground black pepper
- Masa Dumplings (recipe follows)
- Masa Dumplings
- 1 cup instant corn masa flour, such as Maseca
- 3/4 cup lukewarm water
- 1 1/2 tablespoons lard or vegetable shortening
- 1/4 teaspoon ground cinnamon
- 1 teaspoon kosher or coarse sea salt, or to taste
- 1/2 teaspoon sugar

Direction

- Yellow Mole with Chicken
- TO MAKE THE SAUCE: Heat a comal or large skillet over medium heat until hot. Lay the chiles flat in the pan and toast them for 10 to 15 seconds per side until they become fragrant and pliable and their color darkens. Take care not to let them burn, or they will turn bitter. Remove from the heat.
- In a medium saucepan, combine the toasted chiles with the tomatillos, tomato, and garlic. Add water to cover and bring to a boil, then reduce the heat to a medium simmer and cook for 10 minutes, or until the tomatillos and tomato are soft. Remove from the heat.
- With a slotted spoon, transfer the chiles, tomatillos, tomato, and garlic to a blender or food processor and let cool slightly. Add the cloves, cinnamon, oregano, salt, and pepper and puree until smooth.
- In a large pot, heat the oil over medium-high heat. Add the onion and sauté for 3 to 4 minutes, until soft and translucent. Add the tomatillo puree and cook until it thickens, about 10 minutes, stirring often.
- Add the chicken broth and hoja santa leaves, if using. Bring to a simmer over medium heat and cook for about 15 minutes. Remove from the heat.
- Meanwhile, make the masa for the dumplings.
- In a deep skillet or Dutch oven, heat the 3 tablespoons oil over medium-high heat until hot but not smoking. Sprinkle the chicken pieces with salt and pepper to taste. Working in batches, add the chicken to the pan skin side down and brown on each side for 4 to 5 minutes.
- Return all the chicken to the pan, pour the mole sauce on top, and bring to a simmer. Reduce the heat to medium-low. Make the

dumplings as directed below. One by one, add them to the mole and cook for another 15 minutes, or until the dumplings are cooked through and the mole has thickened enough to coat the back of a wooden spoon. Serve.
- Masa Dumplings
- In a large bowl, mix the masa flour with the water, then knead for about 1 minute, until the dough is smooth and free of lumps. Add the lard, cinnamon, salt, and sugar and mix for another minute, until well incorporated and smooth.
- Roll the dough into 1-inch balls, then, with your little finger, make a dimple in the middle of each dumpling.
- Keep covered until ready to cook.

360. A Simple Chicken & Rice Noodle Bowl.

Serving: Serves 4 | Prep: | Cook: | Ready in:

Ingredients

- 2 chicken breasts, skin-on & bone-in
- 4 cups water
- 1 teaspoon sea salt
- 14 ounces thin rice noodles
- 1 lime, cut into wedges
- 4 scallion, chopped
- 4 tablespoons fish sauce
- 1-2 chilis or jalapenos, chopped (optional)

Direction

- In a stock pot, add chicken, water & salt. Bring to a boil & then simmer for 45 minutes. Take the chicken out & leave the broth on low heat to stay warm. Let the chicken cool on a cutting board for about 10 minutes, then shred the meat off.
- To cook the rice noodles, follow the directions on the package. Then drain & rinse with cold water.
- Add the noodles to the bottom of the bowl, then chicken, scallions & chili. Ladle the broth over the noodles. Then 1 TBL of fish sauce for each bowl, a squeeze of lime & a bit of cracked pepper.

361. Asian Chicken Salad

Serving: Serves 6 | Prep: | Cook: | Ready in:

Ingredients

- for the dressings:
- 5 tablespoons grape seed oil, divided
- 2 large clove garlic, minced, divided
- 2 teaspoons ginger juice (instructions below) from 1 knob of ginger about 2 1/2" long
- zest and juice of one lime
- 1 tablespoon honey
- 1 tablespoon rice wine vinegar
- 1 teaspoon wasabi powder or several dashes of hot sauce (to taste)
- 3/4 teaspoon kosher salt, divided
- 1/4 black pepper
- 6 tablespoons hoisin sauce
- 2 tablespoons fresh lime juice
- for the salad:
- 4 cups shredded or diced cooked chicken breast
- 3 scallions, thinly sliced on a bias
- 1 red bell pepper, cut into 1" matchsticks
- 1 large carrot, peeled and julienned or grated on a box grater
- 1 mandarin oranges, supremed or 1 11-oz. can mandarin oranges, rinsed and well drained
- 1/3 cup roughly chopped cilantro
- 2 tablespoons chopped fresh mint leaves
- 1 6-ounce package baby arugula
- 1/3 cup roughly chopped cashews, plus additional for garnish
- sprinkle of crispy chow mien or rice noodles (for garnish and crunch)
- black sesame seeds (optional)

Direction

- For the dressings:
- Using a micro plane grater, grate the knob of ginger until it has been reduced to pulp. Scoop up the pulp into a fine mesh sieve. Hold the sieve over a bowl and press on the solids with the back of a spoon. Extract as much of the ginger juice as possible, rolling the pulp back onto itself and pressing. Discard the solids. You should have about 2-3 teaspoons of juice. Divide the juice into two small bowls. One is for the hoisin-lime sauce, the other is for the Asian vinaigrette.
- For the Asian vinaigrette: Combine 3 tablespoons grape seed oil, 1 teaspoon ginger juice, lime zest and juice from one whole lime, honey, garlic, vinegar, wasabi powder, 1/2 teaspoon salt and pepper into a small bowl. Whisk to combine. Taste for seasonings, adjust if necessary and set aside.
- For the hoisin-lime sauce: In a small bowl combine remaining 2 tablespoons grape seed oil, garlic, remaining ginger juice, hoisin sauce, lime juice and remaining kosher salt. Whisk to combine - sauce will be thick and creamy. Taste for seasonings and adjust if necessary.
- For the salad:
- In a large bowl combine the scallions, bell pepper, carrot, orange segments, cilantro and mint leaves. Toss to combine. Add the chicken and toss to combine. Add the cashews and spoon 2-3 tablespoons of Asian vinaigrette over the salad and toss well to coat. You can add more dressing if necessary, but don't overdress the salad.
- Divide arugula onto four plates. Top the arugula with mounds of the chicken salad. Drizzle scant amount of hoisin lime sauce over the salad and dot along the rim of the plate. Sprinkle the salad with additional cashews, chow mien or rice noodles and black sesame seeds, if desired. Enjoy.

362. Basil Chicken With Brown Rice

Serving: Serves 3 to 4 | Prep: | Cook: | Ready in:

Ingredients

- 4 pieces chicken
- 3 bunches basil
- 3 bunches green parts of beets
- 1 onion
- 1/3 cup lime juice
- 3 tablespoons olive oil
- salt and paper
- 1 cup chopped tomato
- Pinch safron

Direction

- Wash the greens and chopped them with onion and sauté them with olive oil in a pan for about 15 to 20 min.
- Add the chicken pieces and continue sauté.
- add half cup water and the lime juice salt and paper and chopped tomato and cover for half hour or until chicken is cooked at the end add pinch if saffron. Serve with hot steamed rice.

363. Boxing Day Pate

Serving: Makes 4 small terrines | Prep: | Cook: | Ready in:

Ingredients

- 1/4 cup shallots--finely diced
- 1/2 cup salt pork-- diced
- 2 large garlic cloves,smashed but kept whole
- 2 tablespoons olive oil
- 1 pound chicken livers--trimmed
- 1 cup chicken stock or broth
- 1 sprig thyme--leaves only
- 1 pinch black pepper
- 8 tablespoons unsalted butter
- 3 tablespoons cognac--be generous

Direction

- In a sauté pan with non-sloping sides, heat the olive oil and toss in the garlic, the shallots and the salt pork. Cook on low until the shallots begin to soften
- Wash and dry the livers. Toss into the shallots and oil and let brown, but don't cook all the way through. It will only take a few minutes
- Remove from heat and immediately tip everything into a food processor. Add the butter in chunks and process until you have a nice thick paste
- Pour through a fine sieve into a clean bowl. Stir in the cognac and then pour into ramekins or gifting jars. For a nice presentation, you can top with clarified butter and a fresh sprig of thyme

364. Spicy Peanut Butter Bacon Cheeseburgers

Serving: Makes 4 burgers | Prep: | Cook: | Ready in:

Ingredients

- 1 pound ground turkey
- 1/2 teaspoon salt
- 1 jalapeño, seeded and finely chopped
- 1/3 cup creamy peanut butter
- 1 tablespoon vegetable oil
- 4 strips turkey bacon
- 4 slices cheddar cheese
- 4 buns (pretzel or regular)
- 4 lettuce leaves (optional)
- 4 slices tomato (optional)

Direction

- 1. In a large bowl, mix together the ground turkey, salt, chopped jalapeño, and peanut butter. Once combined, separate into 4 equal portions. Form each portion into a patty about 3/4-1 inch thick, and press an indentation into the center of each with your fingers (this will help the burger keep its shape as it cooks).
- 2. Heat the vegetable oil in a skillet over medium heat for 2-3 minutes. Place the patties in the skillet and cook for 3-4 minutes on each side. While the patties are cooking, in a separate pan, cook the bacon according to the directions on the package.
- 3. Reduce the heat on the patties to low. Flip the patties back over to the original side, top with cheese, cover the skillet with a lid, and cook for an additional 3 minutes.
- 4. Place the patties in the buns, top with bacon, lettuce, and tomato slices (if desired).

365. Đuveč

Serving: Serves 8-10 | Prep: | Cook: | Ready in:

Ingredients

- 8 chicken thighs, cut into large pieces
- 4 smoked sausages, sliced
- 1 pound onion, diced
- 1 pound mix peppers, diced
- 4 ounces celery, diced
- 10 cloves of garlic, sliced
- 1/2 cup sunflower oil
- 2 teaspoons sea salt
- 1 cup parsley, chopped
- 2-3 sprigs thyme
- 1 1/2 cups arborio rice
- 3 cups crushed tomato
- 3 cups water
- 1/2 teaspoon black pepper
- 1 teaspoon chili flakes
- 2 cups fresh or frozen peas

Direction

- Position rack in the middle of the oven and preheat to 350°F.
- Add onions, celery, peppers, garlic, thyme and oil in a deep baking dish, mix and cook in the oven for 20 minutes.

- In meantime cut and season the chicken with salt, black pepper and chili flakes, cut sausage and add to the vegetables with chicken, mix and bake for another 20 minutes.
- Take out of the oven and add crushed tomato and rice, mix and add 3 cups of water, 1 tsp salt and cook for additional 30-35 minutes.
- Check for seasoning, add peas and parsley, mix and cover for 10-15 minutes, you don't have to cook peas.

Index

A

Ale 125,158,185

Almond 4,7,8,51,194,227

Angelica 133

Anise 5,112,168

Apple 3,5,7,18,24,99,105,192

Apricot 4,5,6,91,101,118,147

Artichoke 3,6,7,19,150,183

Asparagus 4,53

Avocado 4,6,37,53,59,60,147,214

B

Bacon 3,5,6,8,22,24,105,125,157,231

Balsamic vinegar 101

Barley 3,7,45,179

Basil 3,5,6,8,19,30,44,53,111,160,199,209,212,230

Basmati rice 127

Bay leaf 168,206

Beans 149,219,223

Beef 3,32,44

Beer 3,30

Black pepper 16,158

Blackberry 7,203

Blueberry 3,5,24,35,36,98

Bouquet garni 174

Bran 3,29

Bread 3,5,6,7,37,118,123,131,132,207

Broccoli 3,6,7,20,38,155,198

Broth 8,17,52,151,223

Brown sugar 129

Brussels sprouts 70,99,205

Buns 7,13,40,186,187

Burger 3,10,18,40,44

Butter 3,5,8,10,30,41,42,48,98,103,107,115,136,142,176,178,201,231

C

Cabbage 4,51,86,199

Cake 6,7,148,176,187

Calvados 151

Caramel 106

Cardamom 3,44,133,168

Carrot 3,7,8,12,24,37,40,44,45,52,70,116,142,168,172,202,212,223

Cashew 3,28

Cauliflower 7,205

Celery 40,53,66,70,104,115,142,168

Champ 188

Chard 7,179,188

Cheddar 42

Cheese 3,5,8,23,39,40,42,52,53,103,106,115,131,132,178,231

Cherry 4,36,48,53,64,84

Chestnut 4,49

Chicken 1,3,4,5,6,7,8,9,10,12,13,14,15,16,18,19,20,21,22,23,24,27,29,30,32,33,34,35,36,38,39,40,41,42,43,44,45,47,48,50,51,52,53,54,55,56,57,58,59,60,61,62,63,64,65,66,67,68,69,70,71,72,73,74,75,76,77,78,79,80,81,82,83,84,85,87,88,89,90,91,95,96,97,98,99,100,102,103,104,105,108,109,110,111,112,113,114,115,116,117,118,119,120,121,122,125,126,127,128,129,130,131,132,133,134,135,136,137,138,139,140,141,145,146,147,149,150,151,152,153,155,156,157,158,159,160,161,162,163,166,167,168,169,170,171,172,173,174,175,176,178,179,180,181,182,183,184,185,187,188,189,191,192,

194,195,196,198,199,200,202,203,204,205,206,207,208,209,210,212,213,214,215,216,222,223,224,225,226,227,228,229,230

Chickpea 3,45

Chicory 4,86,87

Chilli 3,9,108

Chipotle 113

Chips 42

Chutney 4,89,101

Ciabatta 12,39,208

Cinnamon 3,36,133,168

Cloves 4,24,53,70,83,133,168,212

Coconut 4,6,7,52,89,90,91,133,152,199,200,212

Cod 133

Coffee 4,86,87

Cognac 4,88,151

Collar 4,92

Coriander 71

Cranberry 105

Cream 4,5,6,7,8,42,55,59,95,96,107,132,185,193,200,215

Crumble 22,34,37,40,196,218

Cucumber 12,32

Cumin 5,36,37,100,108,200

Curacao 56

Curry 3,4,5,6,7,8,18,58,59,70,75,78,89,108,133,134,139,140,152,212,218,220

D

Daikon 12

Date 5,102

Dijon mustard 18,47,54,57,67,70,99,100,142,159,161,162,169,181,186,204

Dill 69

Duck 3,5,6,7,16,105,106,107,147,186,193,197

Dumplings 3,4,7,8,9,75,208,228,229

E

Edam 5,112

Egg 3,4,5,25,37,38,40,53,91,107,115,131,178

F

Fat 5,13,52,97,179

Fennel 4,7,56,83,127,133,183

Feta 4,6,7,55,84,135,200

Fettuccine 3,43

Fish 17,168,212

Flour 76,87,107,178

Fontina cheese 84

French bread 124,174

Fruit 3,5,23,100

G

Game 4,86,87

Garam masala 133

Garlic 3,4,5,7,9,10,12,16,36,37,52,53,70,83,93,94,101,108,113,127,128,129,136,181,182,199,200,201,207,212,214

Gin 5,6,7,108,113,114,128,133,177,197,199,200,209,212

Gnocchi 5,7,95,208

Grain 4,76

Grapes 7,53,180

Gravy 4,6,7,8,70,142,164,165,211,215,216

Guacamole 155

H

Ham 7,40,187

Harissa 5,123

Hazelnut 3,7,18,183

Heart 5,125

Herbs 70,210

Hoisin sauce 42

Honey 3,4,5,7,42,60,99,118,125,126,127,203,204,212

J

Jaggery 16

Jam 3,29

Jerusalem artichoke 112,150,183,184

Jus 37,56,71,141,185

K

Kale 37,136

L

Lamb 6,135

Leek 24

Lemon 3,4,5,6,7,10,16,20,56,63,96,104,111,131,133,136,137,147,157,161,172,199,200,212

Lettuce 3,23,66

Lime 5,6,24,129,138,139,199,212

Ling 112

M

Mandarin 88

Mango 6,132

Marsala wine 62

Matzo 6,143

Mayonnaise 22,66,105

Meat 3,4,5,6,7,8,25,37,44,45,49,62,76,89,106,114,170,184,201,218,219,220

Milk 76,131,179,199,200,212

Mince 36,52,148,199,202

Mint 4,6,55,135

Mozzarella 44,66,201

Mushroom 4,7,36,44,79,201,210

Mustard 4,5,6,7,10,76,100,141,142,185,204

N

Noodles 4,6,52,88,145

Nut 3,4,13,24,28,49,55,179

O

Oil 3,9,10,12,14,16,24,26,36,37,40,44,49,52,53,56,70,111,115,116,127,128,131,149,169,179,184,185,200,214

Olive 6,7,10,12,24,26,29,31,36,37,38,44,48,49,53,56,57,70,77,100,101,107,113,115,116,125,127,128,129,131,136,144,147,168,169,173,179,182,185,194,200

Onion 3,5,6,7,29,36,37,52,53,70,105,106,107,115,128,142,149,153,179,193,194,200,210,212,213

Orange 4,6,7,55,56,66,107,135,182,188,197,213

Oregano 5,37,127,145

Oyster 5,115

P

Paella 3,6,11,12,157

Pancetta 4,44,55,79

Paprika 4,5,6,10,16,64,127,150

Parmesan 4,5,6,8,26,27,34,48,57,58,84,90,96,113,115,131,132,159,160,167,175,200,201,206,220,221

Parsley 115,116,210

Passata 27

Pasta 3,4,5,6,7,27,53,83,84,131,160,200,201

Pastry 107

Peach 3,6,7,24,29,161,198

Peanuts 7,192

Pear 6,7,163,183

Peas 200

Pecan 4,66,85,91

Pecorino 207

Peel 45,58,60,93,95,119,120,142,158,178,182,188,209,212,225

Penne 4,53

Pepper 3,4,5,6,10,12,13,24,28,31,36,42,44,48,52,53,56,64,66,70,73,100,115,116,118,127,128,131,136,138,142,149,153,164,16

8,171,179,200,201,214

Pesto 3,4,6,19,55,56,167

Pickle 4,6,12,73,168

Pie 3,4,5,7,8,13,64,65,102,107,168,210,220

Pineapple 3,6,7,28,128,175,178

Pizza 7,200

Plum 52

Pomegranate 5,7,123,129,181

Porcini 5,93

Pork 3,4,32,49

Port 6,44,172

Potato 3,4,5,6,7,23,67,93,94,102,159,170,185,200,202,212

Poultry 131

Prosciutto 4,5,26,66,106

Pulse 47,50,61,62

Q

Quail 5,125

Quinoa 4,7,52,183,205

R

Radicchio 7,188

Radish 7,178

Rhubarb 4,64

Rice 3,4,5,6,7,8,9,14,15,28,31,32,66,67,89,97,108,111,112,121,126,127,128,129,148,149,166,172,191,221,227,229,230

Ricotta 4,57

Risotto 7,179

Roast chicken 142,166

Roast potatoes 105

Rosemary 4,5,6,10,78,96,157

Rye bread 136

S

Saffron 6,166

Sage 4,60

Salad 3,4,5,6,7,8,13,17,18,22,23,37,39,41,48,51,63,66,88,99,101,104,118,120,131,136,151,163,178,181,183,188,192,196,224,229

Salsa 5,6,42,115,120,121,175

Salt 3,6,10,11,12,16,18,21,22,28,30,31,35,36,41,42,44,48,49,50,53,62,66,69,70,71,75,80,87,89,96,100,102,105,106,108,111,115,116,120,127,128,129,130,131,133,144,147,148,149,150,151,159,164,168,169,172,181,183,194,197,207,210,212,213,214,215,217,221,222

Sausage 3,6,7,27,34,39,135,178,179,185,189

Savory 7,67,186

Sea salt 11,29,173,178,182,194

Seasoning 12,52,131,132,196,218

Seeds 4,7,37,51,127,128,181,190

Sesame oil 14,15,81,186

Shallot 7,180,212

Sherry 7,20,104,183,223

Shortbread 7,197

Sichuan pepper 50,184,185

Soup 3,4,5,6,7,8,40,44,45,67,68,74,84,100,116,126,137,143,172,180,199,209,210,212,216,219,221,227

Soy sauce 191

Spaghetti 8,219

Spices 5,106,129

Spinach 3,4,7,23,44,52,57,83,84,200,201

Squash 3,7,8,35,189,219

Star anise 142

Steak 4,77

Stew 3,4,5,6,7,8,21,45,70,78,102,127,132,133,141,172,199,200,210,225

Stock 5,36,53,99,115,116,168,200,212,223

Stuffing 4,5,6,7,47,49,94,115,123,135,196

Sugar 107,128,191

Sumac 7,205

Syrup 35,36

T

Tabasco 59,176

Taco 5,6,7,119,175,192,199

Tahini 4,77

Tamari 168,212

Tarragon 5,6,93,94,173

Tea 3,7,8,35,36,60,141,175,196,197,207,216

Thyme 120

Tomatillo 4,8,84,216

Tomato
4,5,6,7,26,27,36,44,48,52,53,84,96,160,161,167,171,205

Truffle 4,5,82,98

Turkey
3,4,5,6,7,8,10,18,19,24,31,37,40,44,45,60,92,101,102,105,1
13,123,138,142,154,164,172,198,215,217,218,219,220,221

Turmeric 8,13,70,71,108,133,222

Turnip 116

V

Vegetable oil 126,159

Vegetables 5,7,95,207

Vegetarian 3,32

Vermouth 14

Vinegar 9,12,36,53,128,223

W

Walnut 129

Wasabi 7,193

Wine 4,7,9,12,36,79,93,128,133,201,211

Worcestershire sauce 10,41,98,176,220

Wraps 3,4,7,23,81,210

Z

Zest 53,107,150

L

lasagna 26,27

Conclusion

Thank you again for downloading this book!

I hope you enjoyed reading about my book!

If you enjoyed this book, please take the time to share your thoughts and post a review on Amazon. It'd be greatly appreciated!

Write me an honest review about the book – I truly value your opinion and thoughts and I will incorporate them into my next book, which is already underway.

Thank you!

If you have any questions, **feel free to contact at:** _author@shellfishrecipes.com_

Maria Girard

shellfishrecipes.com

Printed in Great Britain
by Amazon